W9-BCQ-237

Curriculum Development and Evaluation in Nursing

Second Edition

Sarah B. Keating, MPH, EdD, RN, CPNP, FAAN, currently is Endowed Professor, Orvis School of Nursing, University of Nevada, Reno (UNR), where she teaches Curriculum Development and Evaluation in Nursing, Instructional Design and Evaluation, and the Nurse Educator Practicum and serves as interim coordinator of the University of Nevada Doctor of Nursing Practice for the Reno campus. She has taught undergraduate and graduate nursing since 1970 and received her EdD in Curriculum and Instruction in 1982. Dr. Keating served as director of the graduate program at Russell Sage College (Troy, NY) and was the director of the School of Nursing at San Francisco State University. She served as dean of Samuel Merritt-Saint Mary's Intercollegiate Nursing Program (1995–2000) and was chair of the California Strategic Planning Committee for ten years. After retiring from Samuel Merritt-Saint Mary's, Dr. Keating has been associated with Orvis School of Nursing, UNR since 2002. She is the recipient of many awards and recognitions and has published in a variety of journals. She has been the recipient of fifteen funded research grants. Dr. Keating led the development of numerous educational programs including nurse practitioner, advanced practice community-health nursing, clinical nurse leader, case management, entry-level MSN programs, nurse educator tracks, the DNP, and MSN/MPH programs. In addition, she serves as a consultant in curriculum development and evaluation for undergraduate and graduate nursing programs and serves as a reviewer for substantive change proposals for the Western Association of Schools and Colleges (WASC) regional accrediting body.

Curriculum Development and Evaluation in Nursing

Second Edition

Sarah B. Keating, EdD, RN, FAAN

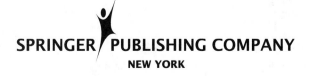

SPRINGER PUBLISHING COMPANY
NEW YORK

Copyright © 2011 Springer Publishing Company, LLC

All rights reserved.

No part of this publication may be reproduced, stored in a retrieval system, or transmitted in any form or by any means, electronic, mechanical, photocopying, recording, or otherwise, without the prior permission of Springer Publishing Company, LLC, or authorization through payment of the appropriate fees to the Copyright Clearance Center, Inc., 222 Rosewood Drive, Danvers, MA 01923, 978-750-8400, fax 978-646-8600, info@copyright.com or on the Web at www.copyright.com.

Springer Publishing Company, LLC
11 West 42nd Street
New York, NY 10036
www.springerpub.com

Acquisitions Editor: Margaret Zuccarini
Production Editors: Rose Mary Piscitelli and Diane Davis
Cover Design: Steven Pisano
Composition: Absolute Service, Inc., Gil Rafanan, Project Manager

ISBN: 978-0-8261-0722-0
E-book ISBN: 978-0-8261-0723-7

14 15 16 / 11 10 9 8

The author and the publisher of this work have made every effort to use sources believed to be reliable to provide information that is accurate and compatible with the standards generally accepted at the time of publication. Because medical science is continually advancing, our knowledge base continues to expand. Therefore, as new information becomes available, changes in procedures become necessary. We recommend that the reader always consult current research and specific institutional policies before performing any clinical procedure. The author and publisher shall not be liable for any special, consequential, or exemplary damages resulting, in whole or in part, from the readers' use of, or reliance on, the information contained in this book. The publisher has no responsibility for the persistence or accuracy of URLs for external or third-party Internet Web sites referred to in this publication and does not guarantee that any content on such Web sites is, or will remain, accurate or appropriate.

Library of Congress Cataloging-in-Publication Data

Curriculum development and evaluation in nursing / [edited by] Sarah B. Keating. — 2nd ed.
   p. ; cm.
  Rev. ed. of: Curriculum development and evaluation in nursing / Sarah B. Keating. c2006.
  Includes bibliographical references and index.
  ISBN 978-0-8261-0722-0 — ISBN 978-0-8261-0723-7 (e-ISBN)
  1. Nursing--Study and teaching. 2. Curriculum planning. 3. Curriculum evaluation. I. Keating, Sarah B. II. Keating, Sarah B. Curriculum development and evaluation in nursing.
  [DNLM: 1. Education, Nursing. 2. Curriculum. 3. Evaluation Studies as Topic. WY 18]
  RT71.K43 2011
  610.73071'1—dc22

                                                     2010042362

Special discounts on bulk quantities of our books are available to corporations, professional associations, pharmaceutical companies, health care organizations, and other qualifying groups.

If you are interested in a custom book, including chapters from more than one of our titles, we can provide that service as well.

For details, please contact:
Special Sales Department, Springer Publishing Company, LLC
11 West 42nd Street, 15th Floor, New York, NY 10036-8002
Phone: 877-687-7476 or 212-431-4370; Fax: 212-941-7842
Email: sales@springerpub.com

Printed in the United States of America by McNaughton & Gunn.

To Arnie, my patient companion.

Contents

Contributors

Lori Candela, EdD, RN, FNP-BC, CNE   Associate Professor, School of Nursing, University of Nevada, Las Vegas

Marilyn E. Flood. PhD, RN   Associate Dean (Emeritus), School of Nursing, University of California, San Francisco

Karen Fontaine, MSN, CMSRN, RN   Director, School of Nursing, Truckee Meadows Community College, Reno, Nevada

Abby Heydman, PhD, RN   Provost and Vice President (Emeritus), Samuel Merritt University, Oakland, California

Melissa Jones, RN, MN   Assistant Professor of Nursing, Linfield-Good Samaritan School of Nursing, Linfield College

Jennifer Richards, PhD, RN   Director of Nursing Education and Research, Renown Medical Center, Reno, Nevada

Patsy Ruchala, DNSc, RN   Professor and Director, Orvis School of Nursing, University of Nevada, Reno

Arlene Sargent, EdD, RN   Associate Dean, School of Nursing, Samuel Merritt University, Oakland, California

Coleen Saylor, PhD, RN   Professor Emeritus, School of Nursing, San Jose State University

Nancy Stotts, EdD, RN, FAAN   Professor, Physiological Nursing, School of Nursing, University of California, San Francisco

Pamela Wheeler, RN, PhD   Associate Professor of Nursing, Linfield-Good Samaritan School of Nursing, Linfield College

Peggy Wros, PhD, RN   Associate Dean for Academic Development, Enhancement and Evaluation, School of Nursing, Oregon Health and Science University

Preface

In the short time since the publication of the first edition of this text, many changes occurred that directly affect nursing curricula now and for the near future. In my view, there are three major changes influencing the development and revision of nursing curricula in this early part of the twenty-first century. They are the rapid initiation of Doctor of Nursing Practice (DNP) programs across the nation, the continuing growth and application of technology to the delivery of nursing programs, and the health care reform legislation that, as of this date, has yet to impact health care, but will certainly change the way care is delivered, with nursing playing a major role in effecting this change. While it is difficult to predict how these changes will play out over the next 5–10 years, they will surely force nursing programs to evaluate and revise their curricula.

The second edition of this text continues to serve nurse educators in schools of nursing and in the practice arena as a practical guide for developing, revising, and evaluating nursing curricula and educational programs. It goes into detail about conducting a needs assessment to determine the extent of revision or development necessary to produce an up-to-date and vibrant curriculum followed by a detailed description of the essential components of the curriculum. Educational evaluation and accreditation are discussed, and directions on how to prepare for an accreditation visit are included.

Contributors to the text are experts in their discipline and provide up-to-date information on curriculum development and evaluation from associate degree to doctoral degree levels. Chapter 13 applies the concepts of curriculum development and evaluation to the practice setting for staff development purposes. The author and contributors review the current literature related to the topics of the text and add their expertise to assist the reader in the application of these concepts to their nurse educator roles.

The final chapter of the text raises current issues facing nurse educators as changes in education and the health care system occur. The critical need for evidence-based practice in education is reviewed with ideas for nurse educator researchers to pursue. The continuing career-ladder and entry-level issues related to nursing are discussed and two proposed curricula are presented for nurse educators to debate. While the DNP is acknowledged as the final degree for advanced practice, will nursing ever see an entry-level doctorate much like other professions? These are the issues to ponder and debate for the future.

Sarah B. Keating, EdD, RN, FAAN

Acknowledgments

The second edition of this text owes its quality and currency to its many contributors. My heartfelt thanks to my colleagues for sharing their expertise with our readers, the students and faculty in schools of nursing, and nurse educators in health care settings who promote the health of clients and the professional development of nurses.

1 Introduction to the History of Curriculum Development and Curriculum Approval Processes

Sarah B. Keating

OVERVIEW OF CURRICULUM DEVELOPMENT AND EVALUATION IN NURSING

This book devotes itself to the processes of curriculum development and evaluation that are critical responsibilities of nurse educators in schools of nursing, staff development, or patient education programs. The curriculum provides the guidelines for how the program will be delivered and the goals within it that are evaluated for effectiveness. The text focuses on curriculum development and evaluation and *not* on instructional design and strategies that are used to deliver the program. Some major theories and concepts that relate to both curriculum development and instructional strategies are discussed but only in light of their contributions to the mission and philosophy of the educational program (e.g., learning theories, educational taxonomies, critical thinking).

To initiate the discourse on curriculum development, a definition is in order. For the purposes of the textbook, the following is the definition: *a curriculum is the formal plan of study that provides the philosophical underpinnings, goals, and guidelines for the delivery of a specific educational program.* The text uses this definition throughout for the *formal* curriculum, while recognizing the existence of the *informal* curriculum. The informal curriculum consists of activities that students, faculty, administrators, staff, and consumers experience outside of the formal planned curriculum. Examples of the informal curriculum include interpersonal relationships, athletic/recreational activities, study groups, organizational activities, special events, academic and personal counseling, and so forth. Although the remainder of the text will focus on the formal curriculum, nurse educators should keep the informal curriculum in mind for its influence and use it to reinforce learning activities that arise from the planned curriculum.

To place curriculum development and evaluation in perspective, it is wise to examine the history of nursing education in North America and the lessons it provides for current and future curriculum developers. Section 1 sets the stage for the process through an examination of nursing's place in the history of higher education and the role of faculty and administrators in developing and evaluating curricula. Nursing curricula are currently undergoing transformation. Today's emphases on the learner and measurement of learning outcomes; integration into the curriculum of quality and safety concepts, evidence-based practice, and translational research and science; and the application of technology to

1

the delivery of the program provide exciting challenges and opportunities for nurse educators. Nursing faculty and educators must consider all of these factors when examining the curriculum and considering change. Today and tomorrow's curricula call for an integration of processes that are learner- and consumer-based and at the same time ensure excellence by building in outcome measures to determine the quality of the program.

History of Nursing Education in North America

Chapter 1 traces the history of American nursing education from the time of the first Nightingale schools of nursing to the present. The trends in professional education and society's needs impacted nursing programs that started from apprentice-type schools to a majority of the programs now in institutions of higher learning. Lest the profession forgets, liberal arts plays a major role in nursing education and sets the foundation for the development of critical thinking, cultural awareness, and a strong science background so necessary to the nursing process. Included in the discussion is an overview of higher education in the United States, its evolution over the past century, and its structure that includes private and public institutions, land-grant universities, academic health sciences centers, large multipurpose universities, small liberal arts colleges, and sectarian and nonsectarian institutions. Changes in the purpose, mission, and organization of institutions over time in response to society's needs are discussed as well as the role they played in professional education.

Chapter 1 reviews the historical events in society and the world that influenced nursing practice and education as well as major changes in the health care system. The major world wars increased the demand for nurses and a nursing education system that prepared a workforce ready to meet that demand. The emergence of nursing education that took place in community colleges in the mid-20th century initiated continuing debate about entry into practice. The explosive growth of Doctor of Nursing Practice (DNP) programs in recent times and their place in advanced practice, nursing leadership, and education brings the past century happenings into focus as the profession responds to changes in the health care system and the health care needs of the population.

Curriculum Development and Approval Processes in Changing Educational Environments

Chapter 2 discusses the processes for programs undergoing change or creating new curricula. Curriculum committees in schools of nursing receive recommendations from faculty for curriculum changes and periodically review the curriculum for its currency, authenticity, and its diligence in realizing the mission, philosophy, and goals. The chapter describes the classic hierarchy of curriculum-approval processes in institutions of higher learning and the importance of nursing faculty's participation within the governance of the institution. The governance of colleges and universities usually includes curriculum committees or their equivalent composed of elected faculty members. These committees are at the program, collegewide, and/or university-wide levels and provide the academic rigor for assuring quality in educational programs.

Faculty and administrators continually assess curricula and program outcomes and based on the results of the assessment, refine existing curricula through major or minor revisions. An issue of contention during the assessment and development phase is what to take out of the curriculum when new content is indicated. The challenge faculty faces is to preserve critical content and at the same time, bring current and future information into the curriculum. This means that faculty must be willing to compromise and give up outdated (but dear) content to make way for newer knowledge. In some instances, new programs are needed with the same processes of assessment used to produce the justification for and establishment of new programs.

It is a cardinal rule in academe that the curriculum "belongs to the faculty." In higher education, faculty members are deemed the experts in their specific discipline; or in the case of nursing, clinical specialties or functional areas such as administration, health care policy, case management, and so forth. They are the people who determine the content that must be transferred to and assimilated by the learner. At the same time, they should be expert teachers in the delivery of information (i.e., pedagogy or in the case of adult learners, andragogy). Curriculum planning and the art of teaching are learned skills and nursing faculty members have a responsibility to include them in their repertoire of expertise as well as being content specialists.

Nursing faculty must periodically review a program to maintain a vibrant curriculum that responds to changes in society, health care needs of the population, the health care delivery system, and the learners' needs. It is important to measure the program's success in preparing nurses for the current environment and for the future. Currency of practice as well as that of the future must be built into the curriculum, because it will be several years before entering classes graduate. In nursing, there is an inherent requirement to produce caring, competent, and confident practitioners or clinicians. At the same time, the curriculum must meet professional and accreditation standards. Although it is unpopular to think that curricula are built on accreditation criteria, in truth, integrating them into the curriculum helps administrators and faculty to prepare for program approval or review and accreditation by assuring that the program meets essential quality standards.

Chapter 2 discusses the role and responsibilities that faculty and administrators assume in undertaking curriculum development and evaluation. Among the responsibilities is reaching consensus on the mission, philosophy, and organizational framework (of their choice), goals, and setting overall end-of-program objectives for the curriculum. Faculty retains academic freedom in implementing the curriculum and choosing individual methods of instruction; however, the preset goals and objectives of the program that the faculty-as-a-whole developed cannot be changed without faculty's and other review entities' approval.

Formative evaluation strategies such as student examinations and course and teaching effectiveness evaluations can trigger the need for revisions of the curriculum. Faculty is responsible for evaluating program outcomes in addition to the day-to-day activities of curriculum implementation (teaching). Evaluation plays an important role in developing the measures for assessment and responding to the feedback from students, graduates, employers, and other consumers of the program.

Administrators provide the leadership for organizing and carrying out the evaluation activities. To bring the curriculum into reality and out of the "Ivory Tower," faculty and administrators must include students, alumni, employers, and the people whom their graduates serve into curriculum building and evaluation processes. Outcomes from the total program are measured through summative evaluation methods such as follow-up surveys of graduates and National Council Licensure Examination (NCLEX) and certification exam results. Chapter 2 introduces the role of accreditation in curriculum development and evaluation. Section 5 continues the discussion on the processes that relate to accreditation and its related activities of program review.

Best-Laid Plans: A Century of Nursing Curricula

Marilyn E. Flood

OBJECTIVES

Upon completion of Chapter 1, the reader will be able to:

1. Compare the nursing curricular events of the 1890s with those of the 1950s.
2. Identify at least two reasons why the 1965 position paper occasioned so much controversy.
3. Describe significant milestones identified in the development of one program type (i.e., diploma, baccalaureate, associate degree, master's, or doctoral).
4. Provide a rationale for identifying the decade most pivotal to the development of one program type (i.e., diploma, baccalaureate, associate degree, master's, or doctoral).
5. Explain the sense in which the Cadet Nurse Corps (CNC) phenomenon and period was transitional (i.e., continuing characteristics of preceding decades with a shift into a direction foundational to the next period).
6. Evaluate the impact of the history of nursing education on current and future curriculum development and evaluation activities.

OVERVIEW

The roots of current curricular arrangements are entwined with the development of nursing as a distinct occupation focused on providing health-related care to strangers. Nursing developed to improve existing institutions and then made new hospitals workable. As a consequence, hospital characteristics, from the social class of patients to the architecture of buildings, influenced nursing's roots. Medicine gradually became a dominant influence in hospitals. Nursing curricula had to take medicine's developing science and technology into account, reflect the changing boundary with medicine, and clarify the nature of nursing within medicine's hegemony.

Although postsecondary education had increasingly centered in collegiate institutions before and after World War I, nursing education remained substantially responsible for hospital service (diploma programs) through the 1950s. However, both baccalaureate and associate degree programs were noticeably visible by the end of that decade. Baccalaureate preparation in nursing, which in the 1920s was envisioned as a goal for the leaders of the profession, gradually transmuted into a basic expectation for nurses. Associate degree programs, coming on the scene as junior or community colleges multiplied after World War II. Compared to diploma programs associate degree programs married the advantages of decentralized, locally based preparation with the advantages of higher education funding, the ethos of an educational environment, and shorter elapsed time from enrollment to graduation.

Master's curricula evolved in this same period, folding into their offerings some of the formerly freestanding postbasic specialist courses in teaching, administration, and public health. They gradually became truly postbaccalaureate curricula and subsequently, came to be oriented primarily around specialized nursing content in clinical areas. As nursing's central disciplinary identity became distinct and differentiated, the need for the capacity to train nurse researchers became pressing. Doctoral curricula were born of this need.

The 1940s, including the activity fomented in connection with the CNC and the optimistic post-War planning, was a transitional decade. Certain forces promoting the post-War changes began their influence before 1940 and change came gradually in the following decades, but the 1940s were pivotal.

The triangulation of subject, setting, and student characteristics served to frame curriculum planning for several decades (Bevis, 1989; Bevis & Watson, 1989; Schubert, 1986). This is an equally useful framework for seeking the "why" and "whither" of nursing curriculum evolution over time. That is, conceptions of nursing, the subject, changed substantially over time. Both health care and educational settings, to say nothing of the larger social order around them, changed from era to era. Students brought different qualifications, expectations, and characteristics to interact with the curricula. Almost nothing happened just because "nursing decided it". However, it is equally true that organized nursing and grassroots nurses played a significant part in shaping ideas that came to be reflected in curricula.

IN THE BEGINNING

The U.S. Civil War was a catalyst for the eventual development of nursing as a paid occupation. During the War, women gave life-saving care under trying circumstances. Other women gained experience and visibility in their home cities by organizing war support efforts related to the health and welfare of soldiers. After the War, these organizing skills were brought to bear on the state of hospitals (Smith-Rosenberg, 1985). Although there were important earlier training efforts of various kinds in the decades prior to the Civil War, the "standard story" usually begins with the founding in 1873 of three training schools (in New Haven, New York, and Boston), which were modeled after the Nightingale School in London (Goodnow, 1934). By 1880, there were 15 nursing schools, and by 1890 there were 35. Most of these schools, including the 2,000 more that were founded in the next 30 years, consisted primarily of on-the-job training mixed with regimented living and working. This "curriculum" was intended to develop proper character traits and habits (Tomes, 1984). The "pupils" were the nursing service for the hospital, which offered its imprimatur in the form of diplomas and pins for enduring this training for the stipulated time. The length of the programs grew from 1 year, to 2, and then to 3 years by the mid-1890s. The hours of work were like those of women in households (i.e., from rising in the morning to retiring to sleep at night). Students came one-by-one as they were available and their services were needed. The patients were mostly poor, without families and/or homes to provide care. From the institution's standpoint, graduates were a byproduct rather than a purpose for the training school. "Trained nurses" generally gave private care in wealthy homes, administered/trained pupils in a training school, or cared for the poor in their homes after graduation (Reverby, 1984).

Despite the existence of the training schools and some public awareness of the abilities of the "trained nurse," the domestic roots of nursing were still very much in evidence. Every woman expected to nurse family members. Older women who had extensive family experience and needed to earn a living, would care for neighbors or contacts referred by word-of-mouth (Reverby, 1987). In some places, short courses in nursing were offered and advertised both to women who wanted to learn better in-family care and those who were preparing to take care of strangers in a hospital (D'Antonio, 1987, 1993). The title of the Clara Weeks-Shaw's *A Text-book for Nursing: For the Use of Training Schools, Families, and Private Students*, first published in 1885, clearly reflects the breadth of the nursing audience in that era. Inside its pages, the hospital context receives considerable attention, and the third edition in 1902 identifies the primary audience as "professional" nurses rather than "amateurs". It assumed an elementary acquaintance with anatomy and physiology, which is now a fundamental part of training.

Physician-authored texts about nursing and for nurses were commonplace and nurse authorship was pioneered in Britain. Clara Weeks (later Weeks-Shaw), a graduate of the New York Hospital School of Nursing in 1880 and founding superintendent of the Paterson General Hospital School from 1883 to 1888, wrote the first widely disseminated text in the United States ("Obituaries," 1940). The possession of such a text led to decreased dependence of graduates on their course notes, supplied information that would otherwise have been missed because of cancelled lectures or note-taking student exhaustion, reinforced the idea that nursing required more than fine character, and exerted a subtle standardizing effect on training school expectations. Such a text today, with its reference to managing the fire in the fireplace during the night and candles as light sources, jars readers into considering the difference in settings. The approximately 100 names in the comprehensive list of medicines, including ether, oxygen, topical agents, and multiple names for the same substance, subverted efforts to keep nurses ignorant of the names of medicines they were administering. Although the topics of venesection and transfusion are listed, venesection was by cutdown at the elbow and transfusion referred to administration of a quart of normal saline over a half hour by glass canula placed in the vein (Weeks-Shaw, 1902).

The 1890s

The International Congress of Charities, Correction, and Philanthropy met in Chicago as part of the Columbian Exposition of 1893. Isabel Hampton, the founding principal of the training school and superintendent of nurses at Johns Hopkins Hospital, played a leading role in planning the nursing sessions for the Congress. At a plenary session, she presented a paper, "Educational Standards for Nurses," that overtly argued the responsibility of hospitals to provide actual education for students and the urgent need for superintendents to work together to establish standards (James, 2002). The paper included her proposal to extend the training period to 3 years in order to allow the shortening of clinical work to 8 hours per day, and to make it possible to admit students in groups rather than one-by-one and for the 3 years of study divided into academic terms (Robb, 1907). During the week of the Congress, Hampton instigated an informal meeting of nursing superintendents that laid the groundwork for the formation of the American Society of Superintendents of Training Schools in the United States and Canada (ASSTS), which later, in 1911, was renamed the National League of Nursing Education (NLNE). Certainly a landmark event within nursing, this was also the first association of a professional nature organized and controlled by women. (Bullough & Bullough, 1978)

The year 1893 also marked the publication of Hampton's *Nursing: Its Principles and Practice for Hospital and Private Use.* The first 25 pages are devoted to a description of a training school, including physical facilities, contents of a reference library, a 2-year curriculum plan—for both didactic content and planned, regular clinical rotations from service to service—and examinations. Hampton notably omitted reference to the pupil nurse residence as a character-training instrument in the training school system, although she noted in other contexts the importance of the residence for the health and social development of students (Dodd, 2001). Clearly she was pushing for a progressive professional education and a professional identity for nursing.

In this century, professionhood seems like an obvious direction for the efforts of Hampton and others such as Lillian Wald and Lavinia Dock who were canonized as early leaders. But throughout the first 75 years of nursing's history as an intentional occupation, many nurses would have deeply disagreed with this as a goal. Barbara Melosh (1982) aptly describes the image many held of nursing as "not merely a profession," but a calling, or an expression of true womanhood. Coexisting with these ideals, she acknowledges, were nurses who intended to give good care but who primarily needed a means of livelihood. A part of Hampton's genius was her ability to embody the womanly service ideals and to talk in the language of calling, while focusing her efforts toward professionalization and arguing for the health and welfare of nurses. For her, these were not divergent goals, but rather, aspects of an integrated whole.

Hampton's Johns Hopkins was absolutely atypical of training schools and was sometimes spoken of as a normal school for nursing. It offered a model of what might have been had other training schools been as well resourced socially, educationally, and financially (Baldwin, 2002). Although an organizational mechanism (the ASSTS/NLNE) had been initiated that was to set standards and provide a network of likeminded superintendents with high educational aspirations, the momentum for hospital founding with corequisite training schools drove the demand for pupils and their 12-hour days or nights of work on the wards. Many schools gave just enough on-the-job training to adequately meet their hospital's own needs. In 1890, there were 35 training schools. By 1900 there were 432, and by 1905, there were 862. The number of training schools peaked at 2,155 in 1926 and then, began a long contraction. Hampton's proposal for the 3-year program length was rapidly adopted by hospitals large and small, but without the 8-hour day.

Retrospective From 1940

From the vantage point of administrator educators in 1940, the 1890s were a world away. They had just lived through a decade of the Depression that resisted governmental fixes. The immediate circumstances of the prior decade demanded innovation to meet new problems. Patients who formerly hired private nurses to care for them in the hospital had come to the wards, now often 4- to 10-bed rooms rather than 30-bed halls, where student services provided care. Students came as members of a class and attrition was hard to predict, thus the ballooning census on the wards made it necessary to hire graduate nurses temporarily. These graduates were often unemployed private duty nurses. The most notable change since 1890 was that people who had homes and families came to hospitals for care (Vogel, 1980). In scattered local areas, systems of health insurance were now available making this a factor for both insured patients and hospitals. Surgery and its aftercare were now hospital events except in remote places. Nurses still did private duty nursing in homes, but increasingly they cared for their individual patients in the hospital setting. Public health nursing attracted graduates who wanted more autonomy and an engagement with broader health concerns. Increased expectations for cognitive learning by students were brought about by several factors, for example, hospital architecture, physician expectations, nursing efforts, and general culture change. With markedly increased numbers of applicants during the Depression, more schools were able to select capable students and to grant diplomas that signified both cognitive learning and character.

National Reports and Standards 1911–1937

The Grading Committee worked from 1926 to 1934 to produce "gradings" based on answers to survey forms. Each school received individualized feedback about its own characteristics in comparison to all other participating schools (Committee on the Grading of Nursing Schools, 1931). The NLNE's 1927 *A curriculum for schools of nursing* provided the implicit framework for the surveys and reports. Although the original hope was that the Committee would rank schools into A, B, and C categories as the Flexner Report had, the Committee pointed out that the work and cost of visiting the many nursing schools (as compared to Flexner's 155) made this impossible.

Even without this actual "grading," it provided more data than nursing had ever had about its schools. For example, it found that the median U.S. nursing school had 10 faculty: the superintendent of the hospital, the superintendent of nurses, the night supervisor, the day supervisor, 2 heads of special departments—usually operating room and delivery room, 1 assistant in a special department, 2 other head nurses, and 1 instructor. This median varied by region from 4 to 17 faculty members. Forty two percent of the faculty had not completed high school. Forty five percent of the superintendents of nursing came to their positions more recently than the senior students' admission dates. Hospital schools in the inter-World-War period presented a highly variable picture. Some still offered only apprenticeship learning, but without "master craftswoman" nurses and with a social milieu more consonant with turn-of-the-century culture. This gave nursing a backward, rigid quality that was susceptible to caricature. Others were pushing their limits to provide stimulating learning and an environment more akin to other educational institutions (Egenes, 1998).

The Grading Committee's reports joined a series of reports dating back to 1910, when the American Hospital Association formed a committee to make recommendations regarding the length of the nurse training course, a model curriculum, and the training of nurse helpers. The resulting model curriculum for large general hospitals, and small hospitals that could affiliate with larger, was a graded 3-year curriculum (i.e., different subjects to be taught in each of the 3 years) intended for students who had had at least 1 year of high school. It included a plan for a 3-month preliminary period that was primarily educational with a secondary emphasis on practice. Notably, it took the position that specialty hospitals should not have training schools (with the exception of psychiatric hospital schools that could affiliate with general hospitals), and it completely ignored the charge to deal with the subject of nurse helpers or assistants. This report included a topical listing of curriculum content with broad ranges of possible hours per topic (Aikens, 1911/1985).

In 1917, 1927, and 1937, the NLNE published a series of curriculum recommendations in book form. The reaction to the title of the first, *Standard Curriculum . . .* led to naming the second *A Curriculum . . .* and the third, *A Curriculum Guide . . . .* The first was developed by a relatively small group, but the second and third involved a long process with broad input, which, even apart from the product, served an important function. The published curricula were intended to set the pace, that is, to reflect a generalization about what the better schools were doing or aimed to do. As such, they give a picture of change over the 20-year period, but they cannot be regarded as providing a snapshot of a typical school. Each volume represents substantial change from the previous and where the same course topical area exists in all three, the level of detail and specificity increases with each decade. Indeed, the markedly increased length and wordy style of the 1937 volume appropriately carries the title, "Guide."

Each *Curriculum* book increased the number of classroom hours and decreased the recommended hours of patient care, in effect making nursing service more expensive. Each *Curriculum* also increased the prerequisite educational level: 4 years of high school, but temporary tolerance of 2 years in 1917, 4 years of high school in 1927, and 1 to 2 years of college or normal school in addition to high school by 1937 (NLNE, 1917, 1927, 1937). This was a selective standard, which was more easily met by students from urban homes. In 1920, only 16.8% of the age cohort graduated from high school; in 1930, 20%, and in 1940, 50.8% graduated (Tyack, 1974). It was not until the 1930s, with the depressed labor market and enforcement of child labor and mandatory attendance laws, that one third of the age cohort nationally attended high school. With the beginnings of a nursing school accreditation mechanism before World War II and the post-War National Nursing Accrediting Service, the function that the *Curriculum* books were intended to serve were now incarnated by consultants and supplanted by concise written standards (Committee of the Six National Nursing Organizations on Unification of Accrediting Services, 1949).

Nursing and Higher Education

Starting in the early 1900s, universities began to enfold such nontraditional fields as education, business administration, and engineering. These were originally taught in freestanding, single-purpose institutions (Veysey, 1965). By the inter-War period, the university had become the dominant institution in the postsecondary landscape (Graham, 1978). From 1920 to 1940, the percentage of women attending college from the 18-to-21 year-old cohort rose from 7.6% to 12.2%. Men's college-going rates rose faster, so that the percentage of women in the student body dropped from 43% in 1920 to 40.2% in 1940 (Eisenmann, 2000; Solomon, 1985).

Nursing made overtures to a few colleges and universities prior to World War I. In 1899, the ASSTS developed the Hospital Economics course for nurses who had potential as superintendents of hospital and training schools. The program involved 8 months of study, using many courses existing in the Domestic Science department, but with a custom-designed course on teaching, and a Hospital Economics course that would be taught by nurses. It was expected that the nurse students could earn sufficient money doing 3 to 4 months of private duty before or after the 8 months to cover the $400 cost of the course (Robb, 1907). This relationship with Teachers College, Columbia University (TCCU) grew and was cemented by the endowment in 1910 of a chair in Nursing, occupied for many years by M. Adelaide Nutting. The nursing faculty at TCCU continued to be unusually influential in nursing education through the 1950s, when other centers began to share influence.

In the first decade of the 1900s, technical institutes such as Drexel in Philadelphia, Pratt in Brooklyn, and Mechanics in Rochester, as well as Simmons College in Boston and Northwestern University in Chicago offered course work to nursing students in the preliminary period (Robb, 1907). The designers of the 1917 *Standard Curriculum . . .* gave some thought to the relationship of nursing education to the collegiate system. In an appendix, they provided their calculations that led them to suggest that the theoretical work in a nursing school was equivalent to 36 units, or about 1 year of college, and the clinical work another 51 units. Also in 1917–1918, with popular patriotism running high and nursing the only entrée for women to direct involvement in World War I, more than 400 college graduates who attended a 12-week preliminary course on the Vassar campus in 1918 subsequently attended schools of nursing across the country. Participating schools committed to a program of just 2 additional years study. Student motivation waned with the early armistice and the rigid atmosphere in some of the schools, so only 42% of the original group graduated from schools of nursing (Armeny, 1983; Gage, 1918; Roberts, 1954).

Over time, a number of ideas were put forward for changing the organization and sponsorship of nursing instruction, among them the idea of aligning nursing within institutions of higher education. But few voices actively campaigned for this idea even as late as the 1930s, despite the recommendation of the Rockefeller-funded Goldmark Report, *Nursing and Nursing Education in the United States* in the early 1920s (1923). Initially such a program was envisioned solely for the leaders of training schools.

Educators who wanted a university context for nursing, and thereby concentration on educational goals and emancipation from dependence on the hospitals' student work–study schemes, looked hopefully at the Yale University School of Nursing, funded by the Rockefeller Foundation starting in 1924, and headed by the determined and respected Annie W. Goodrich. Similarly encouraging was the program at Western Reserve University, endowed by Francis Payne Bolton in 1923, following considerable prior work within the Cleveland civic community. Vanderbilt was endowed by a combination of Rockefeller, Carnegie, and Commonwealth Funds in 1930. The University of Chicago established a school of nursing in 1925 with an endowment from the distinguished but discontinued Illinois Training School in 1925 (Hanson, 1991). Dillard University established a school in 1942 with substantial foundation support and governmental war-related funds. Mary Tennant, nursing adviser in the Rockefeller Foundation, pronounced the Dillard Division of Nursing "one of the most interesting developments in nursing education in the country, irrespective of race" (Hine, 1989, p. 79). Although these were milestone events, endowments did little to dissipate the caution, if not hostility, toward women on American campuses. Neither did they cure all that was ailing in nursing education. They funded significant program changes, but even these would not meet the accreditation standards of later decades (Faddis, 1973; Kalisch & Kalisch, 1978; Sheahan, 1980).

According to the Journal of the American Medical Association (1927), 25 universities granted bachelor's degrees to nurses by 1926. By the end of the 1930s a bewildering array of "collegiate" programs existed, partly because baccalaureate programs were being invented by trial and error within the combinations of opportunities and constraints presented in each local hospital and university pair (Petry, 1937).

THE CADET NURSE CORPS

World War II, with its demands for all able-bodied young men for military service, mobilized available women for employment or volunteer service. Indeed every resident was engaged in the effort by the mandates of food, clothing, and gasoline rationing, and by persuasion toward everything from tending victory gardens to buying savings bonds. From mid-1941 to mid-1943, with the help of federal aid, nursing schools increased their enrollments by 13,000 over the baseline year and 4,000 postdiploma nurses completed postbasic course work to enable them to fill the places of nurses who enlisted. Some inactive nurses returned to practice (Roberts, 1954). Despite the effort necessary to bring about this increase, hospitals were floundering and more nurses were needed for the military services.

Congress passed the Bolton Act, which authorized the complex of activities known as the CNC in June 1943. It was conceived as a mechanism to avoid civilian hospital collapse (in the absence of the one fourth of all active nurses who went to War), to provide nursing to the military, and to ensure an adequate education for student nurse cadets. The goal was to recruit 65,000 high school graduates into nursing schools in the first year (1943–1944) and 60,000 the next year. This represented 10% of girls graduating from high school and the whole percentage of those who would expect to go to college! The program exceeded the goals for both years (Kalisch & Kalisch, 1978).

Hospitals sponsoring training schools recognized that CNC schools would outrecruit non-Cadet schools, thereby almost certainly guaranteeing their closure or radical shrinkage. Thus, they signed on, despite the fact that hospitals had to establish a separate accounting for school costs, literally meet the requirements of their state boards of nurse examiners to the satisfaction of the CNC consultants, and allow their students to leave for federal service during the last 6 months of their programs, when they would otherwise be most valuable to their home schools. Schools received partial funding from a separate appropriation for the modifications necessary to build classrooms and library space, and to secure additional student housing. Visiting consultants looked at faculty numbers and qualifications, clinical facilities available for learning, curricula, hours of student clinical and class work, the school's ability to accelerate course work to fit into 30 months, and the optimal number of students the school could accommodate (Robinson & Perry, 2001). Only high school graduates could qualify to become cadets (Petry, 1943). Schools were pressed to increase the size of their classes and number of classes admitted per year, to use local colleges for basic sciences to conserve nurse instructor time, and to develop affiliations with psychiatric hospitals, both for educational reasons, and secondarily to free up dormitory space for more students to be admitted. Consultants could give 3-, 6-, or 12-month conditional approval to the schools while deficiencies were corrected (Robinson & Perry, 2001). Given the pressure to keep CNC-approved status, schools made painful changes.

Students, who were estimated to be providing 80% of care in civilian hospitals, experienced a changed practice context. They now had to decide what they could safely delegate to Red Cross volunteers and any paid aides available. Extra responsibility for nursing arose from the shortage of physicians. With grossly short staffing, nurses had to set priorities carefully. All of these circumstances altered student learning, whether or not they were codified in course content or lesson plans. The intense work of the consultants, who provided interpretation and linkage between the United States Public Health Service (USPHS) in Washington and each school, and their strategy of simultaneously naming deficiencies and identifying improvement goals were a critical factor in the success of the programs as well as improvement in nursing education. Without the financial resources of the federal government to defray student costs, to assist with certain costs to schools, and to provide the consultation, auditing, and public relations/recruitment functions, the goals could not be met. Lucile Petry, the Director of the Division of Nursing Education in the USPHS, combined a sense of the social significance of nursing with firsthand experience in nursing education, a humility that equipped her to work with all kinds of people, and generously give credit to everyone involved in the massive undertaking. Opinions differed on such questions as the cutoff point for irredeemably weak schools, but overall, the effort was pronounced a substantial success for nursing (Roberts, 1954).

After the end of the War in 1945, much of the remainder of the decade was devoted to reversing the changes occasioned by mobilization and absorbing the new post-War reality. Among the benefits for returning military—including nurses—was funding for higher education. This gave nurses unexpected access to colleges and universities and expanded public aspirations for higher education.

1950–2000

Nursing curricula were transformed in the years from 1950 to 2000. Change in the intervening years has been at least as great as from 1890 to 1940. Consider, for example, the gradual sorting out of the wildly idiosyncratic arrangements that were forged between hospital schools and colleges in the preceding decades and the bewildering array of postbasic courses for nurses offered by various units of colleges and universities. Even degree-granting programs, both baccalaureate and master's programs, were variable in sequencing, unit value and scheduling, and terminal expectations in the 1950s. Experiments involving junior or community colleges in sponsorship of nurse programs were underway in the 1950s. Even the hospital-sponsored diploma programs, which dramatically decreased in number during these years, were substantially transformed into educationally focused efforts. By the early 1970s, the rich but disorderly profusion of the 1950s had been regularized, most immediately through the influence of accreditation processes. By the late 1960s, master's programs were beginning to prepare clinical nurse specialists, and the literature described nurse practitioner roles. Coronary care and intensive care units required staff nurses to exercise judgment and to take action in a far wider range of clinical situations than formerly acknowledged within nursing's scope of practice and educators were trying to sort out the implications for both graduate and undergraduate programs. These developments in practice, together with educators' decisions to focus graduate preparation on nursing rather than on teaching and administration, transformed master's programs. Research capacity grew and research training in doctoral programs developed.

The relentless drumbeat of talk about "the hospital nursing shortage" continued through much of these 50 years, with a hiatus only in the early 1990s. Given the expansion in bed capacity fueled by Hill-Burton legislation and subsequent similar funding, expanded private insurance coverage, the advent of Medicare and Medicaid, and the development of technology to treat a wider range of patients intensively, the increased demand for nurses was not surprising. Supply-side solutions could not keep up with demand, even though nurses gradually increased their workforce participation rates to a very high level. Nurse wages did not rise sufficiently to give hospitals incentives to treat nurses as a scarce resource and thus, bring supply and demand into equilibrium. (Lynaugh & Brush, 1996)

ACCREDITATION

From the standpoint of the ordinary nursing school, the possibility of actual accreditation became a reality in the 1950s. The NLNE developed standards for accreditation and made pilot visits from 1934 to 1938. By 1939, schools could list themselves to be visited in order to qualify to be on the first list published by NLNE. Despite the greatly increased work, turnover, and general disruption created by the War, 100 schools had mustered both the courage and the energy required to prepare for accreditation evaluation and judged creditable by 1945. Many schools that had qualified for provisional accreditation, however, were due for revisiting by the end of the War. The Association of Collegiate Schools of Nursing (ACSN), formed in 1932, exercised a kind of "accreditation" via its requirements for full and associate membership, but its standards primarily influenced schools that aspired to be part of this group or that attended conferences it cosponsored. Only 26 schools were accredited by ACSN in 1949. The National Organization for Public Health Nursing (NOPHN) had been accrediting postbasic programs in public health since 1920 but more recently had considered specialty programs at both baccalaureate and master's level, and the public health content in generalist baccalaureate programs (Harms, 1955). By 1948, these organizations, along with the Council of Nursing Education of Catholic Hospitals, ceded their accrediting role to the National Nursing Accrediting Service (NNAS), which published its first combined list of accredited programs just 1 month before the survey-based interim classification of schools was published by the National Committee for the Improvement of Nursing Services (NCINS) in 1949 (Petry, 1949). The classification put schools in either Group I, the top 25% of schools, or Group II, the middle 50%, leaving other schools unlisted and unclassified.

The NNAS, much like the Cadet Nurse program before it, elected a strategy designed to entice schools with at least minimal strengths to improve. It published the first list of temporarily accredited schools in 1952, giving these schools 5 years to make improvements and qualify for full accreditation. During the intervening time, it provided many special meetings, self-evaluation guides, and consultant visits to the schools. By 1957, the number of fully accredited schools increased by 72.4% (Kalisch & Kalisch, 1978). Changes in hospital school programs were catalyzed and channeled by accreditation norms (Committee of the Six National Nursing Organizations on Unification of Accrediting Services, 1949). But ultimately, the forces that drove change were primarily external, ranging from public expectations of postsecondary education mediated through hospital trustees and physicians to competition among programs for potential students, who now had access to information about accreditation and who were recruited heavily by schools, which still had substantial responsibility for nursing service. By 1950, all states participated in the State Board Test Pool Examination, another measuring rod that induced improvement or closure of weaker schools.

Despite the influential Carnegie- and Sage-funded *Nursing for the Future* in 1948, which recommended a broad-based move of nursing education into general higher education, nursing's earliest centralized accreditation mechanism concentrated considerable energy on improving diploma schools, as had the Grading Committee before it (Brown, 1948, Roberts, 1954). Why this seeming mismatch between aspirations and effort? Partly, it sprang from realism: Students were in hospital schools, whether ideal or not, so they needed the best possible preparation because nursing services would reflect this quality. (Postgraduation learning via staff development or socialization into the traditions of a service was not considered a significant factor.) Further, the quality of many of the baccalaureate programs left a great deal to be desired and their capacity for more students was limited, so these could not be promoted as an immediate or ideal substitute for diploma programs. Although by 1957 there were 18 associate degree programs (Kalisch & Kalisch, 1978), no one foresaw the speed of their multiplication in the next decade. Finally, nursing's collective sense of social responsibility burdened it with finding ways to continue to provide essential services, both within the hospital and elsewhere, as its educational house moved from the base of the hospital to the foundation of higher education (Lynaugh, 2002).

BACCALAUREATE EDUCATION

By the 1950s, the diverse baccalaureate curricula of the 1930s multiplied. As one educator wrote in 1954, "Baccalaureate programs still seem to be in the experimental stage. They vary in purpose, structure, subject matter content, admission requirements, matriculation requirements, and degrees granted upon their completion. Some schools offering baccalaureate programs still aim to prepare nurses for specialized positions. Others, advancing from this traditional concept, seek to prepare graduates for generalized nursing in beginning positions" (Harms, 1955, p. 285).

Although a few programs threaded general education and basic science courses through 5 years of study, the majority structured their programs with 2 years of college courses before or after the 3 years of nursing preparation, or book-ended the nursing years with the split 2 years of college work (Bridgman, 1949). Margaret Bridgman, an educator from Skidmore College who consulted with a large number of nursing schools, made favorable reference to the "upper division nursing major" in her volume directed toward both college and nursing educators (Bridgman, 1953). However, the paramount issues, she said, were whether or not (a) the academic institution and academic goals had meaningful involvement and influence in the program as a whole, and (b) degree-goal and diploma-goal students were co-mingled in nursing courses. Programs that failed the first test criterion were termed the "affiliated" type. In 1950, 129 of 195 schools offering a basic (prelicensure) program were of the affiliated type. In 1953, 104 of the 199 schools still offered both degree and diploma programs (Harms, 1955) and given the pragmatics of programs, probably co-mingled the two types of students in courses. To further complicate the situation, only 9,000 of the 21,000 baccalaureate students in 1950 were prelicensure students. The remaining 12,000 postdiploma baccalaureate students were not evenly distributed among schools, so some programs found themselves with a sprinkling of prelicensure students among a class of experienced diploma graduates.

Bridgman recommended that postdiploma students be evaluated individually and provisionally with a tentative grant of credit based on prior learning, including nursing schoolwork, and successful completion of a term of academic work. The student's program would be made up of "deficiencies" in general education and prerequisite courses and then courses in the major itself. Credit-granting practices varied considerably from place to place, so a nurse could easily spend 1.5 to 3 years earning the baccalaureate (Bridgman, 1953). National nursing organizations elected not to update the curriculum guide in the late 1940s, perhaps because the 1937 Guide still presented challenges. However, Bridgman provided "suggestions for content" using the categories of

1. Knowledge from the physical and biological sciences,
2. Communication skills,
3. The major in nursing,
4. Knowledge from social science (sociology, social anthropology, and psychology), and
5. General education, all of which she thought should ideally be interrelated throughout the program.

Of the 199 colleges and universities offering programs leading to bachelor's degrees in 1953, the National Nursing Accrediting Service accredited 51 basic programs.

Given the constant expansion of knowledge relevant to nursing, it was doubly difficult for programs with a history of a 5-year curriculum to shrink to 4 academic years in the 1960s and early 1970s. The expanded assessment skills expected of coronary and critical care nurses, together with the master's-level clinical content emphasis in clinical nurse specialist and certificate nurse practitioner programs, stimulated the inclusion of more sophisticated skills in baccalaureate programs in the early to mid-1970s (Lynaugh & Brush, 1996). In response to nursing service agitation to narrow the gap between new graduate organizing skills and initial employment expectations, and the much talked about "reality shock," baccalaureate programs structured curricula to allow a final experience in which students were immersed in clinical care to focus on skills of organization and integration, stimulated by a multipatient assignment.

Associate degree-prepared nurses of the early 1980s found expectations and mechanisms for matriculating into baccalaureate programs much more clearly defined than described by Bridgman 30 years earlier, and indeed, some baccalaureate programs were designed specifically for associate degree graduates. The ever-expanding body of nursing knowledge forced repeated decisions about which content was most essential and what clinical settings would bring about the best learning. By the 1990s, as hospital censuses plummeted and sick patients shuttled back and forth between home and ambulatory settings, programs were forced to consider increasing community-based clinical experience with its attendant challenges to find placements and provide geographically dispersed instruction.

ASSOCIATE DEGREE PROGRAMS

Programs of the 1950s in senior colleges had to cope with the entrenched traditions of both hospitals and universities as they struggled to make changes. By contrast, associate degree nursing programs began with a clean slate. They were initially welcomed by community colleges. The lure of having an additional supply of nurses promoted at least grudging cooperation from clinical agencies, although hospital nursing staff and administrators in many places had misgivings about the curricular arrangements and limited clinical experience of students.

At the height of the government-supported access to college for veterans after World War II, the President's Commission on Higher Education projected that a much higher proportion of young Americans had the ability to do postsecondary work than had actually completed it before the War. The Commission envisioned low-cost-to-student education at both the community colleges and the former normal schools that were increasingly redesignated as colleges (President's Commission on Higher Education, 1948). Junior colleges had existed for some time and California developed many public junior colleges, which had dual classification as grades 13 and 14 of secondary education and years 1 and 2 of college (Lavine, 1986). Emphasis formerly had been on preparing students to transfer to senior colleges with junior year standing. The postwar conversation in educational circles, however, focused on transforming the "junior" college into a "community" college, which would provide preparation for fields that required only 2 years of postsecondary study, while continuing to fulfill the transfer function. In this period the excitement and the new thinking in junior college circles was about development of terminal programs to serve the needs of local students and local employers (Haase, 1990).

In early 1950, representatives of NLNE approached their counterparts at the American Association of Junior Colleges (AAJC) suggesting that they form a joint committee, including the Association of Collegiate Schools of Nursing, to study nursing education. The focus was to be the Brown Report, (i.e., *Nursing for the Future*) authored by Esther Lucille Brown, a social anthropologist with the Russell Sage Foundation (Brown, 1948). The immediate context for the committee, from the nursing side, was significant. In 1947, the Board of NLNE adopted the policy goal that nursing education should be located in the higher education system. Also in 1947, the faculty at TCCU launched a planning process that involved Eli Ginzberg, a young economist, who asserted that nursing could be thought of as a whole set of functions and roles rather than a single role or type of worker. He posited that nursing needed at least two types of practitioners, one professional, and one technical (Haase, 1990).

Starting in fall 1947, Brown began her conferences with nursing leaders and visits to more than 50 schools, completing her report so that it could be disseminated in September 1948. In one section of the report, she compared nursing to engineering with its highly valued technical workers. She believed that perhaps a "graduate bedside nurse" needed more preparation than a practical nurse, but less than a full-fledged professional nurse. In early 1949, NLNE sought funding for the joint work with community colleges and found the Russell Sage and W.K. Kellogg Foundations responsive with substantial support (Haase, 1990)

By May of 1950, nurse members of the AAJE–NLNE–ACSN Joint Committee reported to the NLNE Board that two possibilities were under consideration: (a) A 2-year program in nursing with transfer at the end of the 2 years to a senior university, and (b) a 3-year program leading to an Associate in Arts or Associate in Science degree and qualification to take the state board licensing examination. Later in the year, the Joint Committee indicated its interest in (a) education of practical nurses, (b) providing associate degree study that would form the base for baccalaureate study, and (c) in-service training for hospital staffs. Concurrently in 1950, Mildred Montag, a doctoral student at

TCCU, used her dissertation to work out the philosophy and plan for a new kind of nursing program and designed a plan for testing the viability of such a program. She was subsequently appointed to the Joint Committee in 1951 and became the project director for the anonymously funded Cooperative Research Project (CRP) in Junior and Community College Education for Nursing in early 1952 (Haase, 1990).

The CRP pilot programs were 2 years long, or 2 years plus a summer. Initially, they were one-third general education and two-thirds nursing, but they moved toward equal proportions of each by the end of the project. The curricula, although controlled by faculty in each school, tended to focus on variations in health in their first year, and then deviations from normal (i.e., physical and mental illness) in the second year. These "broad fields" were accompanied by campus nursing laboratory learning and by clinical learning experiences in a wide variety of client- or patient-care settings, but with a major hospital component. Students in the pilot programs were somewhat older than diploma or baccalaureate students, and some were married (a nonstarter in many diploma programs) and had children. Men were a small percentage of the students, but tripled the representation in diploma programs. State board examination pass rates for graduates of the pilot group were comparable to those of other programs.

From the mid-1950s to mid-1970s, when the associate degree program growth rate peaked, the number of programs doubled about every 4 years. By 1975, there were 618 associate degree programs in nursing, comprising 45% of basic nursing programs and graduating a comparable percentage of the new graduates each year. Diploma programs comprised 31% of basic programs; although given the recency of AD program development, the vast majority of nurses in practice still originally came from diploma programs (Haase, 1990; Rines, 1977). By 1959, W.K. Kellogg Foundation assistance to the expansion of associate degree nursing education totaled more than $3,000,000 dollars. The Nurse Training Act of 1964 and subsequent federal legislation funding nursing also contributed to program growth (Scott, 1972).

Over the ensuing years, elapsed time from enrollment to graduation lengthened, partly because of the expanding knowledge base needed to be "a bedside nurse," sometimes because of pressures from elsewhere on campus to expand general education, sometimes because of sequencing requirements of the nursing faculty, and on occasion because of the level of student preparation and ability or to student choice. Much time was devoted to communicating with hospital nursing service representatives to identify students' competencies at graduation so that new graduate orientations and staff development plans articulated with them. Curricular offerings were fine-tuned to ensure that these baseline competencies were met. When "the bedside" noticeably moved out of the hospital in the early 1990s, questions about preparation for practice in the home care context became urgent, but the familiar condition of the hospital "nursing shortage" laid these to rest.

NURSING EDUCATION CIVIL WAR

The cultural upheaval that characterized the mid-1960s through the 1970s had its counterpart in nursing. Within nursing, a rift grew between those who believed an incremental approach would eventually get nursing education situated optimally, undefined although that was, and those who believed that the eventual goal should be clearly specified far in advance so that changes could take the goal into account. Nurses involved in day-to-day patient care and many diploma nurse educators tended to cluster in the first group, and those, particularly educators, who were in national or regional leadership positions were in the second group. The latter group focused on the professional end of the nursing continuum, working to achieve the fullest possible academic and professional recognition for nursing so that its advocacy and action would have broad credibility and influence.

From this perspective, the American Nurses Association 1965 position paper, "Educational Preparation for Nurse Practitioners and Assistants to Nurses", seemed like the next logical step (ANA, 1965). After all, for more than 15 years the NLNE, reconstituted and combined with the NOPHN, ACSN, and National Association of Industrial Nurses (NAIN) in 1952 to be the National League for Nursing (NLN), had been saying that education for nursing belonged in institutions of higher education. The idea that nursing was a continuum, comprised of vocational, technical, and professional segments, had been talked about intermittently in those same circles during that entire period.

Unfortunately, the Position Paper dropped like a bomb on people who had never heard these conversations. It was said to ignore diploma schools and nurses altogether, classify associate degree-prepared nurses as technical nurses, and downgrade vocational/practical nurse preparation. Fundamental questions, such as the "fit" of the three-part typology with the range of nursing work, the location and nature of the boundaries between the segments of the continuum, and the regulatory and licensure implications of such a plan could hardly be debated because of the emotionality that surrounded the specter of the loss of access to the "RN" title for associate and diploma nurses and what appeared to be the hijacking of the term "professional".

Regardless of nursing program background, the term "professional" had been applied to all that was good. General usage, likewise, cast "professional" in positive terms. A person who did a project or handled a situation "professionally" knew it was well done; a student who "looked professional" knew she had met certain standards (however little clean shoelaces may have had to do with actual professionalism); and a student who studied to be a "professional nurse" would qualify to take the state board examination, and in the years just before the position paper, thought she would give comprehensive, individualized care to patients. "Technical" just did not have the same ring to it; "technical" sounded limited and mechanical; "technical" sounded "less than". However knowledgeable, talented, and essential technical workers were in the discourse of educational macroplanners and economists, the word translated poorly to the world of nursing. Immense amounts of creative and emotional energy were diverted into this conflict.

The crisis was gradually defused, partly by action on the recommendations of the next committee to study nursing, "The National Commission for the Study of Nursing and Nursing Education" (1970), which was commonly known as the Lysaught Commission, which reported in 1970. Among the recommendations in *Abstract for action* were (a) statewide planning for the number and distribution of nursing education programs, (b) career mobility for individual nurses, and (c) cooperation of nursing service and education in working to improve patient care. As the world around community colleges changed so that more and more people, particularly women, resumed formal education after a hiatus, and senior colleges had good experience with community college graduates who sought baccalaureate degrees, the concepts of "career mobility" and "articulation" came into nursing discourse. By 1972, the NLN prepared a collection titled, "The Associate Degree Program—A Step to the Baccalaureate Degree in Nursing". However, according to Patricia Haase, a historian of associate degree programs, it was also true that "(i)t was assumed by some in baccalaureate education that the curricula of the two nursing programs were not related, that they occupied two separate universes" (Haase, 1990). Rapprochement was gradually achieved, but sensitivities, which have their roots in this conflict, exist to this day.

MASTER'S PROGRAMS

Master's programs differentiated from undergraduate programs and developed a distinctive focus in the 30 years from 1950–1980. Initially, the dire need for faculty in all three types of prelicensure programs prompted the impulse to establish first-level graduate programs. Federal funding for traineeships and program development, starting in 1957, provided resources for expansion. The outlines of advanced clinical knowledge and practice gradually emerged, first in the discussion and implementation of preparation for the clinical nurse specialist role in the acute care practice context. Almost concurrent with this, although using a continuing education approach, nursing and medical educators were designing programs for preparation on nurse practitioners for outpatient care.

Master's programs were few and relatively small in the 1950s. The 1951 report of the NNAS Postgraduate Board of Review noted that in some instances, the same set of courses led to a master's degree for students who held a baccalaureate and to a baccalaureate for students who had no prior degree. Some of the clearly differentiated master's programs had so many prerequisites that few students qualified for admission without clearing multiple "deficiencies" by taking additional course work. The Report opined that few programs focused on nursing "in its broadest sense," as contrasted to teaching and administration. Even this narrower focus seemed to be designed for the 2,000 hospitals with schools of nursing rather than the 4,500 hospitals without schools (NNAS Postgraduate Board of Review, 1951).

A work conference on graduate nurse education sponsored by the NLN Division of Nursing Education in fall of 1952 concluded that master's graduates needed competencies in interpersonal relations, communication skills, their selected functional area (e.g., teaching or administration), promotion of community welfare, and "sufficient familiarity with the principles and methods of research to conduct and/or participate in systematic investigation of nursing problems and evaluate and use research findings" (Harms, 1955, p. 297). However, a 1954 study comparing six leading schools' master's curricula identified wide variability in actual practice. Program lengths were nominally 1 year for students without deficiencies; however, this actually ranged from 24 to 38 semester credits. Although research was an agreed-upon master's focus, only one of the six schools had one course that by title could be identified as addressing this area. And names of degrees varied widely (Harms, 1955).

Given the relatively few students seeking admission and the small size of programs, regional planning became important, particularly in the South and the West.

In regional activity that was the precursor to the formation of the Southern Council on Collegiate Education for Nursing (SCCEN), it was agreed in 1952 that six universities—University of Alabama, University of Maryland, University of North Carolina, University of Texas, Vanderbilt University, and Emory University—would come together to plan five new master's programs to serve the South. This Regional Project in Graduate Education in Nursing garnered funding from both the W.K. Kellogg and Commonwealth Foundations. By 1955, all six programs were admitting students (Reitt, 1987).

In the West, the Western Conference of Nursing Education was convened in early 1956 by the Western Interstate Commission for Higher Education (WICHE). Nursing educators, nurse leaders in various other positions, and nonnurse representatives from higher education from the western states gathered to advise WICHE on the development of nursing education programs in the area. A 2-month study of nursing education in the West conducted by Helen Nahm laid the groundwork for the meeting. This report provided the group with the essence of hundreds of interviews conducted with educators in nursing and related fields in the eight states, as well as nurse manpower data by state for 1954. Respondents reportedly believed that graduate programs in nursing should contain more work in social science fields, advanced preparation in physical and biological science fields, strong foundations in education, courses basic to research, courses in philosophy, research in some area of nursing, and "graduate courses in a clinical nursing area which are truly of graduate caliber . . . " (WICHE, 1956, p. 16). Subsequently, the Western Interstate Council for Higher Education in Nursing (WICHEN) sponsored joint work that developed early master's level clinical content and terminal competencies in the early and mid-1960s (Brown, 1978; WICHE, 1967).

Enrollment in master's programs almost doubled between 1951 and 1962, growing from 1,290 to 2,472 (Harms, 1955, Kalisch & Kalisch, 1978). During the 1960s, clinical area emphases replaced functional specializations as the organizing frames for curricula. This shift in focus to nursing itself not only clarified and enriched baccalaureate curricula in later decades (Lynaugh & Brush, 1996), but it also freed doctoral level training to focus directly toward nursing knowledge development.

The clinical specialist role, idealized by educators, combined advanced clinical area knowledge with sophisticated care giving, care integration, and care improvement skills. The concept of such a master's-level role was discussed as early as 1949 and the first program embodying the concept was developed in 1954 (Smoyak, 1976). A number of papers on the subject came into the literature in the 1960s. The NLN Council of Baccalaureate and Higher Degree Programs devoted its third annual meeting in 1968 to the topic of clinical nurse specialist (CNS) preparation. Plenary papers, reflecting the flux of the period, blurred the concepts of clinically expert knowledge and the CNS's role and described preparation for the role variously as master's and doctoral work. The published proceedings of the meeting closed with a summary role description that bears striking resemblance to the current general outlines of the role (National League for Nursing Council of Baccalaureate and Higher Degree Programs, 1969). Although this idealized role description existed, the circumstances of each employing agency differed in actual practice, so the mix and emphasis of responsibilities varied from place to place, and various agencies combined clinical specialist functions with others, such as supervision or staff development, in actual practice.

Political pressure for access to care, interacting with the shortage and maldistribution of physicians and recognition that nurses could competently do a subset of physician work led to federal support for the spread of nurse practitioner (NP) programs (Bullough, 1976; National Commission for the Study of Nursing and Nursing Education. 1971). Until the mid-1970s most nurse practitioner preparation was designed and offered as non-degree-related continuing education. The first national conference on family nurse practitioner curricula convened in January 1976. At that point, programs ranged from 4-month certificate level offerings to specialties set within master's programs, with divergent characteristics depending upon rural or urban settings. Certificate programs accounted for 71% of NP program grants funded by the Division of Nursing of the USPHS that year. Just 9 years later, in 1985, 81% of NP program grants went to master's level programs without any change in the authorizing law and presumably the award criteria (Geolot, 1987). Multiple factors drove or accommodated this change. Practice settings had higher expectations, fears of nurse educators about preserving the essence of nursing subsided, sufficient numbers of potential students saw value in a graduate degree, and faculty members who reconceptualized the curricula were persuasive. Not insignificantly, federal funds were available to assist with the costs of transition. Curricular trends over the 20-year period included a proportionate decrease in time spent on health assessment and medical management, movement of pharmacology from freestanding courses to integration in medical management courses—and back again to freestanding, increased emphasis on health promotion and chronic illness management, and development of common clinical core courses in schools where multiple nurse practitioner specialty tracks existed (Geolot, 1987).

Although graduate education in the 1960s and 1970s appears inventive and creative in retrospect, educators at the time found the simultaneous and sometimes conflicting changes difficult to reconcile. Clinical specialists were easiest to see as a development on the familiar base of nursing. But wariness, if not suspicion, greeted nurse practitioners, that seemed tainted by too-close associations with medicine and the work of medicine. Outside of academia, critical care nurses, an example of practice-born specialists, formed their own specialty association, raising questions about the fragmentation of nursing. Regional Medical Programs spearheaded continuing education efforts for both nurses and physicians that furthered nurse competence, but outside of standard nursing education channels. And then, from within nursing, came the idea of primary nursing. The recurrent question, "What is nursing?," sometimes shaded into a pessimistic "nursing will soon disappear" lament in this period (Gunter, 1966). Clinical specialization, whether at the advanced practice or staff nurse level, signaled a fundamental shift within nursing, occasioning uneasiness or frank antagonism because of the deeply held valuing of "sameness" in nursing. This sameness was equated to "equity," which was at odds with "expertness." For some to be "special[ized]" implied that others were not (Smoyak, 1976).

Most large master's programs had multiple specialties by the mid-1980s, but these only weakly correlated with the major specialty organizations and with certification mechanisms (Styles, 1989). The clinical expertise and interest of nursing faculty, links to local resources, community needs for a particular specialty, and federal/state/local voluntary organization financial initiatives to address specific health problems all drove the pattern of specialty development (Burns et al., 1993). Nursing specialty organizations, reflecting current practice perspectives, exerted a substantial shaping influence on specialty curricular content in their respective areas. The rapid expansion—27%—in the number of master's programs in the last half of the 1980s (Burns et al., 1993) may have spurred creative naming of specialties for purposes of student recruitment. Efforts to rationalize the relationships of the specialties to one another and where possible to achieve common use of resources were the natural response to this proliferation.

By the 1990s, permutations of what had been considered clinical specialist content were being combined with nurse practitioner approaches. Advanced practice nurses of both types were beginning to question whether the two roles were, after all, so different from one another (Elder & Bullough, 1990). Changes in health care financing and delivery were prompting clinical nurse specialist programs to include content to prepare graduates to deal with cost and reimbursement dimensions of care for populations (Wolf, 1990) and pressuring practitioner programs to prepare graduates to care for patients with less stable conditions. By the end of the first decade of the 21st century, this trend has coalesced into an advanced practice regulatory model that will have standardized graduate-level educational requirements if it is implemented as envisioned (Trossman, 2009).

The *Essentials of College and University Education for Professional Nursing* (AACN, 1986), with its ambitious goals for a substantial liberal arts and sciences background, reflected both nursing self-understanding and changing external circumstances. Applicant interest and professional vision converged to support the development of programs at the master's level for nonnurse college graduates. Students completed prelicensure generalist preparation before focusing in a specialty or delimited area, leading to the master's as the first professional degree (Wu & Connelly, 1992). Very few such programs had existed in the prior 2 decades (Diers, 1976; Plummer & Phelan, 1976). The *Essentials of Master's Education for Advanced Practice Nursing* codified the broad areas of agreement about master's preparation among educators (AACN, 1996) and this, together with accreditation mechanisms and a shared external environment, nudged programs toward common curricular characteristics.

The 1986 *Essentials* document foreshadowed another turning point in the long evolution of organized nursing thinking about the placement of basic generalist professional preparation within the standard degree structures of higher education. Given projections of health care system demand for nurses over the next 3 decades, the need for more comprehensively prepared nurses at the microsystem level because of increased care complexity, and concurrent flagging applicant interest in baccalaureate programs with contrasting brisk interest in first professional degree master's programs, it seemed that the time had come to begin to move basic generalist professional preparation to the master's level (AACN, 2002, 2003, 2007a). Early adopter programs began translating the curriculum template in the planning documents into the unique contexts of each school and cooperating nursing service provider(s). Variants were designed for both BSN and nonnurse college graduate applicants (AACN, 2007b). Accreditation and individual graduate certification reinforced curriculum similarity across institutions, and many hope that practice settings will adopt differentiated practice roles that will eventually support regulatory recognition (AACN, 2008, 2010b). Concurrent with this consensus effort, the Carnegie Foundation for the Advancement of Teaching, as part of its multiyear comparative study of professional education in the United States, funded a study of education for nursing practice. Although this focuses more on the "delivery" of the curriculum (i.e., on teaching–learning and the formation of nursing students) than on structures and content, the curricular implications both for basic programs and nurse teacher preparation are clear (Benner, Sutphen, Lonard, & Day, 2009).

DOCTORAL PROGRAMS

Educators began to focus on the hope of developing doctoral work in nursing in the midst of the chaotic educational diversity of the 1950s. The need for doctorally prepared faculty to teach master's students, whom it was hoped would graduate and teach in the multiplying baccalaureate programs, fueled part of the interest in this topic. But for leaders already involved in higher education, it was painfully clear that nursing needed some capacity for its own research that would focus on questions related to nursing interventions to create a coherent body of tested knowledge and improve care.

Both the Nursing Education Department at TCCU and nursing at New York University (NYU) offered arrangements with their education departments for nurses to engage in doctoral level study before the 1950s; however, the numbers of graduates were small. TCCU revised its program in the 1950s but continued to grant the EdD. With the coming of Martha Rogers as Chair of the Department of Nursing Education at NYU in 1954, the doctoral program was redirected to become a PhD in Nursing. University of Pittsburgh established a PhD with a focus in pediatric or maternal nursing in 1954. In contrast to Martha Rogers's view that theory was the starting point that would lead to knowledge development in the "applied" field of nursing, Florence Erickson and Reva Rubin at Pittsburgh believed that extensive exposure to clinical phenomena, along with skilled faculty guidance, would develop a true nursing science (Parietti, 1979). In the West, in the early WICHE/WICHEN conversations, the temporary need for help from other disciplines for research training was posited as a mechanism to build nursing knowledge and a critical mass of investigators (WICHE, 1956). The journal *Nursing Research* became available in 1952 as a mechanism for systematic communication (Bunge, 1962).

In 1955, the nursing research grants and fellowship program of the Public Health Service allocated $500,000 for research grants and $125,000 for fellowships, the first such funding for nursing. From 1955 to 1970, 156 nurses were supported by Special Predoctoral Research Fellowships for doctoral study and from 1959 to 1968, 18 schools of nursing received federally funded Faculty Research Development Grants to stimulate research capacity. The Nurse Scientist Graduate Training Programs, which provided federal incentive funding to disciplines outside of nursing to accept nurses as students and provided fellowships to the students, were designed to create a critical mass of faculty and a climate conducive to establishing doctoral programs in nursing (Grace, 1978). The Program continued from 1962 to 1976 and funded more than 350 nurse trainees (Berthold, Tschudin, Peplau, Schlotfeldt, & Rogers, 1966; Murphy, 1981).

Three additional doctoral programs were established in the 1960s (Boston University, 1960, DNSc, psychiatric/mental health focus; University of California San Francisco (UCSF), 1964, DNSc, multifocus; Catholic University, 1968, DNSc, medical–surgical and psychiatric/mental health foci). The Boston program took a clinical immersion approach analogous to the University of Pittsburgh. UCSF's program was structured as a research degree but identified clinical involvement as the base for knowledge development, influenced both by nurse faculty with a strong clinical identity and by the grounded theory perspectives of the several social scientists who were a part of the faculty.

A federally funded series of nine annual ANA-sponsored research conferences was initiated in 1965 and WICHEN sponsored the first of its annual Communicating Nursing Research conferences in 1968, thus creating space for face-to-face research exchange. MEDLARS made its debut in 1964, the first in a series of databases that would aid dissemination. Essential components for school of nursing research centers were identified (Gunter, 1967). A series of three federally funded conferences in Kansas City on nursing theory in 1969–1970 provided further opportunity to work through the divergent views of the relationships of theory, practice, and research to one another (Murphy, 1981).

In 1971, the Division of Nursing and the Nurse Scientist Graduate Training Committee (NSGTC) convened an invitational conference to address the type(s) of doctoral preparation. In this setting, Joseph Matarazzo, Chair of the NSGTC, presented a paper arguing that nursing was ready as a discipline to launch PhD study, citing its body of knowledge and the qualifications of trainees (Matarazzo & Abdellah, 1971; Murphy, 1981). Comprehensive information about the state of nursing doctoral resources became available by the mid-1970s (Leininger, 1976), and by the late 1970s, National Doctoral Forums, open to schools with established programs, provided a mechanism for exchange of viewpoints about doctoral education. Three additional research journals began publication in 1978 (Gortner, 1991). *The Discipline of Nursing* (Donaldson & Crowley, 1978) was a milestone paper. It differentiated the discipline of nursing from the practice of nursing but related the two as well and proposed a productive interrelationship of research, theory, and practice. It shifted the terms of debate away from the dichotomous basic/applied categories.

The body of knowledge in nursing was still, relative to the old disciplines, rather modest in the late 1970s, but the progress in 2 decades had been amazing, and the infrastructure to support further development was substantial (Gortner & Nahm, 1977). Students were focusing their dissertation research on nursing clinical issues (Loomis, 1984). However, the DNSc and PhD degrees, the two dominant degree titles, although differently named, were indistinguishable in their objectives and end products (Grace, 1978). Finally, themes related to the challenge of mentoring students who are dealing with what is not known, and fostering "humanship" between students and faculty to encourage student growth were beginning to come to print at the end of this decade (Downs, 1978).

Fifteen additional doctoral programs opened their doors during the 1970s (Cleland, 1976; Parietti, 1979). From 1980 to 1989 the number of programs grew from 22 to 50, prompting editorial comment, " . . . as dandelions in spring, more and more doctoral programs are appearing" (Downs, 1984). Other observers surveying the situation recommended regional planning to sponsor joint programs, but conceded that the resources were in individual universities and states, and that the mechanisms for making such efforts were nonexistent. They predicted stormy waters for programs that launched without adequate internal and external supports in place (McElmurry, Krueger, & Parsons, 1982). At the end of the 1980s, doctoral educators were examining the balance between theory and research methods on the one hand and "knowledge" or "substance" in the curriculum (Downs, 1988).

Programs expanded from 50 to 70 between 1990 and 1999. By the early 1990s, as the research programs were more numerous and robust in the older and larger schools, greater emphasis on research team participation (Keller & Ward, 1993) and mentoring into the range of activities doctoral graduates became visible themes (Meleis, 1992; Katefian, 1991). Postdoctoral study became more feasible and attractive (Hinshaw & Lucas, 1993).

The perennial question from the 1960s to the 1980s, that is, whether nursing should adopt the PhD or the DNSc, was answered by the hundreds of individual choices of applicants and the program choices of numerous schools. By 2000, only 12% of nursing doctoral programs conferred the DNSc, or variants thereon (McEwen & Bechtel, 2000). Much less clear, however, was the difference between the two. Concerns about attention to "substance," that is organized analysis of the body of nursing knowledge, the adequacy of research programs to provide student experience, and preparation for the teaching component of graduates' expected academic roles, occupied curriculum planners in research-focused doctoral programs at the end of the century (Anderson, 2000).

Questions about the desirability and feasibility of developing clinical or practice-focused doctoral programs in nursing were perennial but intermittent until the past decade (Mundinger et al., 2000), when the American Association of Colleges of Nursing in 2004 adopted a proposal that would move preparation for advanced practice nursing from the master's degree framework to the doctoral level by 2015 (AACN, 2004, 2009). Such programs are currently designed to articulate with both nursing baccalaureate and nursing master's degree (first professional degree and second). The 4 postbaccalaureate academic years include core areas for all students as well as clinical specialty-focused study. The research-training component emphasizes the translation of research into practice, practice evaluation, and evidence-based practice improvement. Following from that, several possible forms of end-of-program practice-focused projects and project reporting formats demonstrate the student's synthesis and expertise, while laying the groundwork for future clinical scholarship (AACN, 2006). Currently, there are equal numbers of research and practice-focused doctoral programs (AACN, 2010a). What the long-term, steady state allocation of nursing's academic resources should be for the two types of programs is yet to be determined. And the development of combination programs, analogous to the MD–PhD, is also yet to be determined.

BEST-LAID PLANS?

Given this survey of nursing curricula, can one say that the curriculum plans of nursing have indeed been "best-laid"? The answer depends on the angle of the lens through which one views the scene. Certainly with narrow focus, one could point to Isabel Hampton's detailed plan for the Johns Hopkins curriculum, or the ever more specific *Curriculums* of the NLNE, or the endless curriculum massage characteristic of the 1960s and 1970s as examples of planning. But the uncertainties of nursing's external environment, its status as a predominantly women's field, and its limited access to major financial support apart from governmental funding have limited its "planning" in a comprehensive sense. More characteristic has been the incremental or directional planning, together with persistent activity to create openings and constant alertness for the unexpected opportunity. Perhaps in the last analysis, the measure of these plans lies not in the elegance of the plans themselves, but in the outcomes of the plans, measured not solely in educational terms, but in nursing's contribution to health.

SUMMARY

Chapter 1 reviews the rich heritage and development of nursing curricula from the mid- to late 1800s to 2010. It discusses the influence that changes in society and the health care system, the Civil War, and international wars had on nursing education. The role of accreditation and the changes it brought about in nursing curricula are reviewed.

The visions of nurse leader educators over the centuries who called for a unified approach to curriculum development in nursing are reviewed, and the discussion continues with a description of the rapid changes in nursing education during the latter half of 1900s that included the development of nursing programs in community colleges and baccalaureate and higher degree programs. Advanced practice roles at the master's level came about as demands for higher levels of nursing practice evolved, as patterns of physicians' practice changed, and as technological advances created opportunities for the adjustment of nursing boundaries. Doctoral programs developed as nursing consolidated its professional identity and began to build the scientific body of knowledge through research. And in the past decade, programs to prepare advanced practice nurses at the professional doctoral level have mushroomed to equal the numbers of research-focused doctoral programs in nursing.

DISCUSSION QUESTIONS

1. If NLNE had formed a joint committee with the American Association of State Colleges in 1950 (fictional name, but conceptually the group of former normal schools that were becoming comprehensive baccalaureate degree-granting institutions in the post-World War II period), would the characteristics of nursing education be different today? Whatever your answer, explain your reasoning.
2. With the exception of a few years in the early 1990s, the shortage of nurses to provide care in hospitals has been a chronic problem with intermittent acute exacerbations since the 1930s. What effects at both macro level (e.g., public opinion, social policy) and micro level (e.g., individual schools, courses) has this had on nursing education? Has the net balance of positive and negative effects been positive for nursing education? Why?

LEARNING ACTIVITIES

Student Learning Activity

Choose teams and debate the wisdom and feasibility of setting the master's degree as the minimum marker for the professional segment of the nursing continuum. Given our 20/20 hindsight gained from the debacle of the 1965 position paper, how would you advise national nursing organizations to go about changing this definition, if it were to be changed?

Faculty Learning Activity:

Trace your school of nursing's history and link major curriculum changes to events external to the nursing program.

I want to thank Joan E. Lynaugh, University of Pennsylvania Center for the Study of the History of Nursing, for her chapter review comments that drew from her seasoned historical perspective and knowledge.

REFERENCES

Aikens, C. A. (1911). *Hospital management*. Philadelphia: Saunders. (Facsimile copy republished by New York: Garland, 1985.)

American Association of Colleges of Nursing. (1986). *Essentials of college and university education for professional nursing*. Washington, DC: Author.

American Association of Colleges of Nursing. (1996). *The essentials of master's education for advanced practice nursing*. Washington, DC: Author.

American Association of Colleges of Nursing. (2002). Report of the task force on education and regulation for professional nursing practice I. Retrieved from http://www.aacn.nche.edu/Education/edandreg02.htm

American Association of Colleges of Nursing. (2003). Clinical nurse leader: Remarks delivered by AACN President Kathleen Ann Long. Retrieved from http://www.aacn.nche.edu/cnl/history.htm

American Association of Colleges of Nursing. (2004). AACN position statement on the practice doctorate in nursing October 2004. Retrieved from http://www.aacn.nche.edu/DNP/DNPPositionStatement.htm

American Association of Colleges of Nursing. (2006). The essentials of doctoral education for advanced nursing practice. Retrieved from http://www.aacn.nche.edu/DNP/pdf/Essentials.pdf

American Association of Colleges of Nursing. (2007a). White paper on the education and role of the clinical nurse leader February 2007. Retrieved from http://www.aacn.nche.edu/Publications/WhitePapers/ClinicalNurseLeader07.pdf

American Association of Colleges of Nursing. (2007b). Clinical nurse leader education models being implemented by schools of nursing. Retrieved from http://www.aacn.nche.edu/cnl/pdf/CNLEdModels.pdf

American Association of Colleges of Nursing. (2008). CNL frequently asked questions. Retrieved from http://www.aacn.nche.edu/cnl/faq.htm

American Association of Colleges of Nursing. (2009). Fact sheet: The doctor of nursing practice (DNP). Retrieved from http://www.aacn.nche.edu/Media/FactSheets/dnp.htm

American Association of Colleges of Nursing. (2010a). Number of doctoral programs in nursing 2006–2009. Retrieved from http://www.aacn.nche.edu/Media/NewsReleases/2010/enrollchanges.html

American Association of Colleges of Nursing. (2010b). Press release: Amid calls for more highly educated nurses, new AACN data show impressive growth in doctoral nursing programs. Retrieved from http://www.aacn.nche.edu/Media/NewsReleases/2010/enrollchanges.html

American Nurses' Association. (1965). Educational preparation for nurse practitioners and assistants to nurses: A position paper. New York: Author.

Anderson, C. A. (2000). Current strengths and limitations of doctoral education in nursing: Are we prepared for the future? *Journal of Professional Nursing, 16*(4), 191–200.

Armeny, S. (1983). Organized nurses, women philanthropists, and the intellectual bases for cooperation among women, 1898–1920. In E. C. Lagerman (Ed.), *Nursing history: New perspectives, new possibilities* (pp. 13–46). New York: Teachers College, Columbia University.

Baldwin, D. O. (2002). Discipline, obedience, and female support groups: Mona Wilson at the Johns Hopkins Hospital School of Nursing, 1915–1918. In E. D. Baer, P. O. D'Antonio, S. D. Rinker, & J. E. Lynaugh (Eds.), *Enduring issues in American nursing* (pp. 85–105). New York: Springer.

Benner, P., Sutphen, M., Leonard, V., & Day, L. (2009). *Educating nurses: A call for radical transformation.* San Francisco: Jossey-Bass.

Berthold, J. S., Tschudin, M. S., Peplau, H. E., Schlotfeldt, R., & Rogers, M. E. (1966). A dialogue on approaches to doctoral preparation. *Nursing forum 5,* 48–104.

Bevis, E. O. (1989). *Curriculum building in nursing: A process.* New York: National League for Nursing.

Bevis, E. O., & Watson, J. (1989). *Toward a caring curriculum: A new pedagogy for nursing.* New York: National League for Nursing.

Bridgman, M. (1949). Consultant in collegiate nursing education. *American Journal of Nursing, 49,* 808.

Bridgman, M. (1953). *Collegiate education for nursing.* New York: Russell Sage Foundation.

Brown, E. L. (1948). *Nursing for the future.* New York: Russell Sage Foundation.

Brown, J. M. (1978). Master's education in nursing, 1945–1969. In J. Fitzpatrick (Ed.), *Historical studies in nursing* (pp. 104–130). New York: Teachers College, Columbia University.

Bullough, B. (1976). Influences on role expansion. *American Journal of Nursing, 76,* 1476–1481.

Bullough, V., & Bullough, B. (1978). *The care of the sick: The emergence of modern nursing.* New York: Prodist.

Bunge, H. L. (1962). The first decade of nursing research. *Nursing Research, 11,* 132–137.

Burns, P. G., Nishikawa, H. A., Weatherby, F, Forni, P. R., Moran, M., Allen, M. E., Baker, C. M., & Booten, D. A. (1993). Master's degree nursing education: State of the art. *Journal of Professional Nursing, 9,* 267–277.

Cleland, V. (1976). Developing a doctoral program. *Nursing Outlook, 24,* 631–635.

Committee of the Six National Nursing Organizations on Unification of Accrediting Services. (1949). *Manual of accrediting educational programs in nursing.* New York: National Nursing Accrediting Service.

Committee on the Grading of Nursing Schools. (1931). *Results of the first grading study of nursing schools.* New York: Author.

D'Antonio, P. O. (1987). All a woman's life can bring: The domestic roots of nursing in Philadelphia, 1830–1885. *Nursing Research, 36,* 12–17.

D'Antonio, P. O. (1993). The legacy of domesticity. *Nursing History Review, 1,* 229–246.

Diers, D. (1976). A combined basic-graduate program for college graduates. *Nursing Outlook, 24,* 92–98.

Dodd, D. (2001). Nurses' residences: Using the built environment as evidence. *Nursing History Review, 9,* 185–206.

Donaldson, S. K., & Crowley, D. M. (1978). The discipline of nursing. *Nursing Outlook, 26,* 113–120.

Downs, F. S. (1978). Doctoral education in nursing: Future directions. *Nursing Outlook, 26,* 56–61.

Downs, F. S. (1984). Caveat emptor. *Nursing Research, 33,* 59.

Downs, F. S. (1988). Doctoral education: Our claim to the future. *Nursing Outlook, 36,* 18–20.

Egenes, K. J. (1998). An experiment in leadership: The rise of student government at Philadelphia General Hospital Training school, 1920–1930. *Nursing History Review, 6,* 71–84.

Eisenmann, L. (2000). Reconsidering a classic: Assessing the history of women's higher education a dozen years after Barbara Solomon. In R. Lowe (Ed.), *History of education: Major themes, 1* (pp. 411–442). New York: Routledge & Falmer.

Elder, R. G., & Bullough, B. (1990). Nurse practitioners and clinical nurse specialists: Are the roles merging? *Clinical Nurse Specialist, 4,* 78–84.

Faddis, M. (1973). *A school of nursing comes of age.* Cleveland, OH: Howard Allen.

Gage, N. D. (1918). Organization of classwork and student life at the Vassar training camp. *American Journal of Nursing, 19,* 18–22.

Geolot, D. H. (1987). NP education: Observations from a national perspective. *Nursing Outlook, 35,* 132–135.

Goldmark, J. (1923). *Nursing and nursing education in the United States.* New York: Macmillan.

Goodnow, M. (1934). *Outlines of nursing history* (5th ed.). Philadelphia: Saunders.

Gortner, S. R. (1991). Historical development of doctoral programs: Shaping our expectations. *Journal of Professional Nursing, 7,* 45–53.

Gortner, S. R., & Nahm, H. (1977). An overview of nursing research in the United States. *Nursing Research, 26,* 10–33.

Grace, H. (1978). The development of doctoral education in nursing: An historical perspective. *Journal of Nursing Education, 17,* 17–27.

Graham, P. A. (1978). Expansion and exclusion: A history of women in higher education. *Signs, 3,* 759–773.

Gunter, L. M. (1966). Some problems in nursing care and services. In B. Bullough & V. Bullough (Eds.), *Issues in Nursing* (pp. 152–156). New York: Springer.

Gunter, L. M. (1967). Notes on a proposed center for nursing research. *Nursing Research, 16,* 185.

Haase, P. T. (1990). *The origins and rise of associate degree nursing education.* New York: National League for Nursing and Durham, NC: Duke University.

Hampton, I. A. (1893). *Nursing: Its principles and practice; for hospital and private use.* Philadelphia: Saunders. (Facsimile republished by Saunders, 1993.)

Hanson, K. S. (1991). An analysis of the historical context of liberal education in nursing education from 1924 to 1939. *Journal of Professional Nursing, 7,* 341–350.

Harms, M. T. (1955). *Professional education in university schools of nursing.* Unpublished dissertation. Stanford University, CA.

Hine, D. C. (1989). *Black women in white: Racial conflict and cooperation in the nursing profession, 1890–1950.* Indianapolis: Indiana University.

Hinshaw, A. S., & Lucas, M. D. (1993). Postdoctoral education—a new tradition for nursing research. *Journal of Professional Nursing, 9,* 309.

James, J. W. (2002). Isabel Hampton and the professionalization of nursing in the 1890s. In E. D. Baer, P. O. D'Antonio, S. Rinker, & J. E. Lynaugh (Eds.), *Enduring issues in American nursing* (pp. 42–84). New York: Springer.

Journal of American Medical Association. (1927). Hospital service in the United States. *Journal of the American Medical Association, 88,* 789–812.

Kalisch, P. A., & Kalisch, B. J. (1978). *The advance of American nursing.* Boston: Little, Brown.

Katefian, S. (1991). Doctoral preparation for faculty roles: Expectations and realities. *Journal of Professional Nursing, 7,* 105–111.

Keller, M. L., & Ward, S. E. (1993). Funding and socialization in the doctoral program at the University of Wisconsin–Madison. *Journal of Professional Nursing, 9,* 262–266.

Lavine, D. O. (1986). *The American college and the culture of aspiration, 1915–1940.* Ithaca, NY: Cornell University.

Leininger, M. (1976). Doctoral programs for nurses: Trends, questions, and projected plans. *Nursing Research, 25,* 201–210.

Loomis, M. (1984). Emerging content in nursing: An analysis of dissertation abstracts and titles: 1976–1982. *Nursing Research, 33,* 113–199.

Lynaugh, J. E. (2002). Nursing's history: Looking backward and seeing forward. In E. D. Baer, P. O. D'Antonio, S. Rinker, & J. E. Lynaugh (Eds.), *Enduring issues in American nursing* (10–24). New York: Springer.

Lynaugh, J. E., & Brush, B. L. (1996). *American nursing: From hospitals to health systems.* Cambridge, MA: Blackwell.

Matarazzo, J., & Abdellah, F. (1971). Doctoral education for nurses in the United States. *Nursing Research, 20,* 404–414.

McElmurry, B. J., Krueger, J. C., & Parsons, L. C. (1982). Resources for graduate education: A report of a survey of forty states in the Midwest, west, and southern regions. *Nursing Research, 31,* 5–10.

McEwen, M., & Bechtel, G. A. (2000). Characteristics of nursing doctoral programs in the United States. *Journal of Professional Nursing, 16,* 282–292.

Meleis, A. I. (1992). On the way to scholarship: From master's to doctorate. *Journal of Professional Nursing, 8,* 328–334.

Melosh, B. (1982). *"The physician's hand": Work culture and conflict in American nursing.* Philadelphia: Temple University.

Mundinger, M. O., Cook, S. S., Lenz, E. R., Piacentini, K., Auerhahn, C., & Smith, J. (2000). Assuring quality and access in advanced practice nursing: A challenge to nurse educators. *Journal of Professional Nursing, 16,* 322–329.

Murphy, J. F. (1981). Doctoral education in, of, and for nursing: An historical analysis. *Nursing Outlook, 29,* 645–649.

National Commission for the Study of Nursing and Nursing Education. (1970). *An Abstract for Action.* New York: McGraw Hill.

National Commission for the Study of Nursing and Nursing Education. (1971). *Nurse clinician and physician's assistant: The relationship between two emerging practitioner concepts.* Rochester, New York: Author.

National League for Nursing Council of Baccalaureate and Higher Degree Programs. (1969). *Extending the boundaries of nursing education—the preparation and roles of the clinical specialist.* New York: Author.

National League of Nursing Education. (1917). *Standard curriculum for schools of nursing.* Baltimore: Waverly.

National League of Nursing Education. (1927). *A curriculum for schools of nursing.* New York: Author.

National League of Nursing Education. (1937). *A curriculum guide for schools of nursing.* New York: Author.

National Nursing Accrediting Service Postgraduate Board of Review. (1951). Some problems identified. *American Journal of Nursing, 51,* 337–338.

Obituaries. (1940). Mrs. Clara S. Weeks Shaw. *American Journal of Nursing, 40,* 356.

Parietti, E. S. (1979). *Development of doctoral education for nurses: An historical survey.* Ann Arbor, MI: University Microfilms International.

Petry, L. (1937). Basic professional curricula in nursing leading to degrees: A study. *American Journal of Nursing, 37,* 287–297.

Petry, L. (1943). U. S. Cadet Nurse Corps. *American Journal of Nursing, 43,* 704–708.

Petry, L. (1949). We hail an important first. *American Journal of Nursing, 49,* 630–633.

President's Commission on Higher Education. (1948). *Higher education for American democracy: A report of the president's commission on higher education.* New York: Harper & Row.

Plummer, E. M., & Phelan, J. J. (1976). College graduates in nursing: A retrospective look. *Nursing Outlook, 24,* 99–102.

Reitt, B. B. (1987). *The first 25 years of the Southern Council on Collegiate Education for Nursing.* Atlanta, GA: Southern Council on Collegiate Education for Nursing.

Reverby, S. (1984). "Neither for the drawing room nor for the kitchen": Private duty nursing in Boston, 1873–1914. In J. W. Leavitt, (Ed.), *Women and Health in America* (pp. 454–466). Madison: University of Wisconsin.

Reverby, S. M. (1987). *Ordered to care: The dilemma of American nursing, 1850–1945.* New York: Cambridge University.

Rines, A. (1977). Associate degree education: History, development, and rationale. *Nursing Outlook, 25,* 496–501.

Robb, I. H. (1907). *Educational standards for nurses.* Cleveland, OH: E. C. Koeckert.

Roberts, M. M. (1954). *American nursing: History and interpretation.* New York: Macmillan.

Robinson, T. M., & Perry, P. M. (2001). Cadet Nurse stories: The call for and response of women during World War II. Indianapolis, IN: Center Press.

Schubert, W. H. (1986). *Curriculum: Perspective, paradigm, and possibility.* New York: Macmillan.

Scott, J. (1972). Federal support for nursing education, 1964–1972. *American Journal of Nursing, 72,* 1855–1860.

Sheahan, D. A. (1980). *The social origins of American nursing and its movement into the university: a microscopic approach.* Ann Arbor, MI: University Microfilms.

Smith-Rosenberg, C. (1985). *Disorderly conduct.* New York: Oxford.

Smoyak, S. A. (1976). Specialization in nursing: From then to now. *Nursing Outlook, 24,* 676–681.

Solomon, B. (1985). *In the company of educated women.* New Haven, CT: Yale University.

Styles, M. M. (1989). *On specialization in nursing: Toward a new empowerment.* Kansas City, MO: American Nurses' Foundation.

Tomes, N. (1984). "Little world of our own": The Pennsylvania Hospital Training School for Nurses, 1895–1907. In J. W. Leavitt (Ed.), *Women and health in America* (pp. 467–481). Madison: University of Wisconsin.

Trossman, S. (2009). APRN regulatory model continues to advance. *The American Nurse, 41*(6), 12–13.

Tyack, D. (1974). *The one best system: A history of American urban education.* Cambridge, MA: Harvard University.

Veysey, L. R. (1965*). The emergence of the American university.* Chicago: University of Chicago.

Vogel, M. J. (1980). *The invention of the modern hospital: Boston 1870–1930.* Chicago: University of Chicago.

Weeks-Shaw, C. (1902). *A text-book of nursing: For the use of training schools, families, and private students* (3rd ed.). New York: D. Appleton.

Western Interstate Commission for Higher Education. (1956). *Toward shared planning in western nursing education.* Boulder, CO: Author.

Western Interstate Commission on Higher Education. (1967). *Defining clinical content: graduate programs,* 1–4. Boulder, CO: Author.

Wolf, G. A. (1990). Clinical nurse specialists: The second generation. *Journal of nursing administration, 20,* 7–8.

Wu, C.-Y., & Connelly, C. (1992). Profile of nonnurse college graduates in accelerated baccalaureate nursing programs. *Journal of Professional Nursing, 8,* 35–40.

2

Curriculum Development and Approval Processes in Changing Educational Environments

Patsy L. Ruchala

OBJECTIVES

Upon completion of Chapter 2, the reader will be able to:

1. Analyze facilitators for and barriers to effective curriculum development and redesign.
2. Evaluate the effectiveness of a nursing curriculum.
3. Apply knowledge of potential barriers to curricular innovations in obtaining approvals for innovative curricular redesign.
4. Evaluate the impact of regulatory and accreditation agencies in the development and evaluation of nursing curriculum.

OVERVIEW

Faculty members have ultimate responsibility for curriculum development, ongoing evaluation, and redesign and must work together to determine what best practices must be implemented in nursing education so that students can master the knowledge and skills necessary for them to become practicing nurses. The innate complexity of nursing education, the need for collaboration with other disciplines within the college or university, the ever-changing and complex health care systems, and the requirements of regulatory and accreditation agencies can position curriculum development and redesign as a daunting process. The use of technology has exploded in both education and health care settings. The current generation of students embrace technology not only in education, but also as ordinary methods of communication and social networking, and their expectations for the use of technology at an advanced level may far exceed the capabilities of many nursing faculty. In addition to navigating the internal approval processes for curriculum approval, meeting the requirements of regulatory and accrediting agencies can also impact the approaches taken when developing or redesigning nursing curricula. This chapter provides an overview of the preparation and support needed for curriculum development/change, issues and challenges that can arise and impact the curriculum development process, innovations in curriculum development, and approvals and accreditations related to nursing curriculum.

THE PROCESS OF CURRICULUM DEVELOPMENT

Preparation and Support for Curricular Change

Nursing education has evolved using various theories from other disciplines as well as newer middle range theories developed specifically for the application to nursing practice. New roles for nurses have been developed to meet the needs of the practice setting as well as the increasing demand for more emphasis on education, primary prevention, and management of chronic diseases (Ben-Zur, Yagil, & Spitzer, 1999; Long, 2004; Pew Health Professions Commission, 1995). The need for change in health professions education is overwhelming, with an emphasis on evidence-based practice, quality improvement approaches, cultural competence, informatics, and interdisciplinary education (Callen & Lee, 2009; Ehnfors & Grobe, 2004; Giddens, Brady, Brown, Wright, Smith, & Harris, 2008; Greiner & Knebel, 2003; Sullivan, 2010). Given the knowledge explosion in science and the emphasis on major reform of health care education, it is no wonder that Giddens and colleagues (2008) point out that curriculum redesign in nursing "is an overwhelming undertaking."

The support of both faculty and administration is imperative for curriculum change. According to Billings and Halstead (2005), curriculum change is inevitable. The need for curriculum change may be a result of community pressure, policy, or accreditation changes, programmatic funding, personnel changes, or the simple acknowledgment that the existing curriculum is no longer effective for current and future students. For effective change to take place, faculty must realize the need for change. This realization, however, may be more apparent to some faculty members than to others.

In addition to recognizing and embracing the need for curriculum change, faculty need the knowledge and skills to engage in this endeavor. The engagement of faculty in ongoing curriculum development and change should begin with their orientation to the university or college. It is routinely expected that faculty will update courses with cutting-edge information each time the course is taught. Individual course updating over time, however, may impact the overall curriculum, resulting in "content gaps." Faculty benefit from serving on their school's curriculum committee and engaging in ongoing dialogue about and evaluation of the curriculum with their faculty colleagues. New faculty or faculty members who have not engaged in curriculum redesign benefit from mentoring by faculty with more experience in curriculum processes (Sawatzky & Enns, 2009). Support for curriculum change includes administrative assurance of needed resources: physical space, secretarial support, workload considerations, expert consultants, and internal administrative assurance and encouragement that the work toward curricular change is valued and needed by the organization and, most importantly, for successful student outcomes. Successful curriculum change requires support from all levels of the organization, including students. Students bring a unique perspective to curriculum committee discussions, particularly when faculty are charged to design a rigorous program while creating an environment conducive to students' learning preferences (Mangold, 2007; Moch, Cronje, & Branson, 2010). In a study of faculty perceptions of implementation of curriculum change, Powell-Cope, Hughes, Sedlak, and Nelson (2008) found that administrators, other faculty, and students who were "champions for curricular change" were also identified as facilitators of successful implementation of the new curriculum.

Curriculum development and redesign always begin at the level of the school curriculum committee. This may be a formal committee within the school or for very small

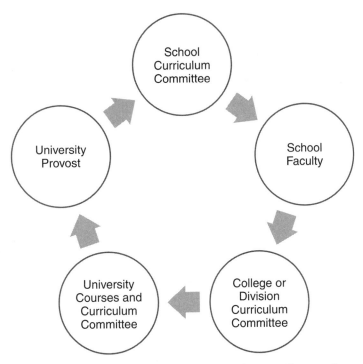

FIGURE 2.1 Example Curriculum Approval Process Sequencing

schools; it may consist of the entire nursing faculty. In most institutions of higher education, curriculum development and redesign must go through an extensive, multilevel approval process. Despite the number of levels in the approval process, a proposal for curriculum approval should be completed with the expectation that it will eventually be sent to the highest review body in the institution, keeping in mind all of the preceding levels of approval and the requirements and appropriate paperwork for routing of the proposal through each level. Although this process will vary at every institution, Figure 2.1 depicts an example for sequencing. Consideration should also be given as to whether this is a proposal for a graduate-level curricular change. If so, there may be another level of approval that would involve the graduate faculty of the school and/or the graduate school within the college or university. No matter what the individual process is, completeness, accuracy, and acceptable institutional formatting are extremely important to successfully navigate all levels of curriculum approval.

ISSUES RELATED TO CURRICULAR DEVELOPMENT OR REDESIGN

Faculty Development

Curriculum development is in itself a faculty development activity (Iwasiw, Goldenberg, & Andrusyszyn, 2009). To be successful in developing and implementing curricular change, Billings and Halstead (2005) indicate that faculty members who understand the problems inherent in the current curriculum and who can effectively evaluate strategies for solving the current problems should be the group initially involved in the change. Faculty who have less experience in curriculum development may need to acquire the knowledge and skills necessary to engage in curriculum work. Working with more experienced faculty, engaging in group discussion and debate, knowing that their contributions to the process will be heard and valued, and providing ongoing administrative support are all part of mentoring less experienced faculty to learn the process for curriculum change.

Budgetary Constraints

Schmitt (2002) and Tanner (2004) postulate that the cost efficiency of clinical nursing education has not been properly assessed, yet nursing has always been considered one of the more costly programs in institutions of higher education. At the time of this writing, the state of the national economy had a significant impact on all aspects of higher education, including nursing. Allen (2008) and Hinshaw (2008) both observed that the retirement of older faculty and the shortage of nursing educators stretches human, fiscal, and physical resources in nursing education. Although the need for more nurses keeps growing, funding for many nursing programs has been significantly impacted. When developing or redesigning nursing curricula, assessment of current and future resources is crucial. Budgetary constraints in hiring faculty along with other resources, such as the availability and use of high-fidelity simulation, will have a major impact on curriculum design/change and implementation of the curriculum (Adams, 2009; Bargagliotti, 2009; Nehring, 2008; Reese, Jeffries, & Engum, 2010). In 2009, almost 55,000 qualified applicants were turned away from U.S. nursing schools as a result of insufficient numbers of faculty, clinical sites, classroom space, clinical preceptors, and budget constraints (American Association of Colleges of Nursing [AACN], 2010). Budget shortfalls and economic declines resulted in scarcer resources available for universities and colleges to support nursing programs, forcing programs to be much more creative in determining strategies to sustain nursing education. Henderson and Hassmiller (2007) encourage the creation of local and regional partnerships with nurse employers, foundations, and other stakeholders as a sustainability strategy needed by the nursing profession.

Amount of Curricular Content

Another issue impacting curriculum development and change is the management of curricular content. The nursing literature provides an overwhelming amount of evidence indicating that faculty and students are besieged with content (Diekelmann, 2002; Giddens & Brady, 2007; Giddens et al., 2008; Ironside, 2004; Powell-Cope, Hughes, Sedlak, & Nelson, 2008). As the information explosion in health sciences education continues to grow, an increasing amount of content is deemed essential to include in all nursing curricula (AACN, 2008; National League for Nursing Accrediting Commission [NLNAC], 2008). One recent example of essential knowledge content to include in nursing curricula relates to a series of reports issued by the Institute of Medicine (Greiner & Knebel, 2003) that generated a great deal of attention to the need to improve the quality and safety of health care delivery. This led to dramatic changes in the practice of nursing, medicine, and other health disciplines. As nursing practice embraced the focus on improved quality and safety, it became clear that graduating nurses were missing critical competencies in this area. The result was a major national initiative, Quality Safety Education for Nurses (QSEN), centered on patient safety and quality topics, with a primary goal to address the challenge of preparing future nurses with the knowledge, skills, and attitudes (KSAs) necessary to continuously improve the quality and safety of the health care systems in which they will work (Sullivan, 2010). As the amount of essential knowledge and content continues to increase, there seems, however, to be an inherent faculty perception that they must teach everything they possibly can to their students in the minutest of detail. Consequently, "content saturation" is a major problem in many nursing curricula. Giddens et al. (2008) surmise that content saturation may be directly related to how faculty teach and that faculty should learn how to teach conceptually and, subsequently, minimize their emphasis on the *amount* of content students must learn.

Technology

Incorporating technology into the curriculum is a must to educate nurses in the 21st century. The advance of technology into our personal and professional lives marched into the arena of higher education, and the lecture method as the gold standard for teaching is rapidly being replaced by technology. The type of technology available for the classroom ranges from very low- to very-high fidelity (Thompson & Skiba, 2008). The methods of curriculum delivery and the use of technology must be addressed in any curriculum development or redesign, including the extent that technology will be used, resources to obtain and sustain technology, and faculty development to use technology effectively. For example, high-fidelity simulators are increasingly being used as an adjunct or replacement to some of the clinical experiences in nursing programs (Nehring, 2009; Reese et al., 2010). However, use of high-fidelity simulation requires a significant up-front investment as well as the cost for ongoing care, use, and replacement of simulators, and staff for simulation centers. In addition, to effectively use high-fidelity simulation, a significant investment must be made for faculty development to use the equipment and for incorporation into the curriculum.

Hartman, Dziuban, and Brophy-Ellison (2007) have identified a number of changes to which faculty must adapt as a result of diffusing technology into teaching and learning:

- Faculty, who are the experts in their respective disciplines, may experience a "balance-of-power shift" when confronted with technologically savvy students who know more about specific technologies than they do.
- Net Generation students use a range of technologies and information sources that are often unfamiliar to their faculty. When faculty communicate through technology, they are likely to use e-mail. Net Generation students communicate with peers through instant messages (IMs) and cell phone text messaging.
- Faculty are reporting a sharp decline in the quality of students' writing, which some attribute to the increasing popularity of IM and text messaging.
- Faculty see students as individual learners and regard students who complete assignments with others as cheaters. Net Generation students value social networking, working in groups, and experiential learning.

- Technology has caused a shift in the way faculty use their time. Traditionally, faculty would be in class, their offices, or their labs, or they would be off campus and inaccessible to students. Students now expect faculty to be accessible via e-mail almost any hour of the day or night and to respond to e-mails within minutes.
- Faculty think of technology as technology. Students think of technology as environment.
- A number of social networking and resource-sharing sites have appeared over the past few years, including Facebook, MySpace, Flickr, YouTube, LiveJournal, Twitter, and Second Life. Students are using these sites as the nexus of their social and even academic universe. Faculty are beginning to use these sites as a means of getting to know their students, as a rapid and reliable way to reach students, and as a method for sharing faculty-produced and student-produced content.

Faculty Issues

The shortage of nursing educators has already been discussed as an issue related to curriculum development and change, yet several other faculty issues arise that can impact curriculum development or redesign. In a study designed to determine nursing faculty perceptions regarding implementing a new curriculum, one of the two barriers determined by Powell-Cope and colleagues (2008) was the challenge of working with faculty colleagues who insisted on keeping the old curricular paradigm. Inherent in curriculum development and redesign is the human dimension of the nursing faculty and subsequently, the interpersonal dynamics associated with every aspect of curriculum redesign.

Fear of and resistance to change are the most influential barriers to progress in curriculum development and redesign. Although not an exhaustive list by any means, the following have been identified as barriers to successful curriculum development and redesign:

1. Differing faculty values about nursing education
2. Fear of losing control of certain aspects of the curriculum
3. Differing views about what needs to be done to the curriculum
4. Lack of embracing the need for curricular change
5. Uncertainty about how to begin the change process
6. Lack of resources
7. Desire to be vindictive so the curriculum committee chair, leader of curriculum change, or program Dean or Director looks bad
8. Lack of rewards
9. Feeling that the curricular change process is too overwhelming given the current resources or time constraints
   (Billings & Halstead, 2005; Cash et al., 2009; Iwasiw et al., 2009)

Faculty work with the curriculum must take into account not only a rapidly changing health care environment, but also the pressures to maintain currency in both clinical expertise and teaching technologies. Cash, Daines, Doyle, and von Tettenborn (2009) identified these pressures as "tensions (that) underpin curriculum and the ways in which knowledge is constructed through the framing of educational (including clinical) experiences" (pp. 318–319). Most nursing faculty members are no longer employed in health care facilities, and, in many instances, this leads to an "education–practice gap." Although clinical supervision of students helps some faculty stay connected to practice, many nursing faculty find it challenging to balance their full-time roles as academicians with the need for ongoing clinical practice. Faculty may find it difficult to access clinical practice experiences even on a part-time basis to maintain current practice knowledge and skills, as complex health care systems and practices, cost implications, and risk management considerations further complicate faculty practice arrangements.

Cultural competence is identified as a critical component of the nursing curriculum. However, not only do students need to be versed in how to care for patients from many cultural backgrounds because of the increased globalization of the nursing profession, but faculty also need to practice cultural competence in their teaching and in curriculum development. Over the past 2 or 3 decades, international experiences in higher education have become increasingly more commonplace. Caldwell, Hongyan, and Harding (2010) assert that nearly 2 million students worldwide are involved in formal education outside of their own country and this figure is likely to reach 5 million over the next 20 years.

Implementation is a critical component to curriculum development and/or redesign. To ensure that the curriculum is implemented as planned, intense oversight is necessary. Although rapid changes in technology and economics, along with the an ever-increasing information explosion and the need for multiculturalism, dictates that ongoing review and redesign of nursing curricula must occur, Giddens and colleagues (2008) caution that the greatest challenge is to resist the temptation to make changes to the new curriculum too quickly before it has been thoroughly evaluated for effectiveness.

Innovations in Nursing Education

A major aspect of the nursing curriculum development and redesign process is the consideration of current and future resources and needs for implementation, including the nature of the health care environment in which future nurses will work. It is widely noted in the literature that because of the complexities of today's health care system and health care delivery, transformation of nursing education is a necessity (AACN, 2008; Bellack, 2008; Coonan, 2008; Greiner & Knebel, 2003). Our traditional methods of nursing education need to give way to more innovative approaches to prepare graduates for the nursing practice of the future. The National Council of State Boards of Nursing (NCSBN; 2009) defined innovation as "a dynamic, systematic process that envisions new approaches to nursing education." Innovations reported in the nursing literature include the use of dedicated education units for clinical education (Moscato, Miller, Logsdon, Weinberg, & Chorpenning, 2007), pedagogical approaches such as "narrative pedagogy" and "deliberate discussion" (Brown, Kirkpatrick, Mangum, & Avery, 2008; Goodin & Stein, 2008), and high-fidelity simulation as an adjunct to or replacement for clinical experiences (Nehring, 2009; Reese et al., 2010). Other innovations in nursing education include partnering with clinical agencies or with other educational institutions to form a consortium for sharing resources for the delivery of nursing education.

Although innovation in nursing education is a must to meet the future need for nurses and the demands of the health care environment, when planning an innovative curriculum, faculty should be aware of potential hindrances that may prolong or even become barriers to the approval and implementation of innovations. First and foremost are the barriers that educational institutions impose on themselves such as multilevel institutional hierarchies and lengthy committee processes to obtain approval of curriculum changes (Bellack, 2008; Coonan, 2008). As a practice profession, nursing education's relationship with health care institutions is critical. Practice settings and educational institutions may not see eye to eye on innovative teaching strategies, and barriers may stem from centralized power bases and linear thinking found in practice (Unterschuetz, Hughes, Nienhauser, Weberg, & Jackson, 2008). In addition, there may be real or perceived regulatory barriers to innovative nursing education. In 2008, the NCSBN established the "Innovations in Education Regulation Committee." The charge to this committee was to identify real and perceived regulatory barriers to education innovations and to develop a regulatory model for innovative education proposals (NCSBN, 2009a). Potential regulatory barriers to innovative nursing education may include specified numbers of clinical or didactic hours in the nursing curriculum, faculty–student ratios, full- and part-time ratios of faculty, and simulation limitations (NCSBN, 2009b). Advance knowledge of potential barriers may assist faculty in negotiating with internal or external stakeholders to overcome these obstacles and create a curriculum that is innovative, resource-friendly, and forward-thinking in educating nurses for the future. Thinking about the consequences of and compliance with the individual state nurse practice act and state nursing regulations before planning innovative curricular changes is very important (Hargreaves, 2008). It is always advisable to consult with the respective state board at the beginning stages of planning for any innovative teaching strategy.

PROGRAM APPROVALS AND ACCREDITATION

After all institutional approvals are obtained for nursing program curriculum development or redesign, external approvals and accreditation processes are critical for implementation and ongoing demonstration of quality and effectiveness.

State Boards of Nursing

Boards of Nursing are state governmental agencies that were established over 100 years ago to protect the public's health welfare. This is done by overseeing and ensuring the safe practice of nursing through regulation of nursing practice (NCSBN, 2010a). For graduates of nursing programs to be eligible to take the national licensure exam (NCLEX-RN) to become registered nurses, the program from which they graduate must be approved by the respective state board of nursing. Although most states in the United States only regulate entry-level nursing education programs, some states do regulate advance-practice programs. The NCSBN has identified five different models that are used by state boards of nursing across the country to approve nursing education programs (Table 2.1). Specific state board regulations for initial and ongoing approval of nursing programs vary, but generally include regulations related to program length, curriculum, number of didactic and/or clinical hours, qualifications of the nursing faculty and the program administrator, program resources, faculty–student ratios, and, more recently, high-fidelity simulation (NCSBN, 2009b; Savers, 2010).

TABLE 2.1 The Five Models of Approval/Accreditation Used by State Boards of Nursing

1. *Boards of nursing are independent of the national nursing accreditors*	These boards of nursing approve/accredit nursing programs separately and distinctly from the national nursing accrediting bodies. Initial approval processes are conducted before accreditation takes place.
2. *Collaboration of boards of nursing and national nursing accreditor*	Boards of nursing share reports with the national nursing accrediting bodies, and/or make visits with them, sharing information. However, the final decision about approval is made by the board of nursing, independent of decisions by the national nursing accreditors. Initial approval processes are conducted before accreditation takes place.
3. *Deem national nursing accreditation as meeting state approvals* 3a. *Deem accreditation as meeting approvals, with further documentation*	Boards of nursing deem CCNE or NLNAC accreditation as meeting state approvals though they continue to approve/accredit those schools that do not voluntarily get accredited. The board of nursing is available for assistance with statewide issues (i.e., the nursing shortage in that state); boards retain the ability to make emergency visits to schools of nursing, if requested to do so by a party reporting serious problems; and the board of nursing has the authority to close a school of nursing, either on the advice of the national nursing accreditors or after making an emergency visit with evidence that the school of nursing is causing harm to the public. Initial approval processes are conducted before accreditation takes place.
	These boards deem CCNE or NLNAC accreditation as meeting state approvals, but they may require more documentation, such as complaints, NCLEX results, excessive student attrition, excessive faculty turnover and lack of clinical sites.
4. *Boards of nursing require national nursing accreditation*	Boards require their nursing programs to become accredited by CCNE or NLNAC, and then they will use Model 3 or 3a to approve them. Initial approval processes are conducted before accreditation takes place.
5. *Boards of nursing are not involved with the approval system at all*	In this model the board of nursing is not given the authority to approve nursing programs. This is usually done by another state authority.

From NCSBN (2010b).

Accreditation

The Council for Higher Education Accreditation (CHEA; 2009) defines accreditation as "the primary means of assuring and improving the quality of higher education institutions and programs in the United States." According to Eaton (2009), accreditation is a "trust-based, standards-based, evidence-based, judgment-based, peer-based process" (p. 5). Institutional accreditation is conducted by regional, national faith-based, national private career, and/or programmatic accreditors. The roles of accreditation include assuring quality, access to federal and state funds (i.e., student aid and other federal programs), engendering private sector confidence, and easing transfer of courses and programs among colleges and universities (Eaton, 2009). Higher education accreditation is a voluntary nongovernmental process and is complementary to federal and state mechanisms that promote quality in higher education. The U.S.

Department of Education (USDE) grants recognition to accrediting agencies that meet its criteria (Commission on Collegiate Nursing Education [CCNE], 2009).

Although steps in the accreditation process differ among agencies, typical steps in the process include:

- The accrediting agency establishes minimum accreditation standards.
- The institution or program seeking accreditation prepares a self-study.
- Volunteer representatives of the accrediting agency conduct site visit for on-site peer review of the institution or program applying for accreditation.
- The accrediting agency takes action regarding whether or not the institution or program meets the established accreditation standards.
- The accrediting agency publishes a list of institutions or programs accredited by the respective agency.
- There is ongoing monitoring of the institution or program for continuing compliance with the established accreditation standards.
  (CCNE, 2009; Eaton, 2009).

Two national accrediting agencies currently provide accreditation for nursing education programs: the NLNAC and the CCNE. Nursing education programs have, however, been accredited since the founding of the American Society of Superintendents of Training Schools for Nurses in 1893. This organization became the National League of Nursing Education (NLNE) in 1912, and in 1917 the NLNE published *A Standard Curriculum for Schools of Nursing* (Kalisch & Kalisch, 1978). In the early 1950s, the National League for Nursing (NLN) evolved from the merging of the NLNE, the Association of Schools of Nursing, and the National Organization for Public Health Nursing. The NLN provided accrediting services until 1997 when the NLNAC was formed as an arm of the NLN specifically for accreditation activities (NLNAC, 2008). The NLNAC accredits various types of nursing programs: practical nursing, diploma nursing, associate degree nursing, baccalaureate degree nursing, and master's degree nursing.

In 1995, AACN appointed its task force on accreditation to examine the feasibility of AACN's assuming accreditation activities for baccalaureate and higher degree nursing programs. Subsequently, in 1998, the CCNE was developed as an autonomous accrediting agency for baccalaureate and higher degree nursing programs. By the summer of 2008, 78% of institutions with baccalaureate and/or master's degree nursing programs in the United States were either accredited by or held new applicant status with CCNE. In the fall of 2008, CCNE conducted its first on-site evaluations of Doctor of Nursing Practice (DNP) programs (CCNE, 2009).

SUMMARY

Curriculum development and ongoing evaluation and redesign are core activities for nursing faculty. Determining how to best facilitate the process, working together as a group to identify and overcome potential barriers inherent in any nursing faculty, and being innovative to meet the challenges of educating future generations of practicing nurses are key elements for successful curriculum development or redesign. Ongoing challenges of the increasing volume of information in nursing and health sciences, the trend toward developing interdisciplinary curricula, the faculty–student gap in today's technologically savvy environment, and meeting the requirements of regulatory and accrediting agencies are all important issues to address in developing nursing curricula for the 21st century.

DISCUSSION QUESTIONS

1. What are ways in which nursing faculty can be motivated to engage in curriculum redesign?
2. What data can be used to convince faculty for the need for curriculum redesign?
3. What real or perceived barriers do regulatory agencies impose on curricular development or redesign?

LEARNING ACTIVITIES

Student Learning Activities

1. Review your state board of nursing regulations for nursing education programs. Describe how these regulations impact the process of curriculum development or redesign in a nursing program in your state.
2. As a small group activity, explore the process for student involvement in curriculum development and/or redesign in your program. In what ways would you change the current level of student involvement in curriculum development?
3. Determine how new or revised curricula of nursing programs are reviewed and acted on by your local state board of nursing. Attend a state board of nursing meeting and describe how the process of nursing program approval relates to the boards mission of protection of the public's health welfare in your state.

Nursing Educator/Faculty Development Activities

1. Review your curriculum to ensure incorporation of accreditation standards.
2. Describe two innovations in curriculum and/or teaching strategies for implementation in your curriculum. What constraints or barriers can you identify that would delay or prohibit you from implementing these innovations?
3. Develop a list of five key facilitators and five key barriers to curriculum development and/or redesign in your school of nursing. How can you as a faculty member assist your school or other faculty members overcome the barriers you have identified?
4. Compare the benefits of having your baccalaureate or master's program accredited by NLNAC or CCNE.

REFERENCES

Adams, L. T. (2009). Nursing shortage solutions and America's economic recovery. *Nursing Education Perspectives, 30*(6), 349.

Allen, L. (2008). The nursing shortage continues as faculty shortage grows. *Nursing Economics, 26*(1), 35–40.

American Association of Colleges of Nursing. (2008, October). *The essentials of baccalaureate education for professional nursing practice.* Washington, DC: Author.

American Association of Colleges of Nursing. (2010, March). *Amid calls for more highly educated nurses, new AACN data show impressive growth in doctoral nursing programs.* [press release]. Retrieved March 31, 2010, from http://www.aacn.nche.edu/media/newsreleases/2010/enrollchanges.html

Bargagliotti, L. A. (2009). State funding for higher education and RN placement rates by state: A case for nursing by the numbers in state legislatures. *Nursing Outlook, 57*(5), 274–280.

Bellack, J. P. (2008). Letting go of the rock. *Journal of Nursing Education, 47*(10), 439–440.

Ben-Zur, H., Yagil, D., & Spitzer, A. (1999). Evaluation of an innovative curriculum: nursing education in the next century. *Journal of Advanced Nursing, 30*(6), 1432–1440.

Billings, D. M., & Halstead, J. A. (2005). *Teaching in nursing: A guide for faculty* (2nd ed.). St. Louis, MO: Elsevier Saunders.

Brown, S. T., Kirkpatrick, M. K., Mangum, D., & Avery, J. (2008). A review of narrative pedagogy strategies to transform traditional nursing education. *Journal of Nursing Education, 47*(6), 283–286.

Callen, B. L., & Lee, J. L. (2009). Ready for the world: Preparing nursing students for tomorrow. *Journal of Professional Nursing, 25*(5), 292–298.

Caldwell, E. S., Hongyan, L., & Harding, T. (2010). Encompassing multiple moral paradigms: A challenge for nursing educators. *Nursing Ethics, 17*(2), 189–199.

Cash, P. A., Daines, D., Doyle, R. M., & von Tettenborn, L. (2009). Quality workplace environments for nurse educators: Implications for recruitment and retention. *Nursing Economics, 27*(5), 315–321.

Commission on Collegiate Nursing Education. (2009). *Achieving excellence in accreditation: The first 10 years of CCNE.* Washington, DC: Author.

Coonan, P. R. (2008). Educational innovation: Nursing's leadership challenge. *Nursing Economics, 26*(2), 117–121.

Council for Higher Education Accreditation (2009). CHEA talking points: Accreditation, students and society. Retrieved April 24, 2010, from http://www.chea.org/pdf/2009_Talking_Points.pdf

Diekelmann, N. (2002). Too much content . . . Epistemologies' grasp and nursing education. *Journal of Nursing Education, 4*(11), 469–470.

Eaton, J. (2009). *An overview of U.S. accreditation.* Retrieved April 24, 2010, from http://www.chea.org/pdf/2009.06_Overview_of_US_Accreditation.pdf

Ehnfors, M., & Grobe, S. (2004). Nursing curriculum and continuing education: Future directions. *International Journal of Medical Informatics, 73*, 591–598.

Giddens, J. F., & Brady, D. (2007). Rescuing nursing education from content saturation: The case for a concept-based curriculum. *Journal of Nursing Education, 46*(2), 65–69.

Giddens, J., Brady, D., Brown, P., Wright, M., Smith, D., & Harris, J. (2008). A new curriculum for a new era of nursing education. *Nursing Education Perspectives, 29*(4), 200–204.

Goodin, H. J., & Stein, D. (2008). Deliberate discussion as an innovative teaching strategy. *Journal of Nursing Education, 47*(6), 272–274.

Greiner, A. C., & Knebel, E. (Eds.). (2003) *Health professions education: A bridge to quality.* Washington, DC: The National Academies Press.

Hargreaves, J. (2008). Risk: The ethics of a creative curriculum. *Innovations in Education and Teaching International, 45*(3), 227–234.

Hartman, J. L., Dziuban, C., & Brophy-Ellison, J. (2007). Faculty 2.0. *Educause Review, 42*(5), 62–76. [Online]. Available: www.educause.edu/apps/er/_erm07/erm0753.asp

Henderson, T. M., & Hassmiller, S. B. (2007). Hospitals and philanthropy as partners in funding nursing education. *Nursing Economics, 25*(2), 95–100.

Hinshaw, A. S. (2008). Navigating the perfect storm: Balancing a culture of safety with workplace challenges. *Nursing Research, 57*(1 Suppl.), S4–S10.

Ironside, P. M. (2004). Covering content and teaching thinking: Deconstructing the additive curriculum. *Journal of Nursing Education, 43*(1), 5–12.

Kalisch, P. A., & Kalisch, B. J. (1978). *The advance of American nursing.* Boston: Little, Brown.

Long, K. A. (2004). Preparing nurses for the 21st century: Reenvisioning nursing education and practice. *Journal of Professional Nursing, 20*(2), 82–88.

Mangold, K. (2007). Educating a new generation: Teaching baby boomer faculty about millennial students. *Nurse Educator, 32*(1), 21–23.

Moch, S. D., Cronje, R. J., & Branson, J. (2010). Part I: Undergraduate nursing evidence-based practice education: Envisioning the role of students. *Journal of Professional Nursing, 26*(1), 5–13.

Moscato, S. R., Miller, J., Logsdon, K., Weinberg, S., & Chorpenning, L. (2007). Dedicated education unit: An innovative clinical partner education model. *Nursing Outlook, 55*(1), 31–37.

National Council of State Boards of Nursing. (2009a). Innovations in education regulation report: Background and literature review. Retrieved March 26, 2010, from https://www.ncsbn.org/Innovations_Report.pdf

National Council of State Boards of Nursing. (2009b). Innovations in education regulation committee: Recommendations for boards of nursing for fostering innovations in education. Retrieved March 26, 2010, from https://www.ncsbn.org/Recommendations_for_BONS.pdf

National Council of State Boards of Nursing. (2010a). Boards of nursing. Retrieved April 23, 2010, from https://www.ncsbn.org/boards.htm

National Council of State Boards of Nursing. (2010b). Approval/Accreditation. Retrieved April 23, 2010, from https://www.ncsbn.org/357.htm

National League for Nursing Accrediting Commission. (2008). *NLNAC Accreditation Manual.* New York: Author.

Nehring, W. (2008). U.S. boards of nursing and the use of high-fidelity patient simulators in nursing education. *Journal of Professional Nursing, 24*(2), 109–117.

Pew Health Professions Commission. (1995). *Critical challenges: Revitalizing the health care professions for the twenty-first century.* UCSF Center for the Health Professions, San Francisco: Author.

Powell-Cope, G., Hughes, N. L., Sedlak, C., & Nelson, A. (2008). Faculty perceptions of implementing an evidence-based safe patient handling nursing curriculum module. *Online Journal of Issues in Nursing, 13*(3).

Reese, C. E., Jeffries, P. R., & Engum, S. A. (2010). Using simulations to develop nursing and medical student collaboration. *Nursing Education Perspectives, 31*(1), 33–37.

Savers, C. (2010). Trends and challenges in regulating nursing practice today. *Journal of Nursing Regulation, 1*(1), 4–8.

Sawatzky, J., & Enns, C. L. (2009). A mentoring needs assessment: Validating mentorship in nursing education. *Journal of Professional Nursing, 25*(3), 145–150.

Schmitt, M. H. (2002). It's time to revalue nursing education research. *Research In Nursing & Health, 25,* 423–424.

Sullivan, D. T. (2010). Connecting nursing education and practice: A focus on shared goals for quality and safety. *Creative Nursing, 16*(1), 37–43.

Tanner, C. A. (2004). Nursing education research: Investing in our future. *Journal of Nursing Education, 43,* 99–100.

Thompson, B. W., & Skiba, D. J. (2008). Informatics in the nursing curriculum: A national survey of nursing informatics requirements in nursing curricula. *Nursing Education Perspectives, 29*(5), 312–317.

Unterschuetz, C., Hughes, P., Nienhauser, D., Weberg, D., & Jackson, L. (2008). Caring for innovation and caring for the innovator. *Nursing Administration Quarterly, 32*(2), 133–141.

II

Learning Theories, Education Taxonomies, and Critical Thinking

Sarah B. Keating

OVERVIEW

Section 2 introduces learning theories, education taxonomies, and the application of critical thinking to evidence-based practice as they apply to curriculum development. Chapter 3 discusses classic and newer learning theories and concepts, whereas Chapter 4 reviews classic and updated education taxonomies and their application to nursing education in addition to the integration of critical and creative thinking skills. These major theories, concepts, and models serve to guide educators as they develop mission and philosophy statements for the program and build the curriculum plan. They are considered again in detail as faculty applies them to the implementation of the curriculum through the processes of instructional design and student evaluation. The latter activities are not a focus of this text rather; this text focuses on faculty's beliefs about them to guide the curriculum plan.

Learning Theories

As discussed in Chapter 2, faculty holds the ultimate responsibility for curriculum development. In that role, faculty members must reach consensus on their beliefs about the learning processes their students undergo to master the knowledge and skills necessary for practicing as nurses. Identifying their beliefs about teaching and learning processes is one of the earliest activities that faculty members take when revising or developing the curriculum. With a preponderance of adult learners in nursing education programs and the need to continue educating the existing and future nursing workforce, it is important that faculty include adult learning theories in their repertoire.

Learning theories are often identified by major categories and include classic theories, newer applications of them to the learning environment, and more recent theories and concepts. Major classifications of learning theories include conditioning, behaviorism, cognitive, social learning, transformational, constructivism, and metacognition. Chapter 3 defines these terms and discusses some of the major learning theorists and their postulates as they apply to the teaching and learning processes, specifically in nursing. It continues with suggestions for their application to various levels of nursing programs and their students and their integration into the mission and philosophy statements of the curriculum.

Education Taxonomies

Chapter 4 reviews the traditional education taxonomies and domains of learning as they apply to nursing education. Although nursing adopted and continues to use modified models of education taxonomies and behavioral models for goals and objectives to organize the curriculum, there is a need to examine newer taxonomies that foster critical and creative thinking processes and metacognition. The continuing issue that faces nursing educators is its reliance on behaviorist theories of learning that focus on the teacher as transmitter of knowledge instead of the learning needs and characteristics of the learner. Behaviorist models of learning are appropriate for students to gain basic knowledge and skills; however, to facilitate the critical and creative thinking skills necessary for clinical decision-making and evidence-based practice, newer models of educational taxonomies and learning theories are necessary. The application of the new taxonomies recognizes the role of the teacher as facilitator, the learner as the focus, and the interactions between the two. They lift the objectives from rote or recall memorization on the part of the learner to higher orders of understanding, conceptualization, and application.

Critical Thinking

An essential part of curriculum planning is the recognition by faculty of critical thinking and the role it plays in the development of clinical decision-making skills and evidence-based nursing practice. Thus, critical thinking must be part of faculty's planning for the curriculum and how it will be integrated into courses and their instructional designs.

Critical thinking is a necessity for students as they apply prerequisite and nursing knowledge to the development of complex thinking skills. The modalities of problem-solving, critical and creative thinking, and decision-making are suited to the current evolving health care system. There is a need for professionals who can respond to health care needs and system changes with strategies that use evidence-based and innovative solutions to health care problems and policies and that foster health promotion and the prevention of disease. The issue raised in the chapter is to what extent nursing curricula should change to meet health care demands and changes in the delivery system and suggestions are offered to meet this challenge.

Learning Theories Applied to Curriculum Development

Coleen Saylor

Coleen Saylor

OBJECTIVES

Upon completion of Chapter 3, the reader will be able to:

1. Evaluate learning theories as possible foundations to guide nursing program curricula in schools of nursing and staff development settings.
2. Compare learning theory strengths and weaknesses as a conceptual basis for teaching and learning strategies within a nursing curriculum.
3. Analyze various learning theories for appropriateness and congruency with the philosophy and mission of educational institutions, schools of nursing, or health care agencies.
4. Select a learning theoretical approach as an overall guide for developing teaching and learning strategies in a specific curriculum program or course.

OVERVIEW

Curriculum revision or development in nursing programs involves an infinite number of difficult questions. How can the program balance expectations between ideal and practical considerations? Which teaching strategies are most relevant for these particular learners? How much flexibility should be included? A few of the other issues include relevant content, appropriate clinical placements, difficulty level of assignments and learning activities, and budget and time constraints.

As curriculum planners wrestle with these and many other concerns, a conceptual or theoretical foundation for learning provides a consistent rationale for their decisions. That is, learning theories provide explanations of how learners learn and how educators can facilitate the best educational outcomes. Each of the approaches to learning suggests applications in the form of teaching strategies that can be emphasized in the curriculum. Just as clinical nursing actions may be based on an understanding of physiological and pharmacological principles, for example, so teaching strategies are based on principles or concepts of how people learn. Nurses are expected to provide rationale for their actions, and similarly, educators rely on learning theory as a rationale for curriculum decisions.

An essential part of the curriculum development process is a discussion among the curriculum planners of their perspectives about how learning occurs. As educators with varied backgrounds, curriculum planners bring a range of viewpoints about the best way for a curriculum to facilitate learning. To produce the best curriculum for a particular program, its faculty, students, and educators can share assumptions and beliefs, discuss previous experiences, and identify the appropriate explanations for learning, because they are relevant to the program under revision. This collegial discussion, although sometimes difficult, provides a unique opportunity for learning as educators describe why a particular theoretical perspective is appropriate or not, in their view. The inclination to jump quickly to choosing teaching strategies would shortcut this process of using a theoretical foundation as a rationale for the later decisions.

In this chapter, **learning** is defined as a "relatively permanent change in mental processing, emotional functioning, and/or behavior as a result of experience" (Bastable, 2008, p. 52). Changes caused by maturation, such as growing taller, do not qualify. Temporary changes such as fatigue or drugs, do not qualify. The changes must take place in the learner's knowledge or behavior (Woolfolk, 2010). A **learning theory** is defined as a "coherent framework of integrated constructs and principles that describe, explain or predict how people learn" (Bastable, p. 52). Learning theories and concepts have much to offer the practice of health care and nursing education, whether used alone or in combination. In the real world of complex clinical sites and busy classrooms, educators draw from various learning theories for the teaching strategies that are appropriate for a particular course, learner, and content. Although everyone has favorite theoretical approaches, all of them have the potential to contribute strategies to teaching and learning situations. Rewards and reinforcement (behaviorism), role modeling (social cognitive), organization of content (cognitivism), peer collaboration (constructivism), and positive regard for students (humanism) all have important benefits. An educator can use strategies from several theoretical models at the same time. For simplicity, this chapter discusses each learning paradigm separately, but remember that the boundaries between theoretical paradigms are somewhat artificial! Further, within each paradigm, there is often controversy and disagreement, and newer researchers may argue for a different point of view, which are all outside of the scope of this discussion.

This chapter reviews the principal psychological learning theories that are most commonly used and have proved useful in academic and health care settings; behaviorist, social cognitive, cognitivist, constructivist, adult, and humanistic perspectives are included. The concepts of *metacognition* and *transformative learning* are included within the cognitive perspective.

In no way does this overview take the place of a more thorough understanding of the many researchers and schools of thought who have contributed to knowledge of how people learn and how educators can use those theoretical understandings for improved learning outcomes. There are many print and electronic resources available for further study in each of these paradigms and others not included here.

BEHAVIORIST LEARNING THEORY

Behaviorism, or **behaviorist learning theory**, is a group of learning theories, often referred to as *stimulus–response*, that view learning as the result of the stimulus conditions and the responses (behaviors) that follow, generally ignoring what goes on inside the learner. Behaviorism is primarily concerned with observable and measurable associations made by the learner (Standridge, 2002). Behaviorists view learning as the result of the stimulus conditions and the responses (behaviors) that follow. For this reason, the theories are often referred to as stimulus–response or behavioristic theories (Huitt & Hummel, 2006). This perspective asserts that behaviors, rather than thoughts or emotions, are the focus of study because behavior is affected by its consequences (Skinner, n.d.; Standridge, 2002). To change people's responses, this perspective changes either the environmental stimulus conditions or what happens after the response occurs. Currently, behavioral educational perspectives are more likely to be used in combination with other learning theories, especially cognitive theory, instead of being used alone; and they are an effective adjunct to these other points of view about learning (Bastable, 2008).

Classical Conditioning

"new math gave me a dislike for math"

Respondent conditioning, also called **classical** or **Pavlovian conditioning**, emphasizes the stimulus and associations made with it in the learning process, depending on associations that are often unconscious. In this model, prior to the conditioning (learning) a neutral stimulus, with no particular value to the learner, is paired with a naturally occurring unlearned (unconditioned) stimulus leading to the elicited (unconditioned) response. Ivan Pavlov, the Russian physiologist, noticed that the dogs in his lab began to salivate before their feeding when they saw the keeper or heard his feet, but before they could see or smell the food. To explain this, Pavlov's following experiment paired a bell, a neutral stimulus that would not ordinarily lead to salivation, with the dog food, the unconditioned stimulus that led to salivation, which is the unconditioned response. If repeated enough, the bell alone began to elicit salivation, showing that conditioning (learning) had occurred. After conditioning, the bell was the conditioned stimulus; salivation in response to the bell was the conditioned response (Green, 2009; Hauser, 2006; Huitt & Hummel, 2006). Those with well-trained dogs have many examples of this type of conditioning.

Classical conditioning, especially of emotional reactions, occurs in all schools mostly through unconscious processes in which students come to like or dislike school, subjects, and teachers. A particular school subject is neutral, evoking little emotional response in the beginning. But the teacher, the classroom, or some other stimulus in the environment that is repeatedly associated with the subject can become a conditioned stimulus. Repeated pairing of math with a teacher who makes fun of student questions may result in the emotions associated with the teacher's responses and also, associated with the subject. In addition to teaching math, the educator is teaching the students to dislike math (LeFrancois, 2000).

One of the processes in classical conditioning is **generalization** (i.e., a conditioned response that spreads to similar situations). After Pavlov's dogs learned to salivate to one particular sound, they would also salivate after hearing other higher or lower sounds. The conditioned response of salivating *generalized* or spread to similar situations (Huitt & Hummel, 2006). These findings have implications for teachers and all educational settings. Students with previous unpleasant or embarrassing educational experiences may well be reminded of them in a new classroom. In one particular class, college students who did not know the answer to the teacher's question had to stand by their chair while the teacher asked another student, then another, until finally someone had the correct answer. During this process the standing students felt shamed. Imagine their feelings years later when a different instructor called upon them, trying to encourage participation in a nursing education class. The embarrassment of the previous experience had generalized to the new classroom. Fortunately, one of the students described the previous process and the resulting discussion of the best ways to facilitate discussion without causing stress to students made a "teachable moment."

Two explanations for why associations form between stimuli and response are contiguity and reinforcement. Watson and Pavlov favored *contiguity*, arguing that the simultaneous pairing of neutral and unconditioned stimuli (the bell and the food) is enough for learning to occur. The **principle of contiguity** states that two or more sensations occurring together often enough will result in association (Woolfolk, 2010). In contrast, Skinner and Thorndike argued that *reinforcement* of the consequences of the response leads to learning. In this case the salivation is reinforced by the dog food appearing as expected. As Thorndike's work progressed from animals to humans, he developed the law of effect, which states that responses just before a *satisfying state of affairs* are reinforced and more likely to be repeated. This work provided the basis for later definitions of reward and punishment, one of the most important contributions of this learning theory upon today's academic settings (Woolfolk).

Operant Conditioning

B. F. Skinner (n.d.) made a distinction between the behavior in classical conditioning and a second, much larger and more important, class of behavior known as operant conditioning. In classical conditioning, responses are brought about by a stimulus and could become conditioned to other stimuli. However, Skinner believed that the principles of classical conditioning account for only a small portion of learned behaviors (Hauser, 2006). He labeled these responses as *elicited responses* and the behavior *respondent* because it occurs in response to a stimulus. The second class of behaviors is not elicited by any known stimuli, but they are simply *emitted responses*. These responses are called *operants* because they are operations performed by the individual. In the case of respondent behavior, the person is reacting *to* the environment, whereas in operant behavior the person acts *upon* the environment. Another distinction is that respondent behaviors are largely involuntary, whereas operants are voluntary (Woolfolk, 2010). **Operant conditioning** is rewarding a desired behavior or random act to strengthen the likelihood of it being repeated (Standridge, 2002). The rat in the Skinner box pressed a lever as a random behavior and was rewarded by a pellet of food. Most rats will quickly learn to press the lever for food as their initially random acts are reinforced (Skinner).

Reinforcement

Reinforcement is commonly understood to mean *reward*, but in this case it means any consequence that strengthens the behavior it follows. Whenever a behavior persists or increases, one can assume that its effects are reinforcing for the individual involved. However, individuals vary greatly in their perceptions of whether consequences are rewards or not. Students who repeatedly misbehave may be indicating that the consequence is reinforcing, even if it hardly seems desirable to another (Standridge, 2002; Woolfolk, 2010). **Positive reinforcement** is a (usually) pleasant stimulus presented following a particular behavior, such as a good grade for an excellent project. However, inappropriate behavior can also be positively reinforced if, for example, an inappropriate student comment elicits laughter in the classroom. **Negative reinforcement** involves the removal of an unpleasant stimulus. If a behavior allows a student to avoid something unpleasant, that is a negative reinforcement. A common example is the car seatbelt buzzer. As soon as the seatbelt is buckled, the annoying noise stops. A tendency to repeat the desired behavior of buckling the belt exists because it was reinforced by the disappearance of the noise (Woolfolk, 2010). Both types of reinforcement strengthen behavior.

In contrast to reinforcement, **punishment** decreases or suppresses behavior; therefore, behavior followed by a punishment is less likely to be repeated. One type of punishment is called **presentation punishment**; the appearance of the stimulus following the behavior suppresses or decreases that behavior. Extra work assigned is an example of this type of punishment following unacceptable classroom work. In contrast, **removal punishment** removes a stimulus following the behavior in question. Taking away privileges after inappropriate behavior is using removal punishment to decrease the likelihood of that particular behavior (Standridge, 2002; Woolfolk, 2010).

Instructional implications of the work on reinforcement, particularly that of Thorndike, focus on the belief that learning results from correct responses being rewarded. Therefore, schools and teachers should provide many opportunities for the desired responses and subsequent reinforcements. Students respond to satisfying experiences; preferring even the simple but important reinforcements of acknowledgement, praise, and smiles. Rewards that are appropriate to the situation and the learner include teacher attitudes, acknowledgment of good questions, praise of work well done, grading policies that reward effort and excellence fairly, flexibility in assignments, a safe classroom emotional climate, regard for the students and their goals (Standridge, 2002), and positive comments on returned papers in any color of ink besides red.

Behaviorist perspectives recommend that teachers be sensitive to this phenomenon and minimize the unpleasant aspects of their courses, the subjects, and of being a student, as much as possible (Woolfolk, 2010). Increasing the number of parking facilities may not be possible, but the teacher's awareness of student inconveniences goes a long way in establishing a more positive experience. Look carefully for assignments seen as "busywork," as each assignment that requires student time and effort should have a clear purpose in meeting the course objectives. Teachers can never know the complete history of students' past anxiety-producing situations, but they can often minimize negative aspects of the classroom environment.

In addition to reinforcement, contracts and behavior modification provide common behaviorist techniques. Contracts can be used to change specific behaviors such as not completing an independent project or meeting clinical assignments. The contract is mutually agreed upon and signed by all relevant parties. Behavior modification is application of positive rewards systematically to improve performance. Skinner (n.d.) stated that behavior modification is simply changing the consequences of behavior. Reinforcement of the behavior pattern then continues until the student has established a pattern of success, at which time the reinforcement is gradually decreased and stopped. In contrast, ignoring an undesirable behavior tends to lead to extinction, according to this perspective (Standridge, 2002).

Behaviorist learning theory is relatively easy to understand and can be effectively used with other learning paradigms. However, some criticisms include this being a teacher-centered model in which learners are considered to be passive and easily manipulated. Further, the rewards are usually external ones rather than promoting intrinsic satisfaction (Bastable, 2008).

SOCIAL COGNITIVE THEORY/SOCIAL LEARNING THEORY

Social cognitive theory emphasizes the importance of observing and modeling behaviors, attitudes, and emotional responses of others. This theory is largely attributed to Bandura (1986) who described how learning takes place with consideration of personal learner characteristics, behavior patterns, and the social environment. Over time, Bandura changed the name of his theory from social learning to social cognitive theory to distance it from the social learning theories of that time, and to emphasize the importance of cognition in people's behavior (Bandura, 1986; Pajares, 2002; Schunk, 2004). This chapter will not differentiate between social learning and, social cognitive theory, and for simplicity, will use the term *social cognitive theory*.

According to the social cognitive theory, people are not driven by inner forces nor controlled by external stimuli. Rather, human functioning is explained in terms of interaction among cognitive, behavioral, and environmental influences and stresses the idea that much learning occurs in a social environment. People learn rules, skills, beliefs, attitudes, and strategies by observation. They learn from models and act in accordance with beliefs about their skills and the possible result of their behaviors (Bandura, 1986; Schunk, 2004).

Initially, behaviorist features and the imitation of role models were emphasized in this explanation for learning. In some texts, the earlier social learning theory was included within the behaviorist category because it was based partially on behaviorist principles of reinforcement. In later constructions, however, Bandura focused on attributes of the self and internal processing. More recently, the theory focused on social factors and the social context for learning, but it clearly encompasses both cognitive and behavioral frameworks. The self-regulation and control that the learner exercises are considered more critical and more reflective of cognitive principles (Bastable, 2008; Schunk, 2004; Woolfolk, 2010).

This theory and its evolution emphasize the agency of the learner, and therefore, it is important to understand what learners perceive and interpret (Bastable, 2008). People are viewed as able to organize and reflect on their behavior, and therefore, able to regulate themselves, rather than simply reacting to environmental forces. Learners can make things happen by their actions because they possess a measure of control over their thoughts, feelings, and actions. Thus, individuals are both products of and producers of their own environments (Pajares, 2002).

With the three essential components of this theory, personal factors, behavior, and environmental influences, teachers can influence learning by strategies focused on any or all of these. They can work to improve students' self-beliefs and habits of thinking (personal factors), improve academic skills and self-regulatory practices (behavior), and change the classroom procedures that might encourage student success (environmental factors; Pajares, 2002).

Self-Efficacy

One of the most useful constructs of Bandura's theoretical work is the concept of self-efficacy. Perceived self-efficacy is defined as "people's judgments of their capabilities to organize and execute courses of action required to attain designated types of performances" (Bandura, 1986, p. 391). Research shows that beliefs about one's self-efficacy influence persistence, effort, and choice of tasks, all of which influence behavior. This concept is particularly important in academic settings; because progress toward the desired goal and positive feedback from teachers both influence the perception of self-efficacy, further raising persistence and effort (Pajares, 2002).

A strong sense of efficacy enhances individual accomplishment and personal well-being in many instances. People with strong perceived capabilities approach more difficult tasks and see them as challenges rather than threats. People who believe that they will be successful sustain their efforts and quickly recover their sense of efficacy after setbacks, because they assume that failure can be corrected with more effort or acquired skills or knowledge. This high self-efficacy approach of individuals produces more successful outcomes and reduces stress (Bandura, 1986).

Individuals who doubt their ability to be successful do not take on difficult tasks and may see them as threats. When faced with possible failure, they are more likely to focus on personal shortcomings and adverse outcomes, and, as a result, they decrease effort and persistence, assuming that the poorer outcomes are a result of their deficient capabilities (Bandura, 1994). Therefore, self-efficacy beliefs, behavior changes, and outcomes are highly correlated; and self-efficacy is an excellent predictor of behavior. "Clearly, it is not simply a matter of how capable one is, but of how capable one believes oneself to be" (Pajares, 2002, p. 8).

Beliefs about one's efficacy are developed through four main sources. Mastery experiences are the most effective source of beliefs in one's capabilities, as success builds a strong belief that one can be successful in the future. Experiences in overcoming obstacles through sustained effort, perhaps after setbacks, serve to create a strong sense of self-efficacy. Such individuals believe that sustained effort may be needed, but they will be successful if they persevere and confront the challenge (Bandura, 1986; Woolfolk, 2010).

The second source of self-beliefs of efficacy is through the vicarious experiences of others. Seeing similar others succeed by sustained effort increases beliefs that an individual is able to master similar activities, and the greater the similarity, the more persuasive are the models' success or failure (Bandura, 1994). If similar classmates can master software for online teaching, individuals are persuaded that they can, too.

Persuasion by someone is a third source of efficacy and can strengthen individuals' ideas about their potential to master a particular activity. As a result of another's opinion, they will exert greater effort and persistence than they would have otherwise. However, unrealistic encouragement will undermine efforts to be successful, so the persuader must be realistic and authentic (Bandura, 1986). Here is a powerful role for teachers who know their students well enough to encourage them, with realistic language. Teachers can show the skills with which to approach a particular problem, identify resources, give examples of others who have succeeded, and offer relevant feedback. If the persuasion boosts the perception of potential success and increases effort, relevant skills, and persistence, it will promote a sense of efficacy. An important part of being a successful persuader is to structure situations in which individuals are likely to be successful, rather than putting people in situations in which they are likely to fail (Pajares, 2002; Woolfolk, 2010).

The fourth source of self-beliefs of efficacy is bodily and emotional states. Students, like all individuals, rely on their interpretation of these states to judge their capabilities. A stress reaction may be considered a predictor of poor performance by those with a lower sense of self-efficacy. In contrast, those with higher self-efficacy beliefs may interpret the stress or arousal as an energizing facilitator of performance (Bandura, 1994). "Butterflies" in the stomach can be interpreted as a sign that one has a lot of energy and will give a good oral performance in class, rather than a sign that one will fail.

Bandura (1986) suggested that a growing body of evidence exists that self-efficacy is important not only in educational pursuits, but also in human accomplishments and well-being. Ordinary social realities are filled with problems, impediments, adversities, and setbacks. People must have a strong sense of their own self-efficacy to sustain efforts to succeed. Providing instances in which students can succeed in challenging endeavors after a sustained and guided effort may well add to their overall perception of self-efficacy in more than the academic setting.

Role Modeling

People learn not only from their own experience, but also by observing others; therefore, modeling is a critical component of this theory (Woolfolk, 2010). Role modeling is a general term referring to behavioral, cognitive, and affective changes resulting from observation of others, including the processes of attention, retention, production, and motivation (Schunk, 2004). Socially acceptable behaviors vary among cultures, groups, and ages of individuals; one of the most important tasks of the home and school is to nurture youth to appropriate behavior for their social circumstances. Bandura (1986) believed that social learning occurs principally by imitation. This type of learning is considered one of the important capabilities of the human species and includes the following steps (Boeree, 2006a):

1. Attention is the observation of the relevant actions of a model.
2. Retention involves processing and organizing the information to be learned so that the image or description can be reproduced with the learner's own behavior.
3. Production or reproduction refers to engaging in the observed behavior.
4. Motivation is required to adopt and repeat the behavior if the behavior produces valued results. (Bastable, 2008; Boeree, 2006a; Pajares, 2002)

Much learning results from imitation as one observes and imitates behaviors of others or symbolic models such as television or book characters. The effects of models are largely informative; that is, observers learn cognitively how to do things and the consequences of their actions. Symbolic models can include written or spoken directions, pictures, or mental images. When this imitation results in positive results or prevents negative results, these behaviors are reinforced and are more likely to be repeated. Reinforcement can be direct, such as praise, or indirect, such as seeing the model rewarded (Bandura, 1986.)

Modeling serves many functions, particularly in academic settings. One of these is **response facilitation**, or providing social prompts for observers to behave in a certain way. The first students to arrive in the classroom or lab can be directed to a desired behavior, such as examining a model or relevant object the instructor has provided. When other students enter the room, they will follow the lead of the earlier students. Another function, **inhibition**, occurs when models receive negative feedback for performing certain actions, such as calling attention to students whose cell phones ring or those who arrive late, and **disinhibition** occurs when these behaviors do not result in negative consequences. So in these instances, the role model was other students, not the teacher or another professional (Schunk, 2004).

Observational learning through modeling occurs when students learn new behaviors that they would not have learned without watching a model. Modeled activities that are perceived to be important and lead to a positive outcome tend to focus student attention and motivation. The perception of model competence such as role and title also commands learner attention (Schunk, 2004). Teachers have many strategies for imparting the importance of an activity or learning experience to the learners such as discussing professional relevance and evaluation of the behavior.

Role modeling is not confined to psychomotor activities. Cognitive modeling includes explanation and demonstration while verbalizing the model's thoughts and reasons for a particular activity (Schunk, 2004). Case studies are only one instance in which teachers can model their problem-solving approach with questions and information processing. "What are the most relevant factors with this client?" "What further information do I need right away?" Educators can "think aloud" while they discuss the case study, ethical dilemma, or other critical thinking example.

Nursing educators may typically think of using role models, nurses in clinical settings, guest speakers, and the instructors themselves, to demonstrate procedures and knowledge. Surely these situations make a powerful impact on students. However, professional role models impart not only procedural or content knowledge, but also attitudes and values. What does it mean to "think like a nurse"? How does a professional nurse treat marginalized individuals? How does a competent nurse say that he or she does not know the answer? How does one handle conflict with other team members? Experienced teachers and nurses often have lasting memories of nurses whom they saw as role models early in their career. Providing the best possible examples for students to observe in their educational experience is a critical part of professional development.

COGNITIVE LEARNING THEORY

Cognitivism, or **cognitive learning theory,** is defined as a group of learning theories focused on cognitive processes such as decision making, problem solving, synthesizing, and evaluating. Decision making, problem solving, synthesizing, and evaluating are cognitive processes and understanding them is the goal of cognitive learning theories (Woolfolk, 2010). Indeed, cognitive processes are the focus of study for this perspective, because mental events are critical to human learning (Huitt, 2006). Historically, educational researchers focused on behavioral objectives and programmed learning from the behavioral perspective, as discussed in a previous section. As that influence declined, however, the focus expanded to the learner and instructional variables in educational settings. Some argue that this focus means a shift from seeing learners as passive products of incoming stimuli from the environment to seeing learners as active agents who have goals, ideas, plans, and actively attend to, select, and organize information. In contrast to the behaviorist approach, cognitivist approaches to learning focus on the human information processing system as it affects cognitive processes during learning and stresses their importance (Bastable, 2008). Huitt (2006) differentiates this viewpoint from other psychological perspectives by saying that whereas the cognitive perspective focuses on cognitive processes, the behavioral view focuses on observable behavior, the humanistic view focuses on personal growth and interpersonal relationships, and the social cognitive view focuses on the social environment as it impacts personal qualities.

The key to learning, according to the cognitive perspective, is the learner's perception, thinking, memory, and information processing and organization. Learning involves the formation of mental connections that may not necessarily be demonstrated in overt behavior changes. This viewpoint has often been compared to computer information processing, with a focus on how people process information from the environment, how they perceive the stimuli around them, how they put those perceptions into memory, and how they retrieve that knowledge (Bastable, 2008; Schunk, 2004).

Educators generally agree that many of these cognitive processes such as concept learning, problem solving, transfer, and metacognition are central to learning (Schunk, 2004). Within these cognitive processes, this theory acknowledges the wide variation in individual learners' perceptions, information processing, and other mental activities as part of the learning process (Bastable, 2008; Woolfolk, 2010). Cognitivist viewpoints focus on the influence of instructional and motivational variables on learners' cognition, creative thinking, critical thinking, and cognitive development (Huitt, 2006; Schunk, 2004). Cognitive theorists share basic notions about learning and memory, but there are differences among specific theorists (Bastable). For curriculum planners differentiating among specific theorists may not be as important as the agreed upon positions and assumptions within the paradigm. However, a few of the theorists central to this paradigm will be discussed here.

First, this section will describe discovery learning, advance organizers, and the importance of content organization; next, metacognition and transformative learning are included. Certainly, both metacognition and transformative learning processes provide essential elements of critical thinking and clinical decision making for nurses and others. Discovery learning is attributed to Bruner who emphasized "hands on" learning and argued that teachers should teach the structure of subjects, examining the real objects whenever possible. **Discovery learning** is obtaining knowledge for oneself by formulating general rules, concepts, or principles through learning activities and assignments rather than studying specific examples by reading or listening to the teacher. By discovery learning, Bruner meant obtaining knowledge for oneself. That is, instead of students studying specific examples by reading or listening to the teacher, they formulate general rules, concepts, or principles through learning activities and assignments. This strategy is not simply letting students do what they want or accidentally discovering something; it is best handled as a directed activity. To facilitate discovery learning, teachers arrange activities in which students search, manipulate, explore, and investigate to form a new insight (Schunk, 2004).

Advance organizers are the major contribution of Ausubel. He disagreed with Bruner, and thought that discovery learning was ineffective because most learning occurred as direct learning. According to this theorist, the **advance organizer** is a means of preparing the learner's cognitive structure for the learning experience about to take place. This teaching strategy involves any activities at the onset of the lesson to help the new information be more readily connected with prior learning or to help direct the learners' attention to important concepts (Schunk, 2004).

Content organization is emphasized by cognitive theorists, as it contributes to memory processing and retrieval of information. Using the cognitive processes, this perspective suggests that memory is enhanced by organizing information and making it meaningful. How learners organize and interpret information is very important. If learners already have some knowledge that is similar, showing connections to previous experience or content makes the new information more easily remembered (Woolfolk, 2010). Similarly, the actual content organization or structure may be remembered. The categories of pharmacology provide an excellent example of this kind of information organization as nursing students learn categories of drugs in which to place new drugs throughout their career, making that learning easier. The following is a sequence of nine specific events for learning using this information processing model of memory (Bastable, 2008):

1. Gain attention;
2. Inform of the objective and expectation;
3. Stimulate recall of prerequisite learning;
4. Present material;
5. Provide learning guidance;
6. Elicit performance;
7. Provide feedback about correctness;
8. Assess performance; and
9. Enhance retention, transfer, and recall.

Metacognition

Metacognition is an important concept in learning cognitive theory and plays a critical role in successful learning. It consists of a student monitoring the learning progress by checking the level of understanding, evaluating the effectiveness of efforts, planning activities, and revising as necessary (Peirce, 2003). It is called **metacognition** because it is cognition about cognition, or thinking about thinking. This activity refers to the deliberate control of thinking activity, or the study of how one develops knowledge about one's own cognitive system (Schunk, 2004).

Educators can acknowledge, cultivate, and enhance metacognitive capabilities of learners by helping them define the learning goal, determine how performance will be evaluated, estimate the time required, plan study time, make a checklist of what needs to happen, and organize materials, as a few of the possible metacognitive activities. Explicitly teaching study strategies in content courses has been shown to improve learning, as students in higher education settings may have only been taught rote memorization skills (Peirce, 2003; Schunk, 2004).

Metacognition can affect motivation because it affects the student's ideas about reasons for success or failure. Good results on academic activities may be attributed to ability and effort, whereas failure may be attributed to the same internal factors, or to external causes such as an overly difficult task or an instructor's unfair testing habits. Attributing success to ability and effort promotes confidence, and the converse is true. Attributing failure to a lack of ability reduces a student's chance to be confident on the next challenging task. Similarly, blaming failure on external causes undermines effort necessary for subsequent academic tasks (Peirce, 2003). Teaching students effective ways of preparing for exams and projects, suggesting valid assessment of readiness, and providing fair, consistent, and transparent grading policies are important metacognitive strategies to promote motivation.

Transformative Learning

A description of how learners construct, validate, and reformulate their understandings of their experience makes up **transformative learning**. This theory is included here as it uses cognitive processes and metacognition, with the specific purpose of transforming one's perspectives. In this perspective, the learner "uses a prior interpretation to construe a new or revised interpretation of the meaning of one's experience to guide future action" (Taylor, 2007, p. 173). First introduced by Mezirow (2000), this explanation for learning is thought to be critical in adult education because adults are expected to make their own interpretations rather than act on the judgments and beliefs of others. Experience and critical reflection are central to the individual's constructing their own beliefs and judgments, rather than uncritically assimilating those of others (Taylor).

The teacher's role in building a trusting climate and being aware of student attitudes is a fundamental element of fostering transformative learning. The classroom should be a community of individuals who are trying, in a shared way, to make meaning of their experience. The teacher acts as a role model with a willingness to learn and change by deepening perspectives (Taylor, 2007). Many sensitive issues within health care, such as social justice, ethnicity, poverty, inequality of access, and physical abuse provide examples in which learners' perspectives may be changed with expanded experiences and information.

General implications of cognitive learning approaches emphasize mental processes and the role of the teacher in terms of effective teaching strategies that facilitate learning. For example, presenting information in an organized manner reflecting students' previous knowledge and its relation to new content helps students understand and make connections, as new information is most easily learned when associated with previous knowledge. Teachers can encourage reflection, sequencing, and can present materials using as many modalities as possible (Schunk, 2004).

Ultimately, this perspective acknowledges that learners determine what is learned, not the teacher. However, teachers can facilitate learning outcomes by using many of the cognitive teaching strategies alone or in combination with strategies associated with other learning perspectives.

CONSTRUCTIVIST LEARNING THEORY

Constructivism is a broad term that includes the work of several different researchers. It is a learning perspective arguing that individuals construct much of what they learn and understand, producing knowledge based on their beliefs and experiences. Although there is not one constructivist theory of learning, most agree on two assumptions: Learners are active in constructing their own knowledge, and social interactions are important in this process (Woolfolk, 2010). This learning perspective argues that individuals construct much of what they learn and understand. That means that learners produce knowledge based on their beliefs and experiences. Knowledge, then, is subjective and personal, emphasizing the importance of culture and context (Kim, 2001). The emphasis on constructivism follows the shift away from environmental factors toward human factors as explanations for learning. Although cognitive theories emphasize learners' information processing, some think that these theories fail to capture the complexity of human learning (Schunk, 2004). *Constructionism* and *constructivism* have been differentiated as different approaches to a common concept, with constructionism more focused on how public knowledge is constructed, rather than individual learning. In contrast, *constructivism*, often referred to as *social constructivism*, emphasizes social interaction and cultural context to explain learning. For curriculum designers, this chapter focuses on constructivism (Kim; Woolfolk).

There are several theorists within the constructivism perspective, but a shared, basic assumption is that active learners construct knowledge as they try to make sense of their experiences. Learners are not passive, "empty vessels waiting to be filled" (Woolfolk, 2010, p. 314). These learners develop mental models and revise them to make sense of their educational experience. These representations are the unique perspective of the learner and, therefore, are unique to the learner. In addition, this type of learning cannot be separated from its context. The way learners interact with their worlds transforms their thinking, and this is known as **situated cognition**. An instructional implication of this idea is that teaching strategies should be consistent with the desired learning outcomes for a particular situation. If the objective is to teach inquiry skills, the curriculum must incorporate inquiry activities (Kim, 2001; Schunk, 2004; Woolfolk). This expectation fits well with nursing courses, as clinical activities provide the necessary situations for learning.

Although constructivism is a more recent perspective, it underlies such educational thinking as the integrated curriculum in which learners study a topic from multiple perspectives. In addition, this perspective emphasizes learner-centered principles such as structuring the learning situation so that learners become actively involved with the content through manipulating materials or social interaction. Observing phenomena, collecting data, generating hypotheses, and working collaboratively are recommended strategies, as examples of hands-on, project-based activities suggested by this approach (Kim, 2001; Schunk, 2004).

Woolfolk (2010) presents five conditions for learning from the constructivist perspective. The first is to provide complex, realistic, and relevant learning environments. Students should not be given "stripped down, simplified problems and basic skills drills" (p. 315) instead of realistic projects, complex situations with many parts, and problems that might have several solutions. Tasks should be authentic, the kind of tasks learners will confront in the real world. For some of these complex procedures, students can initially be supported through a process called **instructional scaffolding**, a process of controlling task elements that are initially beyond the learners' capacity. For example, the teacher might do much of the work in the beginning, after which the learner does an increasing role, leading to independence. This process allows the learner to focus on the parts of the task that are possible at any particular point (Schunk, 2004; Woolfolk, 2010).

The second condition is to provide for social interaction and social responsibility as part of learning. Peer collaboration is, therefore, valued; peers working cooperatively create social interactions that provide an instructional function. One goal of teaching may be to develop students' abilities to establish their own positions and defend them, yet respect other points of view. In the United States, considered to be individualistic and competitive, peer collaboration may be more of a challenge, yet some constructivists believe that higher order mental processes develop through these social interactions (Woolfolk, 2010).

The third condition for learning from the constructivist perspective is to support multiple perspectives and representations of content. Complex content requires more than a simple explanation or one particular approach. This idea is consistent with the spiral curriculum in which teachers introduce fundamental structures of a subject early, and then revisit the subject in more and more complex form over time. Woolfolk (2010) suggests that a single approach to complex content leads to oversimplification by the learners.

Nurturing self-awareness in understanding how knowledge is constructed is the fourth constructivist condition for learning. Students should be aware that their beliefs and experiences shape what each of them "know." Learners with different assumptions and experiences may have different knowledge. If students are aware of the influences on their thinking, they may be more reflective and self-critical while respecting the positions of others. Finally, the fifth condition for learning is to encourage student ownership of learning. This might include encouraging learners to make their own thinking processes explicit through dialogue, writing, or other representations (Woolfolk, 2010).

Another strategy suggested by this model is *apprenticeships*, in which novices work with experts in work-related activities, as they provide the necessary social interaction for effective learning (Schunk, 2004). Knowledgeable guides provide models, demonstrations, and evaluation, and the performances are real life, important, and focused on cognitive objectives. Apprenticeships are one way to keep education relevant to the real world of the practitioner. Suggested features include expert coaching, conceptual scaffolding, learner articulation of knowledge, and reflection on their progress (Woolfolk, 2010). Nursing programs have many examples of apprenticeships, more likely called *preceptorships*.

Problem-based learning is a strategy consistent with this learning perspective that initially grew out of research on expert knowledge in medicine. Learners are confronted with a problem that initiates their inquiry and collaboration to find solutions. Students analyze the problem, generate ideas, identify missing information, apply new knowledge, and evaluate the solutions. During this process, their teacher supports them with *scaffolded* information, if necessary. In true problem-based learning, the problem is real and the students' actions matter (Woolfolk, 2010). Teachers who wish to incorporate constructivist pedagogy in their program face the challenges of providing the necessary complex, collaborative, and relevant learning environments balanced with the practical considerations of a content-heavy curriculum and limits on time and energy.

ADULT LEARNING THEORY

Malcolm Knowles is the central figure in U.S. adult education. First interested in *informal education*, he used the term to refer to informal programs in associations or clubs, pointing to the friendly and informal climate, flexibility of the process, and the enthusiasm and commitment of learners and teachers. He initially differentiated these informal programs at community centers, industries, and churches from the formal programs established by educational institutions (Knowles, 1978; Smith, 2002). The definition of **adult learning theory** and **andragogy** used for this text is: a model of learning using assumptions of adults' autonomy, life experiences, personal goals, and need for relevancy and respect.

Knowles was convinced that adults learn differently from children and his earlier work on informal adult education provided the foundation for his later work on the adult education movement. He assumed that adult learners were different from child learners in self-concept, experience, readiness to learn, orientation to learning, and motivation. Knowles' conception of *andragogy* was the adult equivalent of pedagogy and assumed that individuals become adults at the point at which they were capable of self-direction. Therefore, when an adult individual is in a situation in which self-direction is not possible, a tension arises. Knowles observed that when students enter a professional school, they have made a big step toward becoming self-directing and identifying with the adult role (Atherton, 2009; Knowles, 1978).

Knowles' concept of andragogy was an attempt to build a comprehensive, integrated theory or model of adult learning out of the isolated concepts, insights, and research findings regarding adult learning (Knowles, 1978). However, some believe that Knowles simply provided a set of guidelines for practice rather than as a theory. Therefore, his assumptions can be read as descriptions of the adult learner rather than a conceptual framework (Atherton, 2009; Smith, 2002). This perspective is particularly helpful to instructors because nursing students are adults. In addition, it is clear and easy to understand. The principles or assumptions of learning and learner characteristics fit nicely with other, more comprehensive theories, such as cognitivism or constructivism, thereby providing the instructor with many ideas for projects and assignments with enough flexibility to be interesting and relevant to the adults in their classes. Thus, the ideas that began as relevant to informal education settings can be appropriate strategies within formal academic settings of all kinds.

In addition, Knowles' ideas remind instructors that learning is a continuing process through life, a perspective very relevant for nursing education. He identified characteristics of adult learners, sometimes described as assumptions, as follows (Lieb, 1991):

1. Adults are autonomous and prefer to direct themselves. Teachers act as facilitators, considering the learners' perspectives about topics and projects. The class must be relevant for the learners' needs.
2. Adults have life experiences and knowledge that need to be connected to the learning experience. Teachers can relate the content to the participants and acknowledge the value of their personal experience.
3. Adults desire an organized, well-defined program that is relevant to their personal goals. Instructors can show the participants how the content will help them reach their goals.
4. Adults are concerned with relevancy. They want to see the rationale for learning this content, which should be applicable to their lives. Letting participants choose projects or objectives that they see as relevant helps to meet this need.
5. Adults are practical. Similar to the earlier characteristics, the content and projects should be useful in work or personal life in some way. Instructors can stress how this may be true.

6. Adults want respect. Teachers must acknowledge their life experiences and treat them as capable of self-direction. These participants can often add much to the program and their knowledge and opinions can be freely sought, even when they provide an alternative perspective to the instructor.

Adults have special needs and requirements as learners according to this adult learning perspective. Effective teaching involves understanding how to use the characteristics of mature learners to the best advantage in a particular learning situation. Knowles (1978) reminds us that the accumulated experience of a mature individual provides a rich resource for learning as well as a broader base to which the learner can relate new information. Adults tend to have a problem-centered orientation to learning and want to apply information to today's problems. The more relevant the course work is to the current clinical assignment, the more relevant the material is for a nursing student.

HUMANISTIC LEARNING THEORY

Finally, this chapter discusses the humanistic perspective. **Humanism,** or **humanistic learning theory,** is an approach to teaching that assumes people are inherently good, possess unlimited potential for growth, and, therefore, it emphasizes personal freedom, choice, self-determination, and self-actualization.

As before, humanism and instructional strategies from other approaches such as behaviorism or cognitivism are often compatible to some extent. In the real world, teachers can demonstrate humanistic approaches and still use the knowledge offered by other approaches (LeFrancois, 2000). Schunk (2004) argues that humanistic theory as applied to learning is constructivist and emphasizes cognitive and affective processes, thereby combining important elements of previously discussed theories. This statement reinforces the notion that the real boundaries between the theories discussed in this chapter are somewhat blurred. In addition, most educators do not fall neatly into one perspective or another but combine strategies from several approaches as relevant for their work.

Proponents of the humanistic approach to teaching object to what they perceive as mechanistic approaches to education. This perspective has its roots in the existential philosophy that wonders about the nature and purpose of humanity, sees humans as basically good, and asserts that teachers place far too much emphasis on measurable outcomes such as standardized tests (LeFrancois, 2000). They believe that because people are inherently good, they possess unlimited potential for growth and development (Boeree, 2006b). Humanistic interpretations emphasize personal freedom, choice, self-determination, and self-actualization. They assert that other approaches are concerned with averages and generalizations, whereas humanism is concerned with the uniqueness and individuality of each individual. In addition to the student uniqueness, this view emphasizes the teacher's attitudes toward the learners. Humanism is compatible with nursing's emphasis on caring, an orientation that is challenged by the increasing emphasis on technology, cost efficiency, and time pressure (Bastable, 2008).

Carl Rogers is the most influential theorist in humanistic theory. His theory emerged primarily as a reaction against the dominant views of the 1940s, Freudian theory, and behaviorism. Rogers believed that individuals instinctively value positive regard, love, affection, and attention. His approach allows individuals to grow in self-esteem, self-discovery, and self-directed learning, with the goal of self-actualization, a person's basic overriding tendency. Rogers asserted that individuals are the center of their own personal experience, known as the **phenomenological field**, a reality that can never be completely known by another (Boeree, 2006b).

Maslow, a major contributor to this theory, is perhaps best known for his hierarchy of needs, an important part of motivation. Maslow believed that humans strive to satisfy their needs, which are hierarchical. Lower order needs, such as physiological and safety needs, must be satisfied before higher order needs can influence behavior (Bastable, 2008). The highest level of need is self-actualization or the desire for self-fulfillment. Self-actualization can be expressed in many different ways according to the individual; the desire to be an ideal mother, an athlete, or to attain academic achievement (Schunk, 2004).

In keeping with Maslow's hierarchy, Rogers believed that the tendency toward actualization, or achieving wholeness, was an innate motivation. This actualizing tendency is the source of hunger and thirst, but also of personal growth, autonomy, and freedom according to this approach (Schunk, 2004). Mastering information and facts is not the central objective of this approach to learning, rather fostering curiosity, enthusiasm, and responsibility is more important and should be the goal of the educator. Humanists believe that self-concept and self-esteem are necessary considerations in any learning situation, and what people want is unconditional positive regard, the feeling of being loved without strings attached. Experiences that are coercive or threatening diminish the learning outcomes for individuals. In professional education, the goal is to provide psychologically safe classrooms and clinical settings where humanistic principles can be demonstrated through various instructional strategies (Bastable, 2008).

The preparation of a humanistic teacher devotes as much attention to teacher attitudes as to subject matter and instructional strategies. Spontaneity, the importance of emotions, an individual's choices, and creativity are critical aspects of a humanistic approach to learning, which has the fulfillment of one's potential as its purpose. Students perceive meaningful learning as relevant because they believe it is important and will enhance their lives (Bastable, 2008). Schunk (2004) recommends that humanistic educators act as facilitators who help students clarify and achieve their goals and establish a classroom climate oriented to significant learning. In this perspective, individual contracts and flexible procedures are preferable to lockstep sequences (Schunk).

Humanistic teachers advocate a philosophy of teaching in which students are given an important role in curriculum decisions in a course. In this perspective, teachers should be learning facilitators rather than didactic instructors and they must be sensitive, caring, and empathetic. Humanistic approaches to education emphasize healthy social and personal development and de-emphasize rigorous, performance-oriented, test-dominated approaches to subject matter (LeFrancois, 2000). Humanistic principles have been a cornerstone of self-help groups, wellness programs, and palliative care (Bastable, 2008).

This theory has its weaknesses as well as strengths, as critics assert it is more of a philosophy than a science (Bastable, 2008). Moreover, information, facts, memorization, drill, and the tedious work sometimes required to master knowledge may well be necessary for knowledge building as even the most self-actualized nursing student still needs to know how to take care of patients safely, function as part of a health care team, and pass professional exams.

Important discussions can take place among nursing educators regarding the need to balance preparing professionals for the real world of complex health care settings with the humanistic goal of personal development. Within the content-heavy courses required for accreditation and clinical settings, is it possible to add a degree of student choice about assignments, increase the feeling of safety within classrooms, and encourage self-esteem and personal growth? Can educators demonstrate positive regard, empathic understanding, and genuineness with the heavy demands of academic or professional programs? The focus on helping people maximize their potential provides an important addition to any theory's strategies, while presenting challenges to teachers and courses with high work demand.

SUMMARY

This chapter presented an overview of the six perspectives on how learning occurs. As educators revise or create new curricula, they are encouraged to consider the potential contributions of all of the different explanations to learning processes. They provide the foundation for alternative teaching strategies that are relevant and applicable to particular classrooms, content, and/or students.

Behaviorism emphasizes the importance of environmental stimuli (the bell, the food) rather than internal thinking processes of the learner. Reinforcement of the resulting behaviors increases the likelihood of that particular behavior being repeated. Associations are formed with positive and negative stimuli that often generalize to new situations (Woolfolk, 2010). Attitudes in education are often affected by previous experiences; for example, a teacher making derogatory remarks about a project on which a student spent considerable time and effort may result in negative attitudes toward a subsequent project.

Social cognitive theory moves the emphasis to the context of learning, emphasizing the importance of the interaction among personal characteristics, behaviors, and the social environment. Personal beliefs such as self-efficacy are important contributions of this perspective, providing the foundation for powerful teaching strategies. Role modeling and other kinds of observational learning provide common and influential teaching strategies relevant for nursing students (Schunk, 2004).

Cognitivism focuses attention on internal, mental processes such as thinking, memory, information processing, and information organization. This perspective suggests many strategies for presenting content in ways that foster memory and understanding for the learner. Within this section, this chapter discussed metacognition and transformational learning. Metacognition, or thinking about thinking, provides an essential part of inquiry, ethical dilemmas, and critical thinking generally, and thereby occupies an important place in nursing classrooms. Transformative learning involves constructing or reformulating one's understanding of an experience (Bastable, 2008).

The constructivist perspective says that learners construct their own version of what they learn and understand. That means that learners produce knowledge based on their beliefs and experience, and social interactions are a critical aspect of this process This perspective argues for teaching content from multiple perspectives and providing real-life problems in all their complexity and realism. Apprenticeships, in which learners work in authentic situations with experts, and problem-based learning are two strategies supported by this approach, because they embrace complex situations, perhaps with more than one good approach (Woolfolk, 2010).

The adult learning perspective reminds instructors that adult students bring a reservoir of experiences and knowledge plus a focus on real-world, relevant, practical issues. Relevancy in course work and clinical assignments is particularly important for these mature students. In addition, adults prefer the flexibility to focus on their own goals and want respect for their accumulated experiences (Smith, 2002).

Finally, the humanistic perspective focuses on the development of the individual, with self-actualization as the highest level. Facilitating the learner's positive attitude, self-esteem, responsibility, and enthusiasm are goals of this approach. Teaching strategies in a humanistic classroom considers the desire of all people for unconditional positive regard (Bastable, 2008).

The learning theories discussed here predate technology and other current issues in education. Some authors suggest that newer paradigms are necessary to reflect the current social environment, exponential knowledge growth, and technological models of communication; yet others continue to use traditional models as conceptual underpinnings. As examples of different models, a theory of connectivism was suggested as more relevant for the rapid increase of knowledge (Siemens, 2005); and a combination of learning theories was used as underpinnings for a study of clinical simulation (Waldner & Olson, 2007). In contrast, more traditional learning models were used in studies in which self-efficacy was correlated with personal digital assistants (PDAs) by student nurses (Kuiper, 2010), and role modeling was identified as the primary teaching strategy of medical clinical teachers (Weissman, Branch, Gracey, Haidet, & Frankel, 2006). Time, empirical research, and thoughtful discussion will determine whether traditional theories remain relevant in today's classrooms and academic issues, and whether new paradigms will emerge.

Conceptual models and theories provide the foundation for many curricular decisions, especially the critical choices of teaching strategies. Management of curricular content and pedagogical innovations is necessitated by several factors including the rapid expansion of knowledge, content-saturated curricula, and changes to the health care delivery system (Giddens & Brady, 2007).

A curriculum plan provides guidelines for a specific educational program to be implemented. Today's nursing programs have constraints on resources, clinical settings that are sometimes less than perfect, and too little time. These factors create enormous downward pressure on programs to simplify, eliminate, and generally make things easier. Learning theories remind planners about the importance of complex content, challenging cognitive tasks, self-efficacy, professional role models, information organization, and regard for students. These theories help provide counteracting "upward" pressure for faculty to design an appropriately challenging, yet practical, curriculum for today's health care practitioner.

DISCUSSION QUESTIONS

1. Evaluate learning theories as possible foundations to guide nursing program curricula in schools of nursing and staff development settings.
2. Analyze various learning theories for appropriateness and congruency with the philosophy and mission of educational institutions, schools of nursing, or health care agencies.

LEARNING ACTIVITIES

Student Learning Activities

1. Compare learning theory strengths and weaknesses as a conceptual basis for teaching and learning strategies within a nursing curriculum.

Nurse Educator/Faculty Development Activities

1. Select one learning theoretical approach as an overall guide for developing teaching and learning strategies in a curriculum program or course.

REFERENCES

Atherton, J. S. (2009). *Learning and teaching; Knowles' andragogy: An angle on adult learning* (online) UK: Retrieved February 8, 2010, from http://www.learningandteaching.info/learning/knowlesa.htm

Bandura, A. (1986). *Social foundations of thought and action: A social cognitive theory.* Englewood Cliff, NJ: Prentice-Hall.

Bandura, A. (1994). Self-efficacy. In V. S. Ramachaudran (Ed.), *Encyclopedia of human behavior* (Vol. 4, pp. 71–81). New York: Academic Press. Retrieved January 18, 2010, from http://www.des.emory.edu/mfp/BanEncy.htm

Bastable, S. B. (2008). *Nurse as educator: Principles of teaching and learning for nursing practice* (3rd ed.). Sudbury, MA: Jones and Bartlett.

Boeree, C. G. (2006a). *Albert Bandura.* Retrieved January 18, 2010, from http://webspace.ship.edu/cgboer/bandura.html

Boeree, C. G. (2006b). *Carl Rogers.* Retrieved Feb 21, 2010, from http://webspace.ship.edu/cgboer/rogers.html

Giddens, J. F., & Brady, D. P. (2007). Rescuing nursing education from content saturation: The case for a concept-based curriculum (Electronic version). *Journal of Nursing Education, 46*(2), 65–69.

Green, C. (2009). *Introduction to psychology as the behaviorist views it: John B. Watson. Classics in the history of psychology.* Retrieved February 18, 2010, from http://psychclassics.yorku.ca/Watson/intro.htm

Hauser, L. (2006). Behaviorists and behaviorisms. *Internet Encyclopedia of Philosophy.* Retrieved February 19, 2010, from http://www.utm.edu/research/iep/b/behavior.htm

Huitt, W. (2006). *The cognitive system: Educational psychology interactive.* Valdosta, GA: Valdosta State University. Retrieved February 19, 2010, from http://www.edpsycinteractive.org/topics/cogsys/cogsys.html

Huitt, W., & Hummel, J. (2006). An overview of the behavioral perspective. *Educational Psychology Interactive.* Valdosta, GA: Valdosta State University. Retrieved February 19, 2010, from http://www.edpsycinteractive.org/topics/behsys/behsys.html

Kim, B. (2001). Social Constructivism. In M. Orey (Ed.), *Emerging perspectives on Learning, teaching, and technology.* Retrieved February 20, 2010, from http://projects.coe.uga.edu/epltt/index.php?title=Social_Constructivism

Knowles, M. S. (1978). *The adult learner: A neglected species* (2nd ed.). Houston, TX: Gulf Publishing.

Kuiper, R. (2010). Metacognitive factors that impact student nurse use of point of care technology in clinical settings. *International Journal of Nursing Education Scholarship, 7*(1), Article 5. Retrieved February 10, 2010, from http://www.bepress.com/ijnes/vol7/iss1/art5/

Lefrancois, G. (2000). *Psychology for teaching* (10th ed.). Belmont, CA: Wadsworth.

Lieb, S. (1991). *Principles of adult learning.* Retrieved January 10, 2010, from http://honolulu.hawaii.edu/intranet/committees/FacDevCom/guidebk/teachtip/adults-2.htm

Mezirow, J. (2000). Learning to think like an adult. In J. Mezirow & Associates (Eds.), *Learning as transformation* (pp. 3–33). San Francisco, CA: Jossey-Bass.

Pajares, F. (2002). *Overview of social cognitive theory and of self-efficacy.* Retrieved January 18, 2010, from http://www.emory.edu/EDUCATION/mfp/eff.html

Peirce, W. (2003). *Metacognition: Study strategies, monitoring, and motivation.* Retrieved February 22, 2010, from http://academic.pgcc.edu/~wpeirce/MCCCTR/metacognition.htm#1

Schunk, D. H. (2004). *Learning theories: An educational perspective* (4th ed.). Upper Saddle River, NJ: Pearson, Prentice Hall.

Skinner, B. F. (n.d.) A brief survey of operant behavior. *B.F. Skinner Foundation.* Retrieved February 15, 2010, from http://www.bfskinner.org/BFSkinner/SurveyOperantBehavior.html

Siemens, G. (2005). *Connectivism: A learning theory for the digital age.* Retrieved February 22, 2010, from http://www.elearnspace.org/Articles/connectivism.htm

Smith, M. K. (2002). Malcolm Knowles, informal adult education, self-direction and andragogy. *The Encyclopedia of Informal Education.* Retrieved February 8, 2010, from www.infed.org/thinkers/et-knowl.htm

Standridge, M. (2002). Behaviorism. In M. Orey (Ed.), *Emerging perspectives on learning, teaching, and technology.* Retrieved February 15, 2010, from http://projects.coe.uga.edu/epltt/index.php?title=Behaviorism

Taylor, E. W. (2007). An update of transformative learning theory: A critical review of the empirical research (1999–2005; Electronic version). *International Journal of Lifelong Education, 26*(2), 175–191.

Waldner, M. H., & Olson, J. K. (2007). Taking the patient to the classroom: Applying theoretical frameworks to simulation in nursing education. *International Journal of Nursing Education Scholarship, 4*(1), Article 18. Retrieved February 24, 2010, from http://www.bepress.com/ijnes/vol4/iss1/art18

Weissman, P. F., Branch, W. T., Gracey, C. F., Haidet, P., & Frankel, R. M. (2006). Role modeling humanistic behavior: Learning bedside manner from the experts (Electronic version). *Academic Medicine, 81*(7), 661–667.

Woolfolk, A. (2010). *Educational psychology* (11th ed.). Upper Saddle River, NJ: Merrill.

4 Taxonomies and Critical Thinking in Curriculum Design

Lori Candela

OBJECTIVES

Upon completion of Chapter 4, the reader will be able to:

1. Examine the evolution of educational taxonomies in curriculum development and evaluation.
2. Explore updates in and revisions to educational taxonomies.
3. Analyze the development of critical thinking in the context of educational taxonomies.
4. Categorize objectives to progress cognitive, affective, and psychomotor skills through nursing education levels.
5. Produce learning activities and objectives that demonstrate structured, higher order thinking skills, and exemplify dispositions of critical thinking.

OVERVIEW

The use of educational taxonomy as ways to view, develop, and evaluate learning objectives is well established in American education. For more than 50 years, educators have turned to taxonomies to provide the terminology for objectives that could be behaviorally measured. Initially, the taxonomy focused on the cognitive or thinking aspect of learning. A revised taxonomy discerned levels of knowledge as well cognitive levels. Later, the affective (values) and psychomotor (physical skills) domains were more fully developed.

The role of critical thinking is directly applicable to educational taxonomy. Even in its earliest version, taxonomy developers acknowledged the need to assess reasoning and problem-solving abilities of students. Some argue that only the upper levels of the taxonomy include critical thinking whereas others see all levels as influential in the development process.

Central to the development of critical thinking skills is the degree to which the student engages with the content. This can best be achieved through the use of well-thought-out, structured active learning strategies.

THE USEFULNESS OF EDUCATIONAL TAXONOMIES

Taxonomy provides a common language and framework for classifying, categorizing, and defining educational goals. The use of taxonomy over the past 50 years facilitated a shift in focus from what is taught to what students are expected to learn. Educators at every level use taxonomy to develop, communicate, and evaluate learning objectives. Curriculum developers and evaluators use taxonomy as a method of mapping the progression of student learning toward larger program outcomes.

OBJECTIVES AND OUTCOMES

The use of objectives in education can be traced back to 1949 when Ralph Tyler published a little book with great influence entitled *Basic Principles of Curriculum and Instruction*. Tyler argued that education should center on the learner and that changes in learner behavior be measured by statements or objectives. Prideaux (2000) noted that Tyler had a "broad view of the nature of objectives . . . " (p. 168). Ralph Mager later advocated that those learner behaviors needed to be stated in very specific terms. These became known as behavioral objectives that replaced verbs such as "understand" with verbs like "identify" (Prideaux).

Many terms have been used over the years to describe how and what students should learn. Terms such as learning objectives, behavioral objectives, instructional objectives, and learning outcomes have inadvertently caused confusion among educators. Some have argued that there is no difference between objectives and outcomes (Harden, 2002). Even today, the verbiage used varies among nursing programs.

The outcome-based education movement advanced the need for clearly articulated outcomes. But many educational programs merely tinkered with small word or title changes instead of truly considering the differences. Harden (2002) argued that there are definite differences between objectives and outcomes. Both describe products of learning, but objectives are more specific and detailed, delineated into learning domains (knowledge, skills, attitudes), stated as intentions, and they are more owned by individual instructors. Simply put, "Outcomes relate directly to professional practice; objectives relate to instruction" (Glennon, 2006, p. 55).

THE CONNECTION OF OBJECTIVES TO LEARNING THEORY

Most educational objectives are rooted in behaviorism. The behavioral view posits that learning does not occur if the desired behavior produced by education is not observable or measurable. This served nursing education well, particularly in terms of skill acquisition. However, the complexity and pace of new information assures that not every skill can be taught. Students must learn to construct new knowledge throughout their lives to adapt and thrive in unknown, ambiguous situations.

The constructivist view is that reality is built or constructed by the person. New information that is taken in is then integrated within the context of previous knowledge, experiences, and perceptions to form new learning and insight (Goudreau et al., 2009; Hagstrom, 2006).

DOMAINS OF LEARNING WITHIN TAXONOMIES

Without question, the work of Benjamin Bloom and his colleagues in the late 1940s and 1950s to develop a common taxonomy will forever be viewed as one of the most important achievements in education in the 20th century (Granello, 2001). The ideas behind the taxonomy were first discussed by Bloom and a group of colleagues attending the American Psychological Association conference in 1948. The group was looking to develop a common framework to promote sharing of ideas for examination materials, research on those examinations, and connections to education. The group determined that this framework could best be achieved if it included "a system of classifying the goals of the educational process using educational objectives" (Bloom, 1994, p. 2).

The group continued meeting regularly for the next several years. It became apparent that the best way to develop a comprehensive taxonomy suitable for the evaluation of learning was to consider it through three categories (domains) that affect the *process* of learning: cognitive behavior, affective behavior, and psychomotor behavior (Halawi, McCarthy, & Pires, 2009). Each domain was conceived as categories that were arranged in a simple to complex hierarchical order. Mastery of behaviors in each lower category was prerequisite to mastery of the next level. Also, every level was a part of the next higher level. The first and most complete work occurred in the cognitive domain. This was logical as it was most closely related to the types of examinations occurring at that time (Bloom, 1994). The work product of the group culminated in 1956 with the publication of *The Taxonomy of Educational Objectives, Handbook 1: Cognitive Domain.*

The Cognitive Domain of Bloom

The first level of the taxonomy is knowledge. For Bloom and his group, knowing is foundational to all other levels. It is remembering what is known and demonstrating it by recitation or recall. The next level is comprehension. Comprehension goes beyond knowledge as the person is able to grasp, understand, and make some sense of information. The understanding may not be complete but is indicative of being able to do something with what you know. Bloom (1994) points out three types of comprehension: (a) translation (putting the information into a different language "in your own words"), (b) interpretation (reordering the information, considering the importance of the concepts, summarizing, generalizing) and (c) extrapolation (making predictions or forecasts).

The third level of the six-tier taxonomy is application. At this level, the student can solve a problem or issue that is new by applying what is known and understood from other experiences. Bloom points out that application is different and more complex than extrapolation at the comprehension level. Extrapolation is based on "what is given" versus the abstraction necessary in application, such as applying a general rule or principle to a new situation. The fourth level is analysis, in which one knows, understands, and can apply information well enough to then break it down into component parts, examine how it is organized and the relationships that exist among the parts. Bloom considered this analysis as a necessary "prelude" to the ability to evaluate the sixth and final level.

The next level is synthesis. This involves the ability to take parts, such as pieces of information, and put them together to form something that was not "clearly present" before. This level is most closely linked with creativity. However, it is not viewed as complete freedom of expression because there are generally some set guidelines or restrictions.

The sixth and final level of the taxonomy is evaluation. This level incorporates all of the previous levels in order to judge (quantitatively and/or qualitatively) the value of what is being studied. Criteria or standards are used in making such judgments. This clearly differentiates it from opinions, which may exist without full awareness or conscious use of logical criteria. Bloom did not see evaluation as the last step of the cognitive levels but as the real connection to the affective domain, which is concerned with values. Sousa noted the connection between the affective and cognitive domains as a way of developing the higher order thinking skills of students.

According to Sousa (2005), the lower three cognitive levels involve convergent thinking in which learners apply what they remember and understand to solving new problems. The upper three levels use more divergent or higher order thinking to develop new insights (Sousa, 2005). Bissell and Lemons (2006) believe that higher order thinking is also present at the application level.

Bloom's taxonomy is widely used in primary, secondary, and postsecondary education to both establish and evaluate learning (Athanassiou, McNett, & Harvey, 2003; Cochran, Conklin, & Modin, 2007). The taxonomy is used across various educational levels and disciplines (Manton, English, & Kernek, 2008). It has been translated into at least 22 languages (Krathwohl, 2002) and is referenced in citations nearly 100 times per year (Bloom, 1994). The taxonomy provided a structure for educators to consider learning and the products of learning.

One of the more recurring criticisms of the original taxonomy is that it is simplistic (Kuhn, 2008). The hierarchal structure of the taxonomy is unidirectional and presumes that each simpler category, that is, comprehension, must be "mastered" before the next level; in this case, application (Krathwohl, 2002; Paul, 1993). Another criticism of the taxonomy has revolved around the category of knowledge. The verbs associated with the knowledge category, such as recall and recite, suggested that knowledge was simplistic; little more than memorization (Booker, 2008; Paul, 1993). New information and research into the areas of learning and cognition led to a significant revision to the original taxonomy (Anderson & Krathwohl, 2001).

The Revised Taxonomy by Anderson and Krathwohl

In 2001, Anderson and Krathwohl published a significant revision to Bloom's taxonomy. Rationale for the revision included the need to rethink of the impact of the original taxonomy on education and how visionary it was at the time. Secondly, there was a need to do so as new knowledge regarding thinking and learning became available (Bumen, 2007). Even as the original handbook was being published, Bloom advocated for updates and changes to the taxonomy as new knowledge became available. The revised taxonomy was different in three areas. The first change was one of terminology. The knowledge category was renamed "remember"; comprehension was renamed "understand." The second change was to move the synthesize level to the top and rename it "create." The third change was to add a second dimension. The revised taxonomy retained the cognitive process dimension and added a knowledge dimension (Anderson & Krathwohl, 2001). The knowledge dimension consists of factual, conceptual, procedural, and metacognitive levels (Roberts & Inman, 2007). The revision allowed the cognitive category to focus on the noun aspect of an objective "principles of sterile technique," whereas the knowledge dimension focused on the verb portion "remember" (Krathwohl, 2002).

Factual knowledge includes the basics that students need to know to be acquainted with the discipline such as knowledge of terminology or specific details. Conceptual knowledge involves understanding the interrelationships of parts within a structure (knowledge of classifications or categories, principles and generalizations, theories, and models). Procedural knowledge includes knowing how to do something such as knowledge of criteria for determining which procedure to use, proper steps in performing a procedure, or developing algorithms/concept maps for patient-specific care. Metacognitive knowledge is knowledge of cognition in general as well as having a personal awareness and knowledge of cognition, such as strategic knowledge, knowledge about cognitive tasks within different contexts, and self-knowledge (Krathwohl, 2002).

The first level of the cognitive dimension, remember, involves retrieving relevant knowledge. This is typified by verbs such as recall and recognize. The second level is to understand or be able to discern the meaning of information. Verbs in this category include interpreting, classifying, summarizing, comparing, explaining, inferring, and exemplifying. At the apply level, the learner is able to use what he or she remembers and understands to carry out an action in a given situation (verbs: execute, implement). To be able to analyze (level 4) is to be able to break something down into parts, examine relationships between, and determine how each part relates to the whole (verbs: differentiate, organize, attribute). The fifth level, evaluate, represents the ability to make judgments based on criteria and includes verbs such as checking and critiquing. The final level is create and includes the ability to put elements together to form new, original products (verbs: generate, plan, produce; Krathwohl, 2002).

The Affective Domain of Krathwohl

Krathwohl, who was a member of the original taxonomy group, further delineated the affective domain of the taxonomy. The affective domain is concerned with feelings or emotions that are expressed values and interests. This domain includes ethical and moral behaviors and features five levels.

Receiving involves being conscious of phenomena and to another's expression of ideas or beliefs. Verbs such as attends, shares, selects, prefers, describes, follows, names, observes, and replies are typical in this category. Subcategories include awareness (becoming aware of something), willingness to receive (ability to suspend judgment or maintain neutrality), and controlled or selected attention in which one is able to differentiate and make selections regarding various stimuli, that is, alertness to human values and judgments about living wills.

Responding is the verbal and nonverbal reactions that indicate a response to a phenomenon ranging on a continuum from compliance to satisfaction. The subcategories range from acquiescence (compliance) in responding to a willingness to respond (voluntarily responding without fear of recrimination) to satisfaction with the response (expressing satisfaction with the response). An example objective for this is, "The first level nursing students express enjoyment when participating in student nurse association activities" (Krathwohl, 2002).

In valuing, students make choices and internalize the value of that choice. It implies that something has worth. Subcategories include acceptance of a value by being able to consistently describe it's worth; preference of the value by seeking it out to fulfill a desire for it; and commitment is activated when the learner develops deep convictions about the value to the point of trying to convince others of the value, that is, "right to life" or "right to choose." The final level is organizing, in which the learner is able to examine values, determine the most significant values, and organize them, even if some conflict with others (Krathwohl, 2002).

By the time a person reaches the highest level of the affective domain, he or she has internalized values and placed them into an internal organized system. Behaviors are consistent and in tune with those values. This is a gradual process and may take a lifetime to achieve. One method to help educators assess learner progression is through writing activities, such as articulating a life philosophy. If done early in the program, it could then be repeated near the end of the program to examine development and differences of thought.

The Psychomotor Domain of Simpson, Dave, and Harrow

There are three psychomotor taxonomies in education. The first was proposed by Simpson (1966) and consists of the following:

- Perception—tuning into sensory cues (verbs: distinguish, identify, select)
- Set—readiness to act (verbs: assume a position, demonstrate, show)
- Guided response—occurs early in the skill and indicates that the learner is capable of completing the steps (verbs: attempt, initiate, try)
- Mechanism—can perform a complex skill at an intermediate stage (verbs: do, act upon, complete)
- Complex overt response—involves correctness in performing the skill (verbs: operate, carry out, perform)
- Adaptation—can modify skills in a new situation (verbs: adapt, change, modify)
- Origination—creative ability or develop an innovative, unique skill that replaces one that was learned (verbs: create, design, invent; Oermann, 1990)

Harrow (1972) developed a taxonomy based on reflex movement, basic fundamental movements, perceptual abilities, skilled movements, and nondiscursive communication. The taxonomy is organized on degree of coordination. At the lowest level, reflex movements include automatic reactions. The next level, basic fundamental movement involves simple movements that can build to more complex sets of movements. At the perceptual level, environmental cues are used to adjust movements. Perceptual abilities at this level are described as tactile, visual, kinesthetic, visual, auditory, and coordinated whereas physical abilities are described as agile, flexible, endurance, and strength. The level of nondiscursive communication is expressive and interpretive, as in the use of body language.

In 1970, Dave published a taxonomy on constructivism including imitate, manipulate, precision, articulation, and naturalization. The taxonomy was based on neuromuscular movement and coordination and underlies criteria proposed by Reilly and Oermann (1990), which were based on a developmental approach to competency. The criteria for each level, according to Reilly and Oermann follows:

- Imitation level—occasional errors are apparent in the necessary actions of the skill and are accompanied by some weakness of gross motor actions and the time required to complete the skill is dependent on the learner's need (verbs: attempt, copy, duplicate, imitate, mimic)
- Manipulation level—coordination of movements occurs with some variation and in the time required to complete the actions of the skill (verbs: complete, follow, play, perform, produce)

- Precision level—a logical sequence carries activities through to completion, almost free of errors in noncritical actions, although the speed of completion continues to be a concern (verbs: achieve automatically, excel expertly, perform masterfully)
- Articulation level—logic is evident in the coordinated actions, few, if any, errors are noted, and the time required to execute the skill is considered reasonable (verbs: customize, originate)
- Naturalization level—professional competence is noted in the skill performance that is automatic and well coordinated (verbs: perform naturally, perform perfectly)

The Holistic Taxonomy of Hauenstein

Hauenstein (1998) proposed a taxonomy that synthesized cognitive, affective, and psychomotor learning into a fourth domain he called "behavior domain" (Figure 4.1). He felt the original taxonomy lacked integration and connection, both of which he considered necessary in order to achieve a holistic curriculum that focused on student understanding, skills, and dispositions. He reduced the categories of the first three domains from six to five. The cognitive domain involved the process of knowing and the development of intellectual abilities and skills. The affective domain is directed toward developing dispositions in relation to feelings, values, and beliefs. The psychomotor domain is defined as the development of physical abilities and skills that result from the input of information and content.

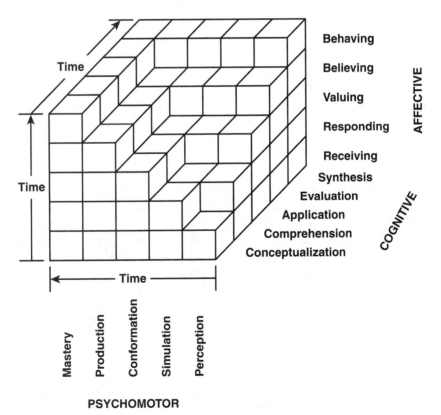

FIGURE 4.1 Hauenstein's Behavioral Domain

The behavioral domain is the "tempered demeanor" that one displays as a reaction to a social stimulus, or an inner need, or both. The behavioral domain consists of acquisition, assimilation, adaptation, performance, and aspiration into the behavioral domain. The acquisition objective is the process of understanding, perceiving, and conceptualizing new information. Assimilation involves comprehending concepts in relation to prior knowledge and explaining it in his or her own terms. Adaptation involves the ability to modify knowledge, skills, or dispositions to conform to an established standard or criterion. Performance is the ability to analyze, qualify, evaluate, and integrate information with personal values and beliefs so that it becomes ingrained and able to be repeated in either new or routine situations (Hauenstein, 1998).

Sipos, Battisi, and Grimm (2008) used the Hauenstein taxonomy in developing a transformative sustainability learning (TSL) unifying framework. The authors used the metaphors of head (cognitive), hands (psychomotor), and hearts (affective) to describe a curriculum in sustainability education. Course objectives and learning activities were developed using all three domains to promote learning, skill acquisition, and a sense of values that could result in "societal transformation."

A New Taxonomy

In 2007, Marzano and Kendall published *The New Taxonomy of Educational Objectives* (2nd ed.). The book provides a detailed description of the theories behind and the use of a two dimensional taxonomy: levels of processing and domains of knowledge. One of the criticisms of the original taxonomy was the hierarchal nature of cognition that indicated the increasing difficulty with each ascending level. Marzano and Kendall disagreed, noting a common psychological principle that even the most difficult mental processes become simple as they become more familiar. The number of steps needed to carry out the mental process and the relationships between steps may not change but the speed at which one can perform them does. For example, a student nurse may take 15 minutes or more to match medications to a medication administration record (MAR) and draw up an injection. That same nurse would likely be able to carry out the task in less than 2 minutes if he or she had performed it many times.

The new taxonomy features six horizontal levels of processing and three vertical rows of knowledge domains. The first four levels of processing are within the cognitive system: retrieval (recognizing, recalling, executing), comprehension (integrating, symbolizing), analysis (matching, classifying, analyzing errors, generating, specifying), and knowledge utilization (decision making, problem solving, experimenting, investigating). The next level is the metacognitive system, which specifies and monitors knowledge in terms of goals, processes, clarity, and accuracy. Self-system thinking is the sixth level of processing. This level is concerned with how motivated a person is in learning a new task given the importance, efficacy, and emotional responses attached to it. Emotions can hinder or facilitate learning (Sousa, 2001) Shulman (2002) discussed the influence of engagement and motivation as both a purpose of education and a "proxy" for subsequent learning.

It is the self-system that decides whether to engage in a new learning task. Internal questions such as how important is this to learn, how much do I believe I can learn it, and how positive or negative do I feel about this new task all affect motivation to learn. Once the self-system decides to engage, the metacognitive system is activated followed by the cognitive system. "All three systems use the students' store of knowledge" (Marzano & Kendall, 2007, p. 12).

The three domains of knowledge are information, mental procedures, and psychomotor procedures. The information domain (declarative knowledge) is represented as hierarchical types. The lower three are described as details (vocabulary terms, facts, time sequences) whereas the higher levels are organizing ideas (principles, generalizations). The mental procedures domain (procedural knowledge) contains two categories: A skills category that uses algorithms, tactics, and single rules and a processes category of macroprocedures. Unlike the procedures in the skills category that can be learned so well as to require little or no conscious thought, macroprocedures are highly complex and require conscious control. The psychomotor domain involves a skill category of simple combination and foundational procedures as well as a processes level of complex combination procedures.

The new taxonomy builds on the work of Bloom's original taxonomy and the Anderson revised taxonomy. According to the authors, new taxonomy differs because it (a) addresses cognitive, affective, and psychomotor learning domains very specifically; (b) places the metacognitive system above the cognitive system; and (c) considers the self-system at the top of the six processing levels. For a more detailed discussion of the new taxonomy, readers are encouraged to consult the Marzano and Kendall book.

CURRICULUM ALIGNMENT USING A TAXONOMY TABLE

The use of taxonomy table (Figure 4.2) is beneficial in assuring that there is alignment among curricular objectives, instruction, and assessment (Anderson, 2002). Educators who assess both cognitive and knowledge dimensions are able to discern a more complete understanding of intended learning (Su, Osisek, & Starnes, 2004). Misalignment of the curriculum may result in assessments and/or objectives that do not reflect instruction. (Airasian & Miranda, 2002).

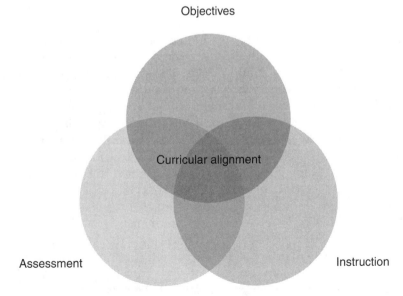

FIGURE 4.2 Curriculum Alignment Using a Taxonomy Table

TABLE 4.1 Taxonomy Table Based on Objectives

The Kowledge Dimension	THE COGNITIVE PROCESS DIMENSION					
	1. Remember	2. Understand	3. Apply	4. Analyze	5. Evaluate	6. Create
A. Factual Knowledge						
B. Conceptual Knowledge	Objective 1	Objective 1			Objective 3	
C. Procedural Knowledge						Objective 4
D. Meta-Cognitve Knowledge		Objective 2			Objective 2	

Key
Objective 1 = Acquire knowledge of a classification scheme of "appeals."
Objective 2 = Check the influences commercials have on students' "senses".
Objective 3 = Evaluate commercials from the standpoint of a set of principles.
Objective 4 = Create a commercial that reflects understandings of how commercials are designed to influence people.

Virtually any objective, activity, or assessment can be plotted in a taxonomy table and can be reviewed and updated regularly to ensure the curriculum is aligned and incorporates concepts that are important for students to learn. As noted in Table 4.1, the horizontal rows of the table represent the cognitive process dimension whereas the vertical rows represent the knowledge dimension.

CRITICAL THINKING AND TAXONOMY

Nurses practice in fast-paced, complex environments in which chaos and change are often the norm (Goudreau, et al., 2009; Rowles & Russo, 2009). Bits of new information bombard us constantly, ensuring that at least some of the content that nursing students learn in school today will be obsolete by the time they graduate. These realities require that nurses quickly assess situations (often with only partial information), make rational clinical judgments, follow with sound clinical decision making, and reflect to assess performance and determine continued learning needs.

Critical thinking requires discernment and a "longing to know—to understand how life works" (Hooks, 2010, p. 7). Critical thinking is important in nursing and in "everyday life" (Valiga, 2009). A single definition of critical thinking has been elusive as evidenced by the numerous definitions that have been advanced over the years. A comprehensive definition advanced by Paul (1993) is presented in Exhibit 4.1.

Valiga (2009) conducted an analysis of 17 definitions on critical thinking and found the following aspects in common: "1) a critical thinker is nonbiased, reasoned and truth oriented; 2) critical thinking involves making judgments; 3) thinking can be judged as critical if it holds up to certain evaluative criteria; 4) tied to a belief or action" (p. 218).

One of the most articulate scholars on critical thinking is Richard Paul. His 1993 book, *Critical thinking: How to prepare students for a rapidly changing world*, challenged educators to fundamentally reconsider how and what content and learning experiences are used in light of developing the thinking skills of students. In 2004, Paul articulated

EXHIBIT 4.1 Definitions of Critical Thinking

Critical thinking is:

- "[A] purposeful, outcome-directed (results-oriented) thinking . . . [that] requires knowledge, skills, and experience . . . [and helps one] constantly reevaluate, self-correct . . ., and strive to improve" (Alfaro-Lefevre, 1999, p. 9).
- "[A] rational investigation of ideas, inferences, assumptions, principles, arguments, conclusions, issues, statements, beliefs, and actions that covers scientific reasoning and includes the nursing process, decision making, and reasoning in controversial issues" (Bandman & Bandman, 1995).
- "[R]eflective and reasonable thinking that is focused on deciding what to do or believe" (Ennis, 1985, p. 45).
- "[P]urposeful, self-regulatory judgment which results in interpretation, analysis, evaluation, an inference as well as explanation of the evidential, conceptual, methodological, criteriological, or contextual considerations upon which that judgment was based" (Facione, 1990).
- "[T]hose skills (or strategies) that increase the probability of achieving a desirable outcome" (Halpern, 1994. p. 13).
- "[A]n investigation whose purpose is to explore a situation, phenomenon, question, or problem to arrive at a hypothesis or conclusion about it that integrates all available information and that can therefore be convincingly justified" (Kurfiss, 1988, p. 2).
- "[T]he intellectually disciplined process of actively and skillfully conceptualizing, applying, analyzing, synthesizing, and/or evaluating information gathered from, or generated by, observation, experience, reflection, reasoning, or communication, as a guide to belief and action" (National Council for Excellence in Critical Thinking, 1992, p. 201).
- "[T]hinking about your thinking while you're thinking in order to make you think better" (Paul, 1993, p. 91).

Principles of Critical Thinking, which includes both characteristics of critical thinkers and needed educational focus. See Exhibit 4.2 for a listing of the Principles of Critical Thinking as articulated by Paul.

Rowles and Russo (2009) discuss the need for critical thinking in nursing programs. They suggest that educators and students have roles in developing critical thinking. Many educators are moving toward a more facilitative role that incorporates active learning strategies. This approach can help to ensure what and how much is taught is associated with how student thinking develops (Anderson, 2002). It also promotes using that knowledge in situations that can then be assessed (Mayer, 2002). Supporting students and acknowledging their accomplishments can promote a learning environment that is safe, comfortable, and positive. This atmosphere promotes self-confidence and courage to explore different and creative ways to consider issues and effects of decisions.

The diversity of previous learning experiences means that students may come from backgrounds in which learning has been passive. Nurse educators see the results of this in students who may come to class unprepared and resist active learning through disengagement or disruption. Critical thinking is complex (Wellman, 2009) and takes time to develop. Nurse educators need to be persistent in engaging students and maintaining expectations for preparation.

Critical thinking is apparent at the higher levels of the taxonomy (Bissell & Lemons, 2006). Friedman et al., (2010) argued that elements of critical thinking exist at every level. Bloom (1994) acknowledged that problem solving associated with critical thinking is based on knowledge and the ability to apply the knowledge "to new situations and problems" (Bloom, 1994, p. 16).

The need for nursing programs to develop and assess critical thinking skills in students was advanced by the National League for Nursing in 1991 (Walsh & Seldomridge, 2006) and the American Association of Colleges of Nursing (1997). The importance of well-developed, critical-thinking skills in those about to enter practice is

EXHIBIT 4.2 Principles of Critical Thinking

Founding Principles from the National Council for Excellence in Critical Thinking

■ There is an intimate interrelation between knowledge and thinking.
■ Knowing that something is so is not a matter of believing that it is so, it also entails being justified in that belief. (Definition: knowledge is justified true belief).
■ There are general as well as domain specific for assessment of thinking.
■ To achieve knowledge in any domain, it is essential to think critically.
■ Critical thinking is based on articulable [sic] intellectual standards and hence is intrinsically subject to assessment by those standards.
■ Criteria for the assessment of thinking in all domains are based on such general standards as clarity, precision, accuracy, relevance, significance, fairness, logic, depth, and breadth, evidentiary support, probability, predictive or explanatory power.
■ Instruction in critical thinking should increasingly enable a student to assess both his or her own thought and action and that of others by reference, ultimately, to standards such as those mentioned previously.
■ Instruction in all subject domains should result in the progressive disciplining of the mind with respect to the capacity and disposition to think critically within that domain.
■ Disciplined thinking with respect to any subject involves the capacity on the part of the thinker to recognize, analyze, and assess the basic elements of thought: the purpose or goal of the thinking; the problem or question at issue; the frame of reference or points of view involved; assumptions made; central concepts and ideas at work; principles or theories used; evidence, data, or reasons advanced, claims made, and conclusions drawn; inferences, reasoning, and lines of formulated thought; and implications and consequences involved.
■ Critical reading, writing, speaking, and listening are academically essential modes of learning.
■ The earlier that children develop sensitivity to the standards of sound thought and reasoning, the more likely they will develop desirable intellectual habits and become open-minded persons responsive to reasonable persuasion.
■ Education—in contrast to training, socialization, and indoctrination—implies a process conducive to critical thought and judgment. It is intrinsically committed to the cultivation of reasonability and rationality (Paul, n.d.).

recognized by the National Council of State Boards of Nursing (NCSBN; Clifton & Schriner, 2010). The main charge of the NCSBN is to protect the safety of the public and the ability to think critically is considered a prerequisite to safe practice. The National Council Licensure Examination-Registered Nurse (NCLEX-RN) aims to assess a candidate's ability to think critically by structuring licensure questions at the higher, analysis levels of the taxonomy. This is the reason why nearly all questions are written at the application and analysis level (Morrison, Nibert, & Flick, 2006).

ACTIVE LEARNING STRATEGIES

Active learning involves strategies to "engage" versus "explain." Educators place more emphasis on facilitating learning than imparting information. Active learning is more likely to involve students in the use of higher levels of cognition where critical thinking is prominent (McConnell, Steer, & Owens, 2003; Scheckel, 2009). Content becomes more relevant as students become more engaged (McConnell, Steer, & Owens). Well-planned active learning strategies can enhance motivation and retention of knowledge for use in other settings (Goudreau et al., 2009).

Active learning involves such strategies as inquiry-based learning, problem-based learning, case studies, team-based learning, discussion, questioning that probes thinking, concept mapping, focused reflection, self-assessment, learning portfolios, projects, simulation, and interactive computer modules, and writing assignments (Friedman et al., 2010;

Leppa, 2004; Luckowski, 2003; Valiga, 2009). Activities may be individual or occur through collaboration within groups. Collaborative activities promote abilities to learn from one another, work within teams, develop social and communication skills, and develop critical-thinking skills through active discourse with one another (DeYoung, 2009).

Developing, implementing, and evaluating active learning strategies take a good deal of thought and time. The activity should correlate with course objectives and connect content to applying and creating new ideas and solutions (Scheckel, 2009). Developing active learning strategies that are reflective and authentic or "world focused" can help to motivate learner engagement and critical-thinking skills (Halstead, 2005; Plack et al., 2007). The many types of active learning strategies allows for assessment of learning beyond multiple choice tests (Tomlinson & McTighe, 2006).

SUMMARY

Nurses today are pressed to know, think, and act quickly in health care settings that are increasingly diverse and complex. Nurse educators are challenged to find ways to sift through ever-growing amounts of information to include as content while considering objectives, learning experiences, and assessments. The use of an educational taxonomy provides a framework for developing, executing, and evaluating course, level, and program objectives and outcomes. A particular benefit to the use of taxonomy is attention to the development of critical thinking at all levels. Critical thinking may be facilitated through the use of active learning strategies that both motivate and engage students.

DISCUSSION QUESTIONS

1. Taxonomies have been in use for over 50 years. In what ways have taxonomies evolved?
2. How can taxonomy used at the program, level, and individual course point?
3. What are the major criticisms associated with the use of taxonomy and how could they be overcome?
4. What does critical thinking look like?

LEARNING ACTIVITIES

Student Learning Activities

1. Write your philosophy of life and why you feel as you do (be specific).
2. Write a five-page position paper describing what the entry level for nursing should be and why. After you develop the draft, develop a reverse outline and revise your paper as needed.
3. Take three multiple-choice questions from a recent examination and rewrite each at the application level.

4. Think about the past 2 weeks in a clinical experience. What is the one thing that sticks out the most in your mind that happened? On the right side of the page, write that situation down with as much detail as you can remember. Now, on the left side of the page, write what you think about what happened. How did it make you feel and why? What would you do if something similar happened and why?

Nurse Educator/Faculty Development Activities

1. How can the taxonomy table illustrate progression toward learning outcomes at the program, year or semester, and course levels?
2. Using a taxonomy table, plot one of your multiple-choice tests (by item number) into a taxonomy table (cognitive level and knowledge domains). Then exchange your test with a colleague and repeat. Now share the results with your colleague and discuss results. In areas where you differ, review the question and determine whether to revise.

REFERENCES

Airasian, P. W., & Miranda, H. (2002). The role of assessment in the revised taxonomy. *Theory Into Practice, 41*(4), 249–254.

Alfaro-LeFevre, R. (1999). Critical thinking in nursing: A practical approach (2nd ed.) Philadelphia: Saunders.

American Association of Colleges of Nursing. (1997). A vision of baccalaureate and graduate nursing education: the next decade. Retrieved from http://www.aacn.nche.edu/Publications/positions/vision.htm

Anderson, L. W. (2002). Curricular realignment: A re-examination. *Theory Into Practice, 41*(4), 255–260.

Anderson, L. W., & Krathwohl, D. R., (Eds). (2001). *A taxonomy for learning, teaching, and assessing: A revision of Bloom's taxonomy of educational objectives.* New York: Addison Wesley Longman.

Athanassiou, N., McNett, J. M., & Harvey, C. (2003). Critical thinking in the management classroom: Bloom's taxonomy as a learning tool. *Journal of Management Education, 27*(5), 533–555.

Bandman, E. L., & Bandman, B. (1995). Critical thinking in nursing (2nd ed.). Norwalk, CT: Appleton & Lange.

Bissell, A. N., & Lemons, P. P. (2006). A new method for assessing critical thinking in the classroom. *BioScience, 56,* 66–72.

Bloom, B. S. (1994). Reflections on the development and use of the taxonomy. In L. W. Anderson & L. A. Sosniak (Eds.), *Bloom's taxonomy: A forty-year retrospective* (pp. 1–8). Chicago: The National Society For The Study Of Education.

Booker, M. J. (2008). A roof without walls: Benjamin Bloom's taxonomy and the misdirection of American education. *Academic Questions, 20*(4), 347–355.

Bumen, N. T. (2007). Effects of the original versus revised Bloom's taxonomy on lesson planning skills: A Turkish study among pre-service teachers. *International Review of Education, 53*(4), 439–455.

Clifton, S. L., & Schriner, C. L. (2010). Assessing the quality of multiple-choice test items. *Nurse Educator, 33,* 12–16.

Cochran, D., Conklin, J., & Modin, S. (2007). A new bloom: Transforming learning. *Learning & Leading with Technology, 34*(5), 22–25.

Dave, R. H. (1970). Psychomotor levels. In R. J. Armstrong (Ed.), *Developing and writing behavioral objectives.* Tucson: Educational Innovators Press.

DeYoung, S. (2009). *Teaching strategies for nurse educators* (2nd ed.). Upper Saddle River, NJ: Prentice Hall.

Ennis, R. (1985). Critical thinking and the curriculum. *National Forum, 65,* 28–31.

Facione, P. A. (1990). Critical thinking: A statement of expert consensus for purposes of educational assessment and instruction (The Delphi Study Report of the American Philosophical Association). Millbrae, CA: California Academic Press.

Friedman, D. B., Crews, T. B., Caicedo, J. M., Besley, J. C., Weinberg, J., & Freeman, M. L. (2010). An exploration into inquiry-based learning by a multidisciplinary group of higher education faculty. *Higher Education, 59,* 765–783.

Glennon, C. D. (2006). Reconceptualizing program outcomes. *Journal of Nursing Education, 45*(2), 55–58.

Goudreau, J., Pepin, J., Dubois, S., Boyer, L., Larue, C., & Legault, A. (2009). A second generation of the competency-based approach to nursing education. *International Journal of Nursing Education Scholarship, 6,* 1–15.

Granello, D. H. (2001). Promoting cognitive complexity in graduate written work: Using Bloom's taxonomy as a pedagogical tool to improve literature reviews. *Counselor Education & Supervision, 40,* 292–307.

Hagstrom, F. (2006). Formative learning and assessment. *Communication Disorders Quarterly, 28,* 24–36.

Halawi, L. A., McCarthy, R. V., & Pires, S. (2009). An evaluation of e-learning on the basis of Bloom's taxonomy: An exploratory study. *Journal of Education for Business, 84*(6), 374–380.

Halpern, D. F. (1994). Critical thinking: The 21st century imperative for higher education. *The Long Term View, 2*(3), 12–16.

Halstead, J. A. (2005). Promoting critical thinking through online discussion. In M. H. Oermann & K. T. Heinrich (Eds.), *Annual review of nursing education, volume 3, strategies for teaching, assessment, and program planning* (pp. 143–163). New York: Springer.

Harden, R. M. (2002). Learning outcomes and instructional objectives: Is there a difference? *Medical Teacher, 24*(2), 151–155.

Harrow, A. J. (1972). *A taxonomy of the psychomotor domain.* New York: David McKay Hauenstein, A. D. (1998). *A conceptual framework for educational objectives: A holistic approach to traditional taxonomies.* New York: University Press of America.

Hooks, B. (2010). *Teaching critical thinking: practical wisdom.* New York: Routledge.

Krathwohl, D. R. (2002). A revision of Bloom's taxonomy: An overview. *Theory into Practice, 41*(4), 212–218.

Kuhn, M. S. (2008). Connecting depth and balance in class. *Learning and Leading with Technology, 36*(1),18–21.

Kurfiss, J. (1988). Critical thinking: Theory, research, practice, and possibilities (ASHE-ERIC Higher Education Report, No 2). Washington, DC: Association for the Study of Higher Education.

Leppa, C. J. (2004). Assessing student critical thinking through online discussions. *Nurse Educator, 29*(4), 156–160.

Luckowski, A. (2003). Concept mapping as a critical thinking tool for nurse educators. *Journal for Nurses in Staff Development, 19*(5), 225–230.

Manton, E. J., English, D. E., & Kernek, C. R. (2008). Evaluating knowledge and critical thinking in international marketing courses. *College Student Journal, 42*(4), 1037–1044.

Marzano, R. J., & Kendall, J. S. (2007). *The new taxonomy of educational objectives* (2nd ed.). Thousand Oaks, CA: Corwin Press.

Mayer, R. E. (2002). A taxonomy for computer-based assessment of problem solving. *Computers in Human Behavior, 18,* 623–632.

McConnell, D. A., Steer, D. N., & Owens, K. D. (2003). Assessment and active learning strategies for introductory geology courses. *Journal for Geoscience Education, 51*(2), 205–216.

Morrison, S., Nibert, A., & Flick, J. (2006). *Critical thinking and test item writing* (2nd ed.). Houston, TX: Health Education Systems

National Council for Excellence in Critical Thinking. (1992). Proceedings of the 12th Annual International Conference on Critical Thinking and Educational Reform (August 9–12, 1992) (pp. 197–203). Rohnert Park, CA: Center for Critical Thinking and Moral Critique, Sonoma State University.

Oermann, M. H. (1990). Psychomotor skill development. *Journal of Continuing Education in Nursing, 21*(50) 202–204.

Paul, R. (n.d.). The National Council for Excellence in Critical Thinking. A draft statement of principles. Retrieved from http://www.criticalthinking.org/page.cfm?PageID=406&CategoryID=48#235

Paul, R. (1993). Critical Thinking: How to prepare students for a rapidly changing world. Santa Rosa, CA: Foundation for Critical Thinking.

Plack, M. M., Driscoll, M., Marquez, M., Cuppernull, L., Maring, J., & Greenberg, L. (2007). Assessing reflective writing on a pediatric clerkship by using a modified Bloom's taxonomy. *Ambulatory Pediatrics, 7*(4), 285–291.

Prideaux, D. (2000). The emperor's new clothes: From objectives to outcomes. *Medical Education, 34.* 168–169.

Reilly, D. E., & Oermann, M. H. (1990). *Behavioral objectives: Evaluation in nursing* (3rd ed.). New York: National League for Nursing.

Roberts, J. L., & Inman, T. F. (2007). *Strategies for differentiating instruction: Best practices for the classroom.* Waco, TX: Prufrock Press

Rowles, C. J., & Russo, B. L. (2009). Strategies to promote critical thinking and active listening. In D. M. Billings & J. A. Halstead (Eds.), *Teaching in nursing: A guide for faculty* (3rd ed., pp. 238–261). St. Louis, MO: Saunders Elsevier.

Scheckel, M. (2009). Selecting learning experiences to achieve curriculum outcomes. In D. M. Billings & J. A. Halstead (Eds.), *Teaching in nursing: A guide for faculty* (3rd ed., pp. 154–172). St. Louis: Saunders Elsevier.

Shulman, L. S. (2002). Making differences: A table of learning. *Change, 34*(6), 36–44.

Simpson, B. J. (1966). The classification of educational objectives: Psychomotor domain. *Illinois Journal of Home Economics, 10*(4), 110–144.

Sipos, Y., Battisi, B., & Grimm, K. 2008). Achieving transformative sustainability learning: Engaging head, hands and heart. *International Journal of Sustainability in Higher Education, 9*, 68–86.

Sousa, D. A. (2005). *How the brain learns* (3rd ed.). Thousand Oaks, CA: Corwin Press

Su, W. M., Osisek, P. J., & Starnes, B. (2004). Applying the revised Bloom's taxonomy to a medical-surgical nursing lesson. *Nurse Educator, 29*(3), 116–120.

Tomlinson, C. A., & McTighe, J. (2006). *Integrating differentiated instruction: Understanding by design.* Alexandria, VA: Association for Supervision and Curriculum Development.

Tyler, R. W. (1949). *Basic principles of curriculum and instruction.* Chicago: University of Chicago Press.

Valiga, T. (2009). Promoting and assessing critical thinking. In S. DeYoung (Ed.), *Teaching strategies for nurse educators,* (2nd ed., pp. 217–235). Upper Saddle River, NJ: Prentice Hall.

Walsh, C. M., & Seldomridge, L. A. (2006). Measuring critical thinking: One step forward, one step back. *Nurse Educator, 31*(4), 159–162.

Wellman, S. S. (2009). The diverse learning needs of students. In D. M. Billings & J. A. Halstead (Eds.), *Teaching in nursing: A guide for faculty* (3rd ed., pp. 18–32). St. Louis, MO: Saunders Elsevier.

Needs Assessment in Curriculum Development

Sarah B. Keating

OVERVIEW OF NEEDS ASSESSMENT CURRICULUM DEVELOPMENT AND EVALUATION IN NURSING

When contemplating a new education program or revising an existing curriculum, a needs assessment is indicated. There are two purposes for conducting an assessment. The first is to validate the currency, academic and professional relevance, and continued need for an existing program. The second is to establish the feasibility for a new nursing program including the demand for it, available resources, academic soundness, and financial liability.

Even though justification for a current program usually exists, it is wise to survey constituents and collect information relative to the same factors that are examined in a needs assessment for a new program. This information either reaffirms assumptions about the curriculum on the part of the program planners or identifies gaps or problems that indicate a need for change. It is also useful for accreditation and program review purposes and can serve as the organizing framework for a master plan of evaluation (see Section 5). Chapters 5 and 6 discuss the essential components of a needs assessment and offer a model for collecting and analyzing information that is preliminary to new program development or expansion and revision of an existing curriculum.

The Frame Factors Model

Johnson (1977) presented a conceptual model for curriculum development, instructional planning, and evaluation that is similar to the nursing process. Although it is a simple and linear model (P [planning] – I [implementation] – E [evaluation]), Johnson expands it into a complex step-by-step logical process for curriculum development and evaluation. The process includes examining the frame factors or context within which the program exists, setting goals, identifying curriculum content, structuring the curriculum, planning for instruction, and finally, evaluation. Johnson speaks of frame factors as the context in which the curriculum exists. Furthermore, he classifies the context into "natural, cultural, organizational, and personal elements" (p. 36). This author chose the term of frame factors, "external" and "internal" from Johnson's discussion and adapted it to curriculum development in nursing. It includes the elements that Johnson identified and adds other components that specifically apply to education, health care systems, and the nursing profession.

Frame factors for this text are defined as the external and internal factors that influence, impinge upon, and/or enhance educational programs and curricula. As a conceptual model, it serves to collect, organize, and analyze information that is useful for the development and evaluation of curricula. There are two major categories of frame factors: external and internal factors. **External frame factors** are those that influence curriculum development in the larger environment and outside the parent institution. **Internal frame factors** are those factors that influence curriculum development and are within the environment of the parent institution and the program itself. Figure S3.1 illustrates the frame factors conceptual model.

Although the principal activities of faculty in curriculum development and evaluation focus on the curriculum plan itself and the need for improvement based on evaluation of the implementation of it (teaching and learning) and program outcomes, faculty should be involved in the needs assessment as well. Even if faculty is not involved in the details of the needs assessment, it needs to be aware of all of the factors that impact and influence the program. Faculty members sophisticated in the assessment of external and internal frame factors have an advantage in viewing the curriculum's place in its financial security, position within the health care system and the profession, and role in meeting the health care needs of the population. Data from the needs assessment are useful to individual faculty seeking grants and other funding to support research and program development.

It is recommended that nurse educators in both the academic and practice settings use this model when evaluating education programs, considering

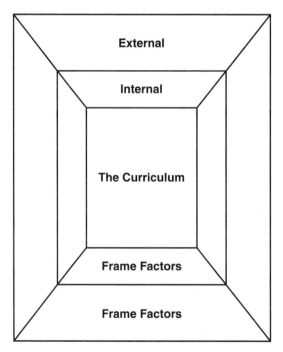

FIGURE S3.1 Frame Factors Conceptual Model.
Adapted from Johnson (1977)

revisions of existing programs, or initiating new ones. Although administrators take the leadership role in conducting needs assessments, faculty should participate in the decision for what type and how much data to collect and what decisions are made that affect the curriculum.

External Frame Factors

Chapter 5 describes the factors in the external environment outside the parent institution and the nursing education program that influence the curriculum. They include the community, population demographics, the political climate and body politic, the health care system and the health needs of the population, the characteristics of the academic setting, the need for the (nursing) program, the nursing profession, regulation and accreditation standards, and external financial support. All of these factors can influence the curriculum in positive and negative ways and although they may not be in the control of the faculty, they are important to recognize and analyze for their impact on the program. They can "make or break" a program. For example, lack of accreditation for a nursing program can prohibit its graduates from career opportunities and continuing education. Each factor is discussed in detail and a table provides guidelines for collecting and analyzing data for informed decision making. Chapter 5 initiates a case study that utilizes the conceptual frame factors model and guidelines and it continues to Chapter 8.

Internal Frame Factors

Chapter 6 discusses the environmental factors within the parent institution and the nursing program that influence the curriculum. The frame factors model identifies the following internal frame factors: description and organizational structure of the parent academic institution; mission, philosophy, and goals of the parent institution; economic situation and its influence on the curriculum; resources within the institution (laboratories, classrooms, library, student services, etc.); potential faculty and student characteristics; and a description of the health care system that supports the curriculum. Similar to the external frame factors, these internal factors influence the curriculum and play a major role in developing, revising, or expanding programs. As with the external frame factors, faculty uses the information gleaned from an assessment of these factors for arriving at decisions regarding the curriculum. The same data collected for a needs assessment are, in fact, related to total-quality management of the curriculum and contribute to the evaluation of the program.

Relationship of Needs Assessment to Total-Quality Management of the Curriculum

Establishing a new program is not an exercise that occurs in a vacuum. Somehow, preliminary information had an impact on the program planners that indicated a possible need for the program. The same is true for the need to revise a program or expand its offerings; that is, there are trigger mechanisms that initiated the change process. Rather than responding to these external stimuli in a reactive way, faculty and nurse educators should have a master plan of evaluation in place that continuously monitors the program and provides the data needed for planning for changes that are both timely and at the same time, look to the future. Such activities are part of a total-quality management process that provides the data for analysis and decisions leading to the continuous improvement and quality of the educational program. The factors discussed in the frame factors model in this section of the text apply to evaluation strategies as well. Although Section 5 discusses program and curriculum evaluation at great length, it is useful to incorporate the notion of evaluation as a process when conducting a needs assessment, not only in terms of the present plans for program start-up and changes, but also for planning for the future.

REFERENCE

Johnson, M. (1977). *Intentionality in education.* Albany, NY: Center for Curriculum Research and Services.

5 External Frame Factors

Sarah B. Keating

OBJECTIVES

Upon completion of Chapter 5, the reader will be able to:

1. Be familiar with the important external frame factors to examine for a needs assessment when developing or revising a curriculum.
2. Analyze external frame factors from the frame factors conceptual model for their application to a needs assessment for curriculum development and evaluation purposes.
3. Examine a case study that illustrates a needs assessment of external frame factors for a curriculum development project.
4. Apply the "Guidelines for Assessing External Frame Factors" in a simulated or real curriculum development situation.

OVERVIEW

Most nurse educators work in an established academic setting or in a health care agency that has a program for staff development and client education. Thus, curriculum development activities usually relate to the revision of the educational program based on feedback from staff, clients, students, faculty, administrators, alumni, and consumers of the program's participants and graduates. It is rather infrequent that new programs are initiated. Whether curriculum development involves a new program or revisions of an existing curriculum, program planners and faculty must evaluate both external and internal frame factors that affect the curriculum, their impact on the current program, and what role they play in forecasting the future.

Chapters 5 and 6 provide detailed information for conducting a needs assessment for the development of a new program and its curriculum or revising an existing curriculum. **A needs assessment for curriculum development** is defined as the process for collecting and analyzing information that contributes to the decision to initiate a new program or revise an existing one. The first step in curriculum development for faculty and program planners is to examine the environmental and human systems factors that influence the curriculum. These factors can be organized into two major categories: external and internal frame factors (Johnson, 1977). Chapter 5 discusses external frame factors that impact an education program, whereas Chapter 6 discusses internal frame factors. **External frame factors** are defined as those factors that influence curriculum development in its environment and outside of the parent institution. **Internal**

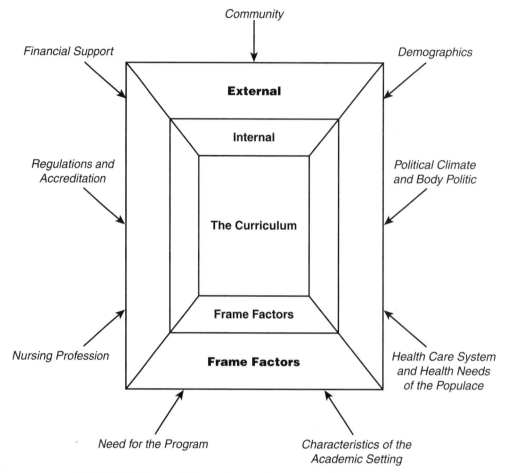

FIGURE 5.1 External Frame Factors for A Needs Assessment for Curriculum Development. Adapted from Johnson (1977).

frame factors are those factors that influence curriculum development and are within the parent institution and the program itself. Figure 5.1 depicts the external frame factors that surround the curriculum to consider when conducting a needs assessment.

DISCUSSION

Description of the Community

The first step in developing or revising a curriculum is to provide a description of the community in which the program exists (or will exist). A needs assessment assures the relevance of the program to a community need and its eventual financial viability. Existing programs often identify the need for revision of their curricula based on recommendations from their consumers or an accreditation report. Whether developing a new program or revising an old one, an examination of the external frame factors is essential to study their impact on the program and its future needs. The program under development or revision is considered in light of its fit to the community that it serves. For the purposes of curriculum development, **community** is defined as "a place-oriented process of interrelated actions through which members of a local population express a shared sense of identity while engaging in the common concerns of life" (Theodori, 2005, p. 662–663).

Depending on the nature of the educational program, the community can be as wide as international to as narrow as a small town within a state. Large universities or colleges with research reputability often attract international scholars, whereas some state-supported programs attract students who live nearby and intend to spend their professional lives in their home community. Both **sectarian** (associated with or supported by a religious organization) and **nonsectarian** (not associated with a religious organization) independent (private) colleges or universities, large and small, face the same challenges when assessing their external environment for curriculum revision or development. Therefore, it is important to identify if the community in which the program is situated as urban, suburban, or rural. Such factors as accessibility to students, faculty, learning resources, and financial support are influenced by the location of the community.

The major industries and education systems in the community are identified as possible sources for students in the program and for potential partnerships for program support and learning experiences. Industry has resources for scholarship and financial aid programs and experts in the field who can serve as faculty or adjunct faculty. Health care industries in particular should be participants in the needs assessment and curriculum planning to bring the reality of the practice setting and the community's health care needs into planning. The major religious affiliations, political parties. and systems such as transportation, communications, government, community services, and utilities in the community are additional external frame factors. These factors have an effect on the curriculum as to its relevance in the community and the support it needs to meet its goal. For example, state-supported schools are very dependent upon government funding, whereas private schools must rely on tuition and endowments.

There are many models in the literature that discuss the major components of a community assessment. Two recent articles discuss the assessment process including Lohmann and Schoelkopf (2009) who discuss the application of a Geographic Information System (GIS) for a community assessment and Williams, Bray, Shapiro-Mendoza, Reisz, and Peranteau (2009) who describe the use of three models including analyses of qualitative and quantitative data, a community participatory model with epidemiological approaches for the analyses of quantitative data, and the third model, a combination of the methods used in the second model.

Demographics of the Population

When considering a new program or revising a curriculum, it is useful to have knowledge of the people who live in the home community of the institution and the broader populace that it will serve. **Demographics** are the data that describe the characteristics of a population, for example, age, gender, socioeconomic status, ethnicity, education levels, and so forth. The demographic information that is vital to program planners includes:

1. the age ranges and preponderance of age groups in the population
2. predicted population changes including immigrant and emigrant statistics
3. ethnic and cultural groups including major languages
4. education levels, and
5. socioeconomic groups.

This information identifies potential students and their characteristics and to some extent, the needs of the population that the students and graduates will serve.

Educational programs and curricula must be geared toward the needs of the learners. If the student body comes from the region surrounding the institution, the characteristics of the students should be analyzed for special learning needs. For example, if there are nurses seeking to advance their careers, the curriculum needs to focus on adult learning theories and modalities. Younger students about to embark on their first professional degree will need curricula that focus on their developmental needs as young adults as well as on the content necessary for gaining nursing knowledge, clinical skills, and socialization into the professional role. Program planners should learn from students coming to the institution from great distances, what drew them to the program, and if those factors are useful for program planning and recruitment. Faculty should identify potential students with needs for learning resources beyond the usual; for example, a need for tutoring for students whose primary language is not English. It is useful to learn about the financial resources of the potential student body and if there is a need for major financial aid programs. Ethnicity and cultural values in the community and their beliefs about higher education have an impact on recruitment strategies and are especially important in light of the need for increasing the diversity of the nursing workforce.

Another consideration related to demographics is the existence of potential faculty and identification of people who have the credentials to teach. Identifying potential faculty through partnerships with industry and the community is helpful if the program needs to recruit new faculty or seek adjunct faculty and preceptors for clinical experiences. Resources for finding demographic information are plentiful. The U.S. Census Bureau (2010) has national and regional statistical and demographic information that is helpful for assessing the population. Its Web site is located at http://2010.census.gov/2010census.

Characteristics of the Academic Setting

Other institutions of higher learning in the nearby community or region have an influence on the program and its curriculum. Identifying other institutions, their levels of higher education (technical schools, associate degree and/or baccalaureate and higher degree), financial base (private or public), and affiliations (sectarian or nonsectarian) gives the assessors an idea of the existing competition for recruiting students, faculty, and staff. Information about the types of programs in nursing that are available from other institutions and their intentions for the future enables developers to understand the gaps in the types of programs and the nature of the competition from other educational programs. For example, if the institution's curriculum offers a nurse practitioner program and two other programs in the region offer similar programs, perhaps the curriculum should be revised to a specialty primary care program such as a Pediatric Nurse Practitioner (PNP) or Geriatric Nurse Practitioner (GNP) track; discontinued, or possibly, entered into a joint venture with the other schools. A private institution that is dependent on tuition and endowments may question whether it should continue to offer a curriculum that is redundant with a state-supported school. Other data to consider are the need for nurses in the area and its surrounds and even though there are multiple programs, the success rates of graduates finding employment in the region.

Benchmarks that the faculty can use to compare its own curriculum against those of its competitors should be identified; for example, the pass rate on NCLEX. Other examples include costs of the program, admission and retention rates, accreditation status, graduate employment rates, reputation in the community, and so forth. It is important to know how the nearby community agencies and health care systems view and hire the graduates of the program. Yet another important factor is the productivity of the faculty members and how their educational credentials, track records in securing grants, publication histories, and research records compare to others.

Suggested resources for collecting data on other academic institutions are as follows. There are seven regional accrediting associations in the United States. They include:

1. Middle States Association of Colleges and Schools
2. New England Association of Schools and Colleges
3. North Central Association of Colleges and Schools
4. The Northwest Commission on Colleges and Universities
5. Southern Association of Colleges and Schools
6. Western Association of Schools and Colleges
    Accrediting Commission for Community and Junior Colleges
7. Western Association of Schools and Colleges
    Accrediting Commission for Senior Colleges and Universities

Addresses and contact information for these associations are found in the "Resources" list at the end of the chapter. The accrediting agencies have directories of all of the schools in their regions. The umbrella organization that lists the agencies may be found at the Council for Higher Education Accreditation (CHEA, 2010) Web site (http://www.chea.org). National databases may be found at the National Center for Education Statistics (NCES, 2010) Web site (http://nces.ed.gov).

Another source for identifying other nursing programs in the region is the list of approved programs provided by the state board of nursing. A listing of the state boards and their Web sites and contact information may be found at the National Council of State Boards of Nursing (NCSBN, 2010; https://www.ncsbn.org/index.htm).

Once the list of other academic institutions is developed, faculty can find descriptions for each school on their individual Web sites or in the library. Libraries or admission departments in most institutions of higher learning have current copies of other college and university catalogs; although, it is becoming increasingly more common to find these descriptions at the institutions' Web sites.

Political Climate and Body Politic

When assessing the community, part of the data describes the public-governing structure. For example, if it is urban, it is useful to know if there is a mayor, a chief executive, and a city-governing board. Likewise, if it is rural or suburban, vital information includes the type of county or subdivision government, who the chief executive is, if the officials are elected or appointed, and what is the major political party.

Equally, if not more important, is information about the **body politic**. A simple definition for the body politic: is the people power(s) behind the official government within a community. It is composed of the major political forces and the people who exert influence within the community. The assessors should identify the major players, their visibility, that is, high profiles or low profiles as the powers behind the scenes. Additional information that reveals the body politic is how those in power influence decisions in the community and how they exert their power by using financial, personal, political, appointed, or elected positions. Specific information that is useful to educators is how the key politicians view the college or university and during elections and other crucial times, if they recognize the power of its people, that is, students, faculty, and staff.

Relative to nursing, the politicians' and the body politic's specific interests in the profession are helpful. For example, if they have family members who are nurses, or they have been recipients of nursing care, they are more apt to support nursing education programs. All educational programs need the support of the community and its power structure. Therefore, the information learned from assessing the political climate is vital to planning for the future and seeking assistance when the call comes for additional resources or for political pressure and support to maintain, revise, or increase the program.

The Health Care System and Health Needs of the Populace

Providing nurses to care for the health care needs of the populace is of critical interest to the health care system and the consumers of care. It is obvious that information about these two factors is essential to education program planning and curriculum development. Schools of nursing expect that the majority of their graduates will remain in the region. However, nursing is a mobile profession, and its members move to other geographic locations far from their alma maters. For example, in California, with one of the largest populations of licensed registered nurses (292,565 in 2009), almost 20% of the nursing workforce lived outside of the state and traveled to work in California (Spetz, 2009).

To assess the health care system, it is necessary to identify the major health care providers, the types of organizations, and financial bases. The following provides a list of major resources that can provide information for an assessment of the health care system. Please note that the U.S. health care system is in a state of flux, thus these data points may change.

- Major health care systems such as Medicare, Medicaid, CHAMPUS, Veterans Affairs, (VA), and so forth.
- Penetration rate of managed care systems (Health Maintenance Organizations [HMOs], Preferred Provider Organizations [PPOs], and Point of Service [POS] insurance plans)

For this discussion, **a managed care system** is defined as a health care system with administrative control over primary health care services in a medical group practice. The intention is to eliminate redundant facilities and services and to reduce costs. Health education and preventive medicine are emphasized. Patients may pay a flat fee for basic family care but may be charged additional fees for secondary care services (Mosby, 2009).

- Other health insurance programs
- Nonprofit or for-profit health care agencies and eligibility for services
- Sectarian and nonsectarian health-related agencies and eligibility for services
- Public health services
- Services for the underserved or unserved population groups
- Major primary health care agencies and providers
- Voluntary health care agencies and their services
- Other community-based health-related services staffed by nurses for example, schools, industry, state institutions, forensic facilities, and so forth.
- Role of nurses in the health care agencies
- Plans to increase or decrease health-related services in the future
- Influence of health care agencies on the curriculum, students' clinical experiences, and graduates' future careers

Information about regional health care systems is available through the following Web sites that contain lists of national, regional, and state health care agencies:

- American Health Care Association (AHCA, 2010; http://www.ahca.org).
- American Hospital Association (AHA, 2010; http://www.aha.org),
- American Public Health Association (APHA, 2010; http://www.apha.org).
- National Human Services Assembly (NHSA, 2010; http://www.nassembly.org).
- National Association for Home Care & Hospice (NAHC, 2010; http://www.nahc.org).

Last but not least, the yellow pages of telephone directories or on the web have listings of regional and local health care agencies and facilities.

The assembled list provides an overview of the health care system within which the program is located. It describes the health care resources that are available or not available to the population including the nursing school and institution's populations. It points out the gaps of services in the community and the possibilities for community partnerships including school-based services for the underserved and unserved populations. It identifies trends in health care services and anticipated changes for the future that can influence curriculum development.

It is useful to know if resources within the system such as health care libraries are available to students and faculty during clinical experiences or as resources for students enrolled in distance education programs. A review of the list pinpoints existing clinical experience sites and the potential for new ones. Personnel in the agencies with qualifications as preceptors, mentors, and adjunct faculty are additional resources for possible collaboration opportunities. Research opportunities for students and faculty may emerge from the review and can influence curriculum development as well as foster faculty and student development.

An overview of the major health problems in the region contributes to curriculum development as exemplars for health care interventions. The Web site of the National Center for Health Statistics (NCHS, 2010), http://www.cdc.gov/nchs, provides general information on leading causes of death and morbidity. Vital statistics, health statistics, and objectives for 2020 are located at the Healthy People 2020 (2010) site (http://www .healthypeople.gov/hp2020/Comments/default.asp)

The Need for the Program

An examination of the external environment informs the faculty about the increased or continued need for nurses. The following data points act as guides to document the need for the program.

- Characteristics of the nursing workforce and the extent of a nursing shortage, if it exists.
- Predictions for future nursing workforce needs.
- Adequate numbers of eligible applicants to the program, currently and in the future.
- Specific areas of nursing practice experiencing a shortage.
- Employers' projections for the numbers of nurses needed in the future.
- Employers' views on the types of graduates needed.

A brief survey of health care administrators can provide this information, although it is sometimes difficult to expect a good return rate in light of the current pressures on administrators. Another strategy is to conduct focus groups that take less than 15 minutes in the health agencies. Instructors who use the facilities for students or clinical coordinators are excellent people for collecting the information. There are several resources to identify the national and regional need for nurses. They are the state nurses' associations that can be located through the American Nurses Association (ANA, 2010; http://www.nursingworld.org/FunctionalMenuCategories/AboutANA/WhoWeAre/ CMA.aspx) and the U.S. Department of Health and Human Services, HRSA Health Professions (2010; http://bhpr.hrsa.gov).

As described previously in the characteristics of the academic setting, knowledge of other nursing programs in the region is useful to avoid curriculum redundancies. The data on the need for the program demonstrate how many of its graduates are needed now and in the future, the level of education necessary to provide the level of care required, and short- and long-term health care system needs. A current nursing workforce demand indicates the possibility for accelerated programs. Shortages in specialties indicate advanced practice curricula and increased opportunities for registered nurses to continue their education.

The Nursing Profession

In addition to the need for nurses, it is important to learn about the nursing profession in the region. Professional organizations are rich resources for identifying leaders, mentors, and financial support such as scholarship aid. Curriculum developers should survey faculty and colleagues for a list of the nursing professions in the region. Such organizations include local or regional affiliates of the ANA; the National League for

Nursing (NLN); Sigma Theta Tau International; educator organizations such as the American Association of Colleges of Nursing (AACN) and the National Organization of Associate Degree Nursing (NOADN); and the plethora of specialty organizations. Questions to gather information about the profession follow: Who are the nurses in the area? Are there professional organizations with which the program can link? What is the level of education for the majority of the nurses in practice? Are there nurses prepared with advanced degrees who could serve as educators or preceptors? Are research activities in nursing and health care underway that present opportunities for students and faculty?

Regulations and Accreditation Requirements

Whether the program is new or under revision, state regulations regarding schools of nursing should be reviewed for their requirements and any recent or anticipated changes in them that affect the curriculum. Information on regulations is available through the state boards of nursing. For a listing of specific state boards of nursing, consult the National Council of State Boards of Nursing (2010) Web site at http://www.ncsbn.org.

National accreditation is not required of schools of nursing; however, it provides the standards for nursing curricula and demonstrates program quality. Sophisticated applicants to the school will look for accreditation. Alumni find it advantageous to graduate from an accredited institution when applying for positions in the job market, for future advanced education, and for positions in the military. Many scholarships and financial aid program require that students enroll in accredited institutions.

Nursing has two major accrediting agencies and a few specialty-accrediting bodies. The National League for Nursing Accrediting Commission (NLNAC) Inc. accredits licensed practical/vocational nursing, associate degree, and baccalaureate and higher degree nursing programs. Detailed information on its accrediting process and standards may be found at its Web site: http://www.nlnac.org (2010). The Commission on Collegiate Nursing Education (CCNE, 2010) accredits baccalaureate and higher degree programs. Information on it may be found at http://www.aacn.nche.edu/Accreditation/pubsguides.htm. In addition to accreditation, there are standards and competencies set by professional organizations that can serve as guidelines or organizational frameworks for curricula. Several examples for prelicensure and graduate level programs are those developed by the AACN for baccalaureate and master's programs and competencies for the Clinical Nurse Leader (CNL) and the Doctor of Nursing Practice (DNP). Access to these documents may be found at the AACN's Web site: http://www.aacn .nche.edu (2010). NLNAC (2010) lists the standards for all levels of nursing education that they accredit including practical/vocational, diploma, associate degree, baccalaureate, master's, and the clinical doctorate in nursing. These standards may be found at its Web site: http://www.nlnac.org/manuals/SC2008.htm.

Another external frame factor that influences the nursing curriculum is regional accreditation. The parent institution of a nursing program undergoes periodic review by its regional accrediting body. Members of the nursing faculty are involved in the regional accreditation process and should be mindful of the standards set by that organization as well as those set by the professional accrediting body. For contact information, refer to the "Resources" list of regional accrediting agencies at the end of the chapter.

Detailed descriptions of accreditation processes and standards for educational programs are described in the Evaluation Section 5 of this text. It is useful to view them for the standards and limitations they impose during the curriculum development process.

Financial Support Systems

An analysis of the finances of the program provides curriculum developers with vital information on the economic health of the program. Indicators of financial health influence how the curriculum will be delivered. Faculty should recognize signs that demonstrate the program's financial viability. If new sources of income for the program are indicated, possible resources need to be identified. The proposed revisions in the curriculum must be realistic in terms of cost. If it is a new program, adequate resources including start-up funds for its implementation must be available. If it is an existing program, faculty and administration should consider whether to continue it at its present level of financial support or increase or decrease support.

Other items of study include how the program is financed and the major sources of revenues such as fees, tuition, state support, private contributions, grants, scholarships, or endowments. Knowing if there are adequate resources to support the program to be self-sufficient is a critical element in the analysis of the financial viability. Although this type of information is within the responsibility of administration, curriculum developers must have a basic understanding of the financial support systems that impact curriculum development.

SUMMARY

This chapter introduced the first step, a needs assessment, in curriculum development and revision. Prior to revising or developing new curricula, an assessment of the factors that influence the education program is necessary. In examining the environment that surrounds the program, curriculum developers look at external frame factors. Table 5.1 serves as a guideline for identifying the external frame factors, collecting the data for an assessment, and analyzing the factors to determine if there is a need for a new program or if changes are necessary for an existing program. Internal frame factors, those within the parent institution and the nursing program that influence curriculum, are considered in Chapter 6.

Analyzing external frame factors in light of proposed new programs or curriculum revisions help faculty and their administrators to determine the type of new program needed or in the case of an existing program, the extent to which changes in the curriculum are indicated. A review of the external frame factors provides a check with reality including the community, in which the program is located, the industry for which the program prepares graduates, and the economic viability of the program.

TABLE 5.1 Guidelines for Assessing External Frame Factors

Frame factor	Questions for data collection	Desired outcomes
Description of the community	Is the community setting conducive to academic programs? Describe its major characteristics, that is, urban, suburban, or rural. What are the major industries, and do they financially support the institution as well employ graduates? Who are the major education systems in the community, and what is the quality of their programs? How do they feed into the parent institution? What are the community services that provide an infrastructure for the institution as well, that is, transportation and communications services?	The institution's campus is located in a safe and supportive environment for its students, faculty, and staff. Industries are stable, have a history of financial support of the institution, and employ its graduates. The public and private school systems, kindergarten through 12 provide graduates for the institution and are of high quality. The school counselors have a strong relationship with the institution's admission department. Community colleges and higher degree institutions collaborate and have articulation agreements for ease of transfer. Students have easy access at reasonable cost to public transportation to and from home (for commuter students) and to stores and other community services. The community has multiple media communication networks of high quality for marketing, public relations, and education purposes. Postal service and other delivery systems are reliable.
	What are the community services that provide an infrastructure for the institution, that is, recreation, housing, utilities, and human and health services? What type of government is in place in the community and what are its politics? Is the government supportive of the institution in its midst and does it recognize its contributions to the community?	There are varied and multiple recreation sites for students' leisure activities. If there are no student health services, the community has quality health and human services for which students are eligible. The government structure is supportive of the parent institution in its community. Key members of the parent institution serve on advisory boards for the local government.
Demographics of the population	What are the characteristics of the general population? What indications are there that the population supports higher education? Within the population, what is the potential for student, faculty, and staff for the program?	The population reflects multicultural and ethnic characteristics with a wide range of age groups. The average income level is at or higher than the average for the region. Poverty levels are low or there are dedicated programs of assistance for the poor. A majority of the population completed high school or higher levels of education and/or there is growing interest in and need for these levels of education. There is an adequate applicant pool for the program(s). There are potential qualified faculty and staff in the locale.

(Continued)

TABLE 5.1 Guidelines for Assessing External Frame Factors *Continued*

Frame factor	Questions for data collection	Desired outcomes
Characteristics of the academic setting	Identify other institutions of higher learning in the region. Within those institutions, what types of nursing programs are offered if any? Are there potential or existing competitors?	Other institutions of higher learning in the region have programs not in direct competition with the curriculum and can serve as feeder schools to the program. There are no known plans that could conflict with the program.
Political climate and body politic	Identify the type of government and its structure. Who are the political power brokers in the community? What are the relationships of the parent institution to the political power brokers?	Key politicians and community leaders support the institution and have working relationships with the people within the educational institution.
The health care system and health needs of the populace	Identify the major types of health care systems and the predominant health care delivery patterns. Describe the major health care problems and needs of the populace in the education program's region. Describe the role of nursing in the health care system.	There are ample spaces currently and for the future for nursing student placements in the various health care systems and settings. The major health cares problems and needs match those foci in the curriculum. Nursing, as the largest health care workforce has a strong representation within the health care system.
The Need for the program	Describe the nursing workforce in the region as well as the state and nation. Describe the numbers and types of nurses needed in the region, state, and the nation for the future.	There is a demonstrated need for nurses in the region, state, and nation currently and in the future. The numbers and types of nurses needed meet the goals and type(s) of preparation available in the education program for the future.
The Nursing profession	List the major professional nursing organizations in the region. Describe the characteristics of nurses in the region.	There are at least two major nursing organizations in the region that can support the program and provide collegial relationships for students and faculty. The types of nurses in the region match the potential applicant pool for continued education and/or faculty and mentor positions.
Financial support	Review an analysis of the present financial health of the parent institution and the nursing program. Develop a list of existing and potential economic resources.	The institution and the nursing program are in solid financial condition and there is either guaranteed state support or substantial endowment funds for the future. There are adequate economic resources for the present and the future of the program.
Regulations and accreditation requirements	Identify the State Board of Registered Nursing regulations for education programs. List accreditation agencies that impact the parent institution and the nursing education program.	The nursing education program meets the state board regulations and has or is eligible for approval. The parent institution is accredited by its regional agency and the nursing program meets the standards of a national professional accrediting body.
Analysis of the data and decision making	Summarize the findings by generating a list of positive, neutral, and negative external frame factors that influence the curriculum.	Make a final decision statement as to the feasibility of the program as it is affected by the external frame factors.

CASE STUDY

*A*case study is presented in this chapter and the next two to illustrate a needs assessment and the development of a proposed curriculum. It includes the collection of external and internal frame factors data, their analyses, and a curriculum decision based on the findings.

Description of the Community

An existing baccalaureate and higher degree nursing program whose home campus is located in a suburban town of 20,000 adjacent to the state capitol with a population of more than 1,000,000 is about to undertake a needs assessment to determine if the program should expand. The home campus is a private, sectarian, multipurpose higher education institution. It has a long history of liberal arts education and over the past 5 decades added several professional schools including business, education, engineering, nursing, and the performing arts. All of the professional schools offer baccalaureate and master's degrees in their majors. There are two doctorate programs, one in education (EdD) and the other, business administration (DBA). The undergraduate population numbers 5,000 with 2,000 graduate students. There are 760 faculty members, 300 of whom work part-time.

Nursing faculty and administrators are aware of the continuing and projected nursing workforce shortage in the nation and in its region, the anticipated legislative changes in the health care system and their effect on the nursing workforce, and the trend for preparing advanced practice nurses at the clinical doctorate (Doctor of Nursing Practice; DNP) level. They have anecdotal information that employers of nurses prefer baccalaureate or higher degree nurses owing to the complexity of the acute care setting and the shortages of nurses prepared to practice in primary care and community settings.

The nursing program has a basic Bachelor of Science (BSN) undergraduate program, (N = 200), a registered nurse (RN) to BSN program (N = 30), and a Master of Science in Nursing (MSN) program with specialties for family nurse practitioners and clinical specialists (adult and family nursing; N = 90). The faculty numbers 30 full-time and 15 part-time with a dean and two associate deans for the undergraduate and graduate programs. There are five faculty members who have released time to coordinate the five tracks in the program. Three administrative assistants and one instructional technology administrator provide management support.

The nursing program is affiliated with a religious-based health care organization of the same denomination as its parent organization. The health care organization is a managed care system and has facilities located throughout the nation and the institution's region. It has been supportive of the nursing program in the past by offering clinical sites for student practice and scholarship or loan forgiveness programs for its staff and students who come to its facilities after graduation. With this information on hand, the dean asks the faculty to conduct a needs assessment for expanding the nursing program by increasing enrollments for entry-level nurses and/or expanding the graduate program to provide additional advanced practice nurses.

Using the "Guidelines for Assessing External Frame Factors" (see Table 5.1), the faculty initiates a needs assessment. The faculty divides the work into teams of two or three, each to collect information on one of the nine external frame factors. Once the data are collected, they will be presented to the faculty group who will refine the data and analyze them according to the need for the proposed program expansion.

The team assigned to community assessment decides to assess the metropolitan area and its surrounds, which includes six major suburban areas and the adjacent three-county rural area. Of the six suburban areas, half are incorporated as town/cities. The team conducts a community assessment using portions of the Kazda et al. (2009) framework that uses interviews of key stakeholders and analyzes Geographic Information System (GIS) data to provide demographic and socioeconomic information according to specific locales. Additionally, the team finds the city, suburban communities, and county Web sites useful in providing much of the information they seek. The major industries and employers in the area include the following:

1. The state government
2. Two small but expanding alternative energy manufacturers
3. Several food-processing plants
4. A large inland port
5. A railroad center that serves the region in the transportation of goods
6. An airplane parts manufacturer
7. A rocket engineering and manufacturing plant
8. Retail and recreation/entertainment industry (including two Native-American–managed casinos)
9. The primary and secondary education systems
10. Several large health care systems that serve the city, suburbs, and rural neighbors

All of the industries have a long history in the area, are financially stable in spite of the recent recession, and the alternative energy manufacturers plan to expand and employ at least 2,000 additional workers over the next 5 years. While the government employee workforce experienced a 15% cut in staffing and the public education system cut 10% of its workforce and services, the two employment systems remain fairly constant in spite of the recession. The non–health-related industries support the business and engineering programs of the parent institution and send many of their workers to the programs for advanced preparation. In the past, two of the manufacturers gave grants to the parent institution for computer engineering scholarships and one manufacturer donated a $25 million grant toward a new business administration building on the home campus.

A state-supported baccalaureate and higher degree program with a nursing program is located in the city. Additionally, there are three state-supported community colleges in or near the city with nursing programs, there is one large university-based medical center that does not have a nursing program, and the closest private college (without a nursing program) is 300 miles distant. The parent institution has existing articulation agreements with all of the community colleges and the state school. There are no DNP programs in the nearby region.

Results from statewide achievement tests reveal that the city's kindergarten through 12th-grade system ranked in the 60th percentile. Most of its students prefer to remain in the local area and the majority of those who continue schooling after high school (40%) go to the local community colleges. Students in the three-county area ranked from the 50th percentile (agricultural areas) to the 82nd percentile (suburban areas) on statewide achievement tests. Fifty-five percent of the suburban students continued their education in either community colleges or higher educational institutions; however, only 15% of students in rural areas continued their education after high school.

The public transportation system within the city includes buses and a light rail system. The light rail system extends into the three surrounding counties with carpool parking lots available for suburbanites to commute to the city. Three major highways intersect with the city providing easy access for automobile travel. There is a middle-sized airport with commuter planes and major airlines and AMTRAK services are available. Greyhound Bus has a terminal in the city with buses providing interstate transportation. The metropolitan buses and light rail system fares are reasonable and there are discounts for students and senior citizens. There is one major daily paper, several suburban papers, at least 25 radio stations, five major television stations, TV cable service, and telecommunication services for computer access. There are many mailing services, in addition to the U.S. Postal Service, such as UPS, FedEx, and Pak Mail located throughout the area.

The capitol city is located on a major river with three surrounding small lakes and there are several state and city recreation parks for picnicking, swimming, boating, and hiking. The city lies between the ocean and mountains; thus winter, summer, and beach sports are no more than 2 to 3 hours away. Low-rent housing facilities are scarce owing to increased demand from people who lost homes in the recession. Utilities are fairly reasonable in cost; however, as mentioned previously, low-rent housing, including utilities are hard to come by. There are municipal systems for the incorporated cities and county services for delivery of utilities that are for the most part, reliable in the delivery of services.

There are four major health maintenance organizations that serve their enrolled members. With a projected modest population growth, two of the health maintenance organizations have plans for expansion. Students and/or their parents who are enrolled in these programs are eligible for services. There are public health clinic services for students who do not have health coverage and who are eligible for state-supported health care programs.

The city has an elected city council with a mayor, whereas the smaller incorporated cites are managed through part-time mayors and city councils with full-time city managers. The counties have elected boards of supervisors and each has a county chief administrator/manager. At the present time, in the urban areas, the Democratic Party has the most representatives in the government. However, the rural areas are more conservative and have elected Republican local governments and representatives to Congress. The three surrounding counties are governed by boards of supervisors with some of the larger suburban communities having local fire department and community services. The three counties have sheriff departments supplemented by state highway patrol services for highway traffic controls and serious felonies.

Although the parent institution's board of regents has only one representative in the public government, the president of the college meets periodically with ad hoc committees of the city councils and boards of supervisors to discuss higher education issues that affect their populaces. He has been in the position of president for more than 15 years and is well known throughout the region. This activity on his part contributes to the presence and image of the parent institution in the region.

Preliminary Conclusions

The location and size of the regional community indicate feasibility for expanding the program. The infrastructure of the city and its surrounds and the population base of the region for potential student and health care services support the existing program and could accommodate additional nursing students and graduates. Housing for students appears to be a major problem. There is only one baccalaureate and higher degree competitor for the nursing program. However, there are three feeder community colleges with potential applicants to the BSN and RN to BSN programs. These issues will be examined in the "Characteristics of the Academic Setting" frame factors.

Demographics of the Population

The faculty team assigned to gathering data on the demographics of the region's population seeks information from the Web sites of the cities and tricounty area. The team learns that the total population of the capitol city is a little over 1.4 million. See Table 5.2 Demographics of the Capitol City and Three Surrounding Counties for a comparison of racial and age groups by city and counties. The major languages spoken at home are English: 67.4% and other languages: 32.6%. (The other major spoken languages are Spanish, Mandarin, or Cantonese.) Forty-two percent of the population has at least one vehicle per household. Of the population, 77.3% hold a high school diploma, and 23.7% have a baccalaureate or higher. The following lists the major occupations for the working population and their percentage distribution: management or professional (including health care): 36.2%; services: 16.2; sales or office work: 28.6%; fishing, forestry, or farming: 0.4%; construction: 7.6%; and production: 11.0%. The unemployment rate is 10.2% and steadily decreasing with the improved economic scene. The median household income is $41,200. There are 11.9% of households below the poverty level. Indications are that the population is growing and that the demographics will remain stable.

In contrast, the populations of the three surrounding counties are quite different. The average median income is $51,000 and less than 5% households were below poverty level. The average age distribution in the counties reveals a

TABLE 5.2 Demographics of the Capitol City and Three Surrounding Counties

Race	Capitol City	Surrounding Counties
White	45.3%	70%
Native American	1.3%	2%
African American/Black	8.6%	7%
Asian	10.9%	9%
Hispanic	12.6%	12%
Two or more races	6.3%	N/A
Other	15%	1%
Age Group		
19 years and under	30.2%	22%
20 to 34	23%	22%
35 to 44	15%	14%
45 to 59	15.9%	21%
60 to 74	10%	13%
75 and over	5.9%	8%

somewhat older population than the city. About 23% of the counties' residents hold a high school diploma, 17% hold baccalaureates, and 31% have some college education but no degree.

Preliminary Conclusions

Overall, this population is growing and, compared to other parts of the state and nation, is economically stable. Its diverse ethnic population meets the program's goal to increase cultural diversity in its student population, while at the same time, there may be need for programs to assist students whose primary language is not English. There are a large percentage of individuals who are educated beyond high school and who are potential faculty and staff for the program and might be interested in second career opportunities. Age breakdowns in the population indicate a large percentage of potential college students between the ages of 18 and 44.

Characteristics of the Academic Setting

The team assigned to identify other institutions of higher learning goes to the regional accrediting body. They find a listing of accredited colleges and universities in the region. They decide to identify those institutions within the selected city and 75 miles outside the radius of the city line. They also look at the city's Web site that lists all of the institutions. Once all schools are identified and they learn which schools have nursing programs, they divide the work among themselves to gather data from the programs' Web sites and interview the administrators of the schools of nursing. The information they seek includes the types of nursing programs and tracks offered, the applicant pool, admission date(s), the enrollments, graduation rates, licensure examination (NCLEX) pass rates, where the majority of graduates work, and the impressions of the administrators for the need for an additional program in the area. The purpose of the interviews is twofold, that is, it gives basic information about other nursing programs in the region, and it also informs them of the potential for another program. The faculty is aware that the interview must be handled delicately with sincere reassurance to the administrators that the proposed program is meant to complement existing programs. This sets the pathway for collaborative relationships in the future should the program begin.

The academic setting team learns that the three community colleges offer associate degree in nursing (ADN) programs and the state-supported school offers a generic BSN program as well as an accelerated RN to BSN program. It has four master's specialty tracks, one in education, one in nursing administration, one in community health nursing, and a nurse practitioner program. Additionally, the faculty learns that the program recently developed an online RN to BSN track that is proving to be very popular. They also note that there is one statewide online RN to BSN program and multiple nationwide programs for RNs.

The three community colleges are about equal in size and their administrators report that their total enrollments approximate 150 with 50 graduates each year. Their qualified applicant pool numbers 350 each, although they believe they may be drawing from the same applicant pool. Their admission rates to fill slots averages 93% to 95% leaving a waiting list each year of about 50 qualified applicants. There are no plans to increase enrollments in the near future owing to the lack of state support for program expansion. The administrators report pass rates on NCLEX ranging from 82% to 100%. The vast majority of their graduates remains in the local area to practice and are in either acute care, nursing home, or home health agencies.

The state-supported BSN and higher degree school administrator reports that they have a total enrollment of 300 students in the basic BSN program, 100 RNs in the RN to BSN program, and 150 in the graduate programs. The MSN nurse practitioner program is the most popular with the community health nursing and education tracks each enrolling approximately 20 students each year. About 75% of the basic BSN students transfer in from the community college, having completed their nursing prerequisites. The remainder enters as freshmen. The basic BSN program graduates approximately 65 each year with an average NCLEX pass rate of 87% for the past 5 years. About 80% of its graduates remain in the area to practice. The qualified applicant pool for the basic BSN program is 350 and again, the administrator believes some of the applicants may be in the same pool as the ADN programs. Owing to constraints on state-supported funds, there are no plans to expand enrollments in the near future.

The RN students come from regional health care agencies and based on the response to the online version of the program, the school may discontinue its traditional RN to BSN program. Most master's students come from the region as well and are seeking additional education for career mobility purposes. Although the MSN applicant pool is small compared to the capacity of the program (200 for 150 slots), the program remains viable. The administrator notes that there have been requests recently from the public who have baccalaureates or higher degrees for a master's or second-degree program. Upon further investigation with the ADN administrators, the faculty learns that they too have experienced these requests, and in fact, have students enrolled in their programs that have bachelor's or higher degrees other than nursing.

Preliminary Conclusions

In addition to its own program, the region has four nursing programs, three ADN, and one baccalaureate and master's degree in nursing program. There appears to be an adequate, qualified applicant pool for these programs and there are waiting lists for the generic programs (ADN and BSN). The RN to BSN pool seems satisfied with the new online program offered by the state-supported school and there are multiple other options for them to complete a baccalaureate in nursing. All of the clinical specialties at the master's level are viable. One tantalizing fact is the interest on the part of college graduates in nursing. There are no fast-track baccalaureate or entry-level master's programs in the region. The faculty team recommends the collection of additional data about this possibility.

Political Climate and Body Politic

The initial description of the community identified the city's government as consisting of a city council and a mayor. At present, the Democrats are the political party in control. The adjacent counties have mayoral and council governments for the smaller cities and boards of supervisors for the county government. The counties are predominantly Republican although recently, there have been some elected posts captured by Democrats. The team assigned to investigate the political climate and body politic decides to attend a board of supervisors meeting in each county and a city council meeting. They also read the local newspapers' metro sections and the editorial pages. They interview faculty and staff who live in the region and the director of extended education to seek opinions on the political climate in the city and counties as they relate to the parent institution. They ask people who live in the three counties to attend a board of supervisors meeting and/or city councils to learn about the major political issues in the region.

The meeting of the city council and mayor of the major city that the team attended happened to have health care issues on its agenda. Citizens were concerned about the pending proposal to close two of the city's public health clinics owing to a shortfall in the state budget and a trickling down effect of less public funds for the clinics. The faculty noted several political action groups in attendance that were vocal in their protests about the closures. It being an election year, the mayor and council members listened carefully to their pleas and by the end of the meeting, assured them that the clinics would remain open. The team observed that the mayor was a strong leader with little dissension among the council members on the various issues.

The survey team was quite interested in learning that the mayor was an RN and knowledgeable about health care issues. They decided to seek an interview with the mayor and were successful in meeting with her for a half hour.

At the meeting, they gained the mayor's support for the possible expansion of the program as long as the other nursing programs in the area supported it. She was well aware of the nursing shortage and the need for preparing additional nurses as well as those for advanced practice.

Faculty and staff who attended county board of supervisors meetings heard many of the smaller issues facing county governments such as the downturn in residential and business development, the need for additional public safety services, and what services to cut when planning for the next fiscal-year budget. Health and nursing-related issues did not come up in the meetings but the people who attended introduced themselves to the board members and identified where they worked. The purpose was to begin to establish recognition of the role of the college and its contributions to the community.

The city's newspaper had several articles on the closure of the public health clinics and the editorial opinion page had a glowing account of the mayor's support for the groups who opposed the closures. The articles discussed the nursing shortage as well, thus, it was concluded that information about the increasing need for nurses was reaching the public. The assessment team scanned local newspapers and decided to continue to do this so that they would keep abreast of the news in the region and also have contact sites if there was a need to publicize the program.

The director of extended education felt that most of the city's and counties' populations were aware of the parent institution from the college's media campaign. The school of extended education runs spot announcements on the radio and even gained some free public service announcement on television, as one of its students is the manager of one of the major stations. The director runs advertisements in the local newspaper, usually a month before the semesters start. The director described his role on the ad hoc committee on higher education for the city council. This role gives him the opportunity to meet other key educators and helps raise the visibility of the institution in the community. It was his overall impression that the reputation of the institution and its quality was gaining in the community.

Preliminary Conclusions

The faculty team concluded that although the parent institution's educational programs are relatively new in the community, key members of the body politic and the public recognize the institution. They felt they had the initial support of the mayor who is a leader in the community, but felt that the nursing program will need to nurture a relationship with her to gain further support. In addition, there is a need to publicize the program in the three-county area and to continue to build relationships with the political leaders. Depending on other findings in the needs assessment, the team felt that there would, at the very least, be no opposition to the program, and at the most, moderate support. One caution was issued and that was the need to work with the administrators and faculty of the existing nursing programs as colleagues. It would be advantageous to develop a program that would complement existing programs and not create a threat to them.

The Health Care System and Health Needs of the Populace

As identified in the community assessment, there are four major health care systems serving the city and its surrounding region. The team assigned to assess this frame factor gathers data through the Web sites of the AHA and the NAHC as well as looking in the yellow pages of the telephone directory. They check the Morbidity and Mortality Weekly Reports (MMWR; Centers for Disease Control and Prevention, 2010; http://www.cdc.gov/mmwr) and the state health department's health statistics and GIS maps (http://www.cdc.gov/mmwr/international/relres.html) for comparisons of the tricounty area's and the capitol city's health indicators with national and statewide data.

One health care system is a nonprofit large, health maintenance organization that has a nationwide network. There are two nonprofit regional health care systems providing enrollees with a wide array of services. One is sponsored by the same religious-based organization as that of the nursing program's parent institution. The other is a federation of former independent nonprofit community, hospitals that merged to share resources for cost savings. There is one moderately sized university-based medical center. There is no public hospital except for the state-supported university medical center; however, there are public health clinics that provide primary care for the medically indigent. The medically indigent receive Medicaid services through the existing health care systems and the Medicaid program (federal and state/county) reimburses the agencies for services provided.

The Veterans Administration has a large medical center with acute care, outpatient services, a nursing home wing, and a rehabilitation center. It prefers RNs with baccalaureates and has master's prepared CNLs, clinical specialists, nurse practitioners, managers, and administrators on staff. It provides clinical practice sites for both undergraduate and graduate students for all of the nursing schools in the area and encourages staff to continue its education with released time or educational stipends.

There are no for-profit agencies except for three for-profit home care agencies that, in addition to patient care services, supply medical equipment. There is one nonprofit visiting nurse association and that agency is under contract with several of the health care systems for home and hospice care. Most school districts have one school nurse; there is a nurse practitioner with four RNs assigned to the city jail, and three of the major industries have occupational health nurses. The predominant pattern of health care is managed care. There are only a few preferred provider organizations and they contract for hospital and other services with one or more of the health care systems.

The major health care problems of the populace match those of the morbidity and mortality statistics of the state and the nation. The population is aging and thus, the need for health services for seniors and chronic diseases are expected to rise. Except for the lack of systemwide health care services for the poor, the systems meet the acute care needs of the populace. For those enrolled in health maintenance organizations, health promotion services seem adequate. The local Women, Infants, and Children (WIC) programs have public health nurses who provide health education and follow-up home visits. The public health clinics do not have a systemwide health education program, providing only immunizations and primary care services in their clinics.

The team interviewed either the chief administrator of nursing or the associate administrator in the major health care systems. The team members learned that the majority of staff nurses are associate degree graduates, whereas a few of the older nurses are graduates of diploma programs. All of the large health care systems employ clinical specialists and those with health maintenance services employ nurse practitioners. A few have staff educators, although those nurses also serve as risk managers. The university-based medical center has an all RN staff and employs more clinical specialists than the other systems. The public health clinics use public health nurses prepared at the baccalaureate level for follow-up visits and nurse practitioners staff the primary care clinics. The visiting nurse organization uses both public health nurses and RNs for home visiting and hospice services. All of the organizations use licensed practical nurses (LPNs) and the administrators report that they have seen an increase in the numbers of LPNs hired to fill the gap created by the RN shortage.

The administrators reported that they welcome nursing students and have existing articulation agreements with the regional nursing schools. The team decided to collect additional information in their interviews to share with the faculty team assigned to the "The Need for the Program" frame factor. The administrators said they could accommodate additional students for learning experiences, particularly if the program were to hold experiences on evening shifts or weekends. The religious-based system was especially open to having additional students in their agencies and indicated that the program's students would receive priority placements. All nursing specialties were represented in the agencies, although some had larger specialty units than others. A list was made of the agencies, their specialty units, and numbers of potential advanced practice and experienced nurses who could serve as preceptors, mentors, clinical instructors, or faculty.

Preliminary Conclusions

The faculty concluded that there are a wide variety of health care agencies with a plethora of potential clinical experiences available for students in an expanded program. Nursing administrators welcomed the idea of an expanded program to increase the numbers of baccalaureate and higher degree nurses in the region. This information would be passed on to the team investigating "The Need for the Program." The health care problems and needs of the populace are not unique and match the existing content of the curriculum. There is a need for health promotion activities, especially for the poor and the aging population, which present opportunities for faculty and student practice.

The Need for the Program

The faculty assigned to the frame factor that describes the need for the program go to the state's board of registered nursing Web site, the Health Resources and Services Administration's (HRSA; 2010) Registered Nurse Population Web site (http://bhpr.hrsa.gov/healthworkforce/rnsurvey04) and the state nurses' association for information on the nursing workforce in the region. They learn that there are 1,450 RNs of whom 1,250 are employed. The four major health care systems report a vacancy rate of 10% and the schools, public health clinics, and home care agency report 50 vacant positions. The team did not include skilled nursing facilities in the survey; however, they learned from a few directors of nursing that they too are experiencing shortages of nurses with a rapid turnover of staff who move to acute care facilities. Calculating the needs for nurses in numbers of vacant positions, the team estimated that there are at least 200 available positions. They note that the existing nursing programs plan to graduate only 125 entry-level nurses. The number of vacancies does not account for the number of nurses in the workforce who plan to retire within the next 5 years, especially in light of the fact that the average age of the nurse in the region is 48.5 years.

In addition to entry-level positions, 100% of the administrators of the nursing services programs told the team that they anticipated increasing their staff owing to the growing demand and complexity of health care. They reported shortages in staff nurses and those in advanced practice, especially clinical specialists and nurse practitioners. The administrators indicated a preference for baccalaureate prepared nurses and when informed about entry-level master's, fast-track RN to master's programs, and DNP programs; their interest increased, especially if the programs are accelerated. They voiced a sense of urgency related to the increased need for nurses. The team's review of state and national studies demonstrated a similar need for nurses and an ever-increasing shortage of nurses over the next decade.

Preliminary Conclusions

There is a documented need for entry-level nurses in the capitol city, the region, state, and nation. In addition, nursing administrators report an increased need for baccalaureate prepared graduates and advanced practice nurses. The needs thus far, match the types of options in the nursing program, that is, basic BSN, RN to MSN, and the advanced practice roles.

The Nursing Profession

The team assigned to describe the nursing profession in the region goes to the Web sites of the major nursing organizations in the nation. They discover that the state-supported baccalaureate and higher degree program sponsors a local Sigma Theta Tau chapter as does the home school of nursing; the state nurses association has a regional affiliate, and there is a Coalition of Specialty organizations in the city. The nurse executive group meets periodically and is loosely affiliated with the American Organization of Nurse Executives (AONE). The administrators of the nursing schools belong to this group and their faculty clinical coordinators have a group of educators who meet twice a year with staff educators in the four major health care systems. There is one health care providers union and that union represents nurses in two of the health care systems.

About 60% of the employed nurses work in acute care; the remainder are in community-based agencies. About 71% of the working nurses have an ADN or diploma; 22% have a BSN; 6% have a master's; and less than 1% have a doctorate. It was difficult to match the educational preparation of the nurses to the type of position they held although anecdotal information demonstrated that the majority of master's prepared nurses were top administrators (vice presidents), clinical specialists, CNLs, or nurse practitioners. The BSN nurses were employed in public health, schools, home care, or as case managers or administrators. Only six nurses with doctorates were found in practice, two were researchers at the university-based medical center, one was a researcher at the VA and another was the staff development/patient education director for the VA, and the remaining two were researchers with the large managed care system. The faculty did not survey faculty of schools of nursing; however, it was acknowledged that there are additional master's and doctorate prepared nurses in the community, some of whom were faculty in other schools of nursing.

Preliminary Conclusions

There are several nursing organizations whose members can serve as preceptors and mentors. There are six known doctorate prepared nurses who could serve as research mentor, preceptors for advanced practice students, and perhaps, faculty. There are master's prepared nurse practitioners, CNLs, educators, administrators, and clinical specialists who are potential students, clinical faculty, preceptors, or mentors.

There is a shortage of nurses in the region, state, and nation. The existing workforce does not meet the preferred need for baccalaureate and advanced practice prepared nurses. The existing schools of nursing cannot meet the current regional demand for nurses and employers of nurses forecast an increasing need in the future. There is a need for programs to increase the numbers of nurses with BSNs and for advanced practice roles.

Regulations and Accreditation Requirements

The dean of the nursing program and the associate deans of the undergraduate and graduate programs act as the team to investigate regulations and accreditation requirements. The program is due for a CCNE reaccreditation visit in 2 years. The nursing program has approval of the State Board of Nursing. A phone call to the executive director of the state board by the dean verifies that the board must approve any expansions of the program that affect any of the licensure or state certification requirements. A proposal for changes in the program must be presented to the board at least 6 months in advance of initiation of the revised program. The board has guidelines for the proposal and will send it to the administrator of the program. Guidelines include a list of qualified faculty, adequate student services, including library facilities, approved clinical facilities, and adequate classroom and learning laboratories. Approval comes through the Education Committee of the Board (ECB) and can be reviewed within 3 months of receipt of the proposal.

The parent institution has regional accreditation. A call to that agency and a review of its standards indicate that new degree programs must be pre-approved by the agency at least 6 months prior to the enrollment of the first class. The criteria for approval are much the same as the State Board of Nursing (SBN). In addition to the requirements of the SBN, the regional agency looks for evidence of infrastructure feasibility and educational effectiveness. The usual turnaround time for a response to a proposal is 2 months.

The nursing program has national accreditation through CCNE. A call to a consultant at that agency finds that education programs must submit a substantive change report no earlier than 90 days prior to implementation or no later than 90 days after its implementation.

Preliminary Conclusions

If the faculty and administrators of the nursing program revise or develop new tracks in the program, the proposal for the changes must be completed and submitted to the Board of Nursing and the regional accrediting agency at least 6 months prior to start-up of the program. A description of the program should be submitted to CCNE 90 days prior to its initiation.

Financial Support

The dean and associate deans of the undergraduate and graduate nursing programs prepare a report and business case on the financial resources of the parent institution and the nursing program. They consult with the comptroller of the institution as well as the director of human resources. The parent institution has an endowment fund of over $120 million. It has an active alumni association and raises at least $2 million each year for scholarships. Its capital operating costs match that of the tuition and fees income each year. It has several million-dollar grants from private and federal sources for research in science and for program development in education. The nursing program has one federal grant ($300,000) for the nurse practitioner program, $10,000 from the federal advanced education nursing traineeships, one managed care system grant for $50,000 for preparing RNs to the MSN, and several scholarship funds totaling $10 million in endowments. The financial-aid programs include a statewide tuition assistance program for needy students, the federally sponsored work–study programs and traineeships, Pell grants, nursing loan programs, and a forgivable loan program from a health care agency for students who agree to work for that agency for 2 years upon graduation. In addition, numerous private scholarships are available to nursing students from external sources.

The comptroller assures the team that the institution will provide a business plan for the nursing program to calculate start-up costs and the economic feasibility of an expanded program. If the program appears to be economically sound, the parent institution will provide the start-up costs. In addition to an analysis of the financial health of the institution, the team examines possible income sources for the expanded program. They contact the nursing administrators of the four major health care systems to discuss possible program development support, physical sites for student classrooms and laboratories, and scholarships or loans for nursing students. The religious-based system has some laboratories that students could use for clinical skills practice, and they are quite interested in scholarship programs or forgivable loans for students who commit to a 2 year contract with that agency upon graduation.

Preliminary Conclusions

The parent institution and the nursing program are financially stable. There is the promise of start-up funds and professional consultation for a business plan if the decision to expand the program is realized. In addition to the traditional economic resources, there are potential sources of income and support from the health care system. See Table 5.3 for an analysis of the external frame factors needs assessment and the conclusions drawn from the findings.

Conclusion

A needs assessment of nine external frame factors revealed a positive external environment for an expanded program when compared to the desired outcomes of the "Guidelines for Assessing External Frame Factors." The faculty recommended that the program continue to study the potential for the program by conducting a needs assessment of the internal frame factors impacting the curriculum. Thus far, findings indicate a demonstrated need to increase the number of nurses in the region at the entry level and advanced practice levels. Nursing administrators in the region are supportive, the community body politic is supportive in the capitol city and there are possibilities for support in the surrounding counties, and there is strong support from one of the key health care systems. The parent institution indicates support by offering to develop a business plan and start-up funds should the faculty recommend an expanded program. Several recommendations were made were made based on the needs assessment thus far:

1. Consider an entry-level graduate program, increase enrollments in the BSN program, accelerate the RN to BSN to MSN program, assess the FNP and clinical specialist tracks for their need in the community to determine if any should be discontinued, remain at present levels, or new ones developed, consider online formats, and possibly develop a DNP program for master's prepared nurses in the region or as an entry-level program.
2. Conduct focus groups of potential entry level and advanced practice students to determine community interest in the proposed programs.
3. Plan meetings with existing nursing education program administrators, health care system administrators, county politicians, and the mayor to nurture relationships.
4. As the work continues, keep records that can eventually be the basis of a proposal, both as an internal document and as a report to regulating and accrediting bodies.

TABLE 5.3 Analysis of the External Frame Factors Needs Assessment Data and Decision Making

Frame factor	Findings			Conclusions
	Positive	**Negative**	**Neutral**	
Community description	Size, location, and infrastructure of the region supports the needs of the college. Industry and services are variable but steady.	Limitation of student housing outside the campus.	Politics vary according to location.	*Positive* The community location and support systems can accommodate an expansion of the program. The political systems support the institution. *Negative* Off-campus students may encounter housing difficulties.
Demographics	Diverse. About 30% with higher degrees. Adequate potential applicant pool.	Possible language barriers.	Middle-income predominates.	*Positive* Applicant pools for entry-level and higher degree are adequate and population is diverse. *Neutral* Socioeconomic variables indicate ability to enroll in private education with some financial aid support. *Negative* Some students whose primary language is not English may need support.
Academic settings	Adequate applicant pool for all five schools. There are three ADN and one BSN program whose graduates are potential applicants for the graduate program. Clinical specialties are viable with FNP popular. Interest in accelerated second baccalaureate or entry-level MSN and DNPs. RNs like online format.	The FNP may be redundant to the existing one in the home nursing program.	Four existing nursing programs in the region.	*Positive* There is interest in online format and accelerated or entry-level master's programs. There are no DNP programs in the region. *Neutral* While there is an adequate applicant pool and there is interest in entry-level programs including the entry-level graduate programs, there are four existing nursing programs. *Negative* FNP track may be in direct competition with state school.

(Continued)

TABLE 5.3 Analysis of the External Frame Factors Needs Assessment Data and Decision Making *Continued*

| Frame factor | Findings | | | Conclusions |
	Positive	Negative	Neutral	
Political climate	The parent institution is recognized in the community. The mayor of the capitol city is an RN, a strong leader and supports the program.	Need to work with existing nursing programs to avoid conflict and redundancies	No opposition to expanded program. The faculty and staff are in the process of developing relationships with community leaders to increase awareness of the program.	*Neutral* The expanded program has a strong potential of success if it works with existing nursing programs and builds positive relationships with the body politic.
Health care system and health needs of the population	There is a wide variety of health care agencies for learning experiences. nursing administrators favor and support BSN or higher degree programs. Health care needs match curriculum content.		There are possible opportunities for student and faculty practice in health promotion activities.	*Positive* The health care system is supportive and offers many learning opportunities for students. Health care needs match curriculum content and there is potential for health promotion practice.
Need for program	There is a need for additional entry-level nurses in light of current and future shortages. There is a demand for BSN prepared nurses. Existing program offerings match the demand.			*Positive* An expanded program could meet the regional demand for additional nurses at the entry-level and advanced practice at the DNP level.
Nursing profession	There are several nursing organizations with nurse leaders that support the program. The majority of nurses are ADN- prepared.		There are six doctorate prepared nurses as potential mentors or faculty. Master's prepared nurses are in advanced roles.	*Positive* Professional nursing organizations and their members are potential supporters, mentors, and faculty for the program. The potential applicant pool for baccalaureate and higher degrees is promising.

(Continued)

TABLE 5.3 Analysis of the External Frame Factors Needs Assessment Data and Decision Making *Continued*

| Frame factor | Findings | | | Conclusions |
	Positive	Negative	Neutral	
Regulations and accreditation			A proposal for the outreach program must be submitted to the regional accrediting body and the State Board of Nursing. A report should be sent to CCNE 90 days prior to its start.	*Neutral* Proposals must be submitted to the accrediting and regulating bodies in advance of initiation if the assessment of external and internal frame factors is favorable toward an expanded program.
Financial support	Financial reports indicate economic health and stability. The parent institution will provide start-up funds. At least one health care system offered financial assistance.		There are other potential financial resources.	*Positive* The financial picture is excellent and there are future potential resources that need to be explored further.
Overall decision	24 positive entries	4 negative entries	11 neutral entries	11 positive conclusions 2 neutral conclusions 3 negative conclusions

DISCUSSION QUESTIONS

1. Conducting a needs assessment is time consuming. Debate the value of conducting the assessment by paid consultants rather than faculty.
2. How does the process of a needs assessment apply to both curriculum development and curriculum evaluation?

LEARNING ACTIVITIES

Student Project

As a student group, examine the community around you for its potential for a nursing program. Use Table 5.1 "Guidelines for Assessing External Frame Factors" to collect data on the external frame factors that you need to consider. After you collect the data, summarize your findings and compare them to the "Desired Outcomes" listed in the table. Based on the findings, justify why or why not a new nursing program is needed.

Faculty Project

Using Table 5.1, "Guidelines for Assessing External Frame Factors," assess your nursing curriculum. Collect data for each external frame factor as it applies to the curriculum. Summarize your findings and compare them to the "Desired Outcomes" listed in the table. In light of your summary, is a curriculum revision indicated? Explain your reasons for the decision to revise or not to revise.

REFERENCES

American Association of Colleges of Nursing. (2010). Retrieved from http://www.aacn.nche.edu

American Health Care Association. (2010). Retrieved from http://www.ahca.org

American Hospital Association. (2010). Retrieved from http://www.aha.org

American Nurses Association (2010). Retrieved from http://www.nursingworld.org/Functional MenuCategories/AboutANA/WhoWeAre/CMA.aspx

American Public Health Association. (2010). Retrieved from http://www.apha.org/

Centers for Disease Control and Prevention. (2010). *Morbidity and Mortality Weekly Reports.* Retrieved from http://www.cdc.gov/mmwr and http://www.cdc.gov/mmwr/international/relres.html

Commission on Collegiate Nursing Education. (2010). Retrieved from http://www.aacn.nche.edu/Accreditation/pubsguides.htm

Council for Higher Education Accreditation. (2010). Retrieved from http://www.chea.org

Health Resources and Services Administration. (2010). The Registered Nurse Population: Findings from the 2004 National Sample Survey of Registered Nurses. Retrieved from http://bhpr.hrsa.gov/healthworkforce/rnsurvey04

Healthy People 2020. (2010). Retrieved from http://www.healthypeople.gov/hp2020/Comments/default.asp

Johnson, M. (1977). Intentionality in Education. (Distributed by the Center for Curriculum Research and Services, Albany, NY.). Troy, NY: Walter Snyder Printer.

Kazda, M., Beel, E., Villegas, D., Martinez, J., Patel, N., & Migala, W. (2009). Methodological complexities and the use of GIS in conducting a community needs assessment of a large U.S. municipality. *Journal of Community Health, 34*(3), 210–215. Retrieved from CINAHL database.

Lohmann, A., & Schoelkopf, L. (2009). GIS—A Useful Tool for Community Assessment. *Journal of Prevention & Intervention in the Community, 37*(1), 1–4.

Mosby. (2009). *Mosby's Medical Dictionary,* (8th ed.). St. Louis, MO: Elsevier.

National Association for Home Care & Hospice. (2010). Retrieved from http://www.nahc.org

National Center for Education Statistics. (2010). Retrieved from http://nces.ed.gov

National Center for Health Statistics. (2010). Retrieved from http://www.cdc.gov/nchs

National Council of State Boards of Nursing. (2010). Retrieved from http://www.ncsbn.org

National Human Services Assembly. (2010). Retrieved from http://www.nassembly.org/nassembly

National League for Nursing Accrediting Commission. (2010). Retrieved from http://www.nlnac.org

Spetz, J. (2009). *Forecasts of the Registered Nurse Population in California. Conducted for the California Board of Registered Nursing. Center for Health Professions and School of Nursing. UCSF. San Francisco.* Retrieved from http://www.rn.ca.gov/pdfs/forms/forecasts2009.pdf

Theodori, G. L. (2005). Community and community development in resource-based areas: Operational definitions rooted in an interactional perspective. *Society and Natural Resources. 18*(7), 661–669.

United States Census Bureau. (2010). *United States Census 2010.* Retrieved from http://2010.census.gov/2010census

U.S. Department of Health and Human Services. (2010). *HRSA Health Professions.* Retrieved from http://bhpr.hrsa.gov

Williams, K., Bray, P., Shapiro-Mendoza, C., Reisz, I., & Peranteau, J. (2009). Modeling the principles of community-based participatory research in a community health assessment conducted by a health foundation. *Health Promotion Practice, 10*(1), 67–75.

RESOURCES

Middle States Association of Colleges and Schools
Middle State Commission of Higher Education (MSCHE)
3624 Market St. 2nd Floor Annex
Philadelphia, PA 19104-2680
Phone 267-284-5000 Fax 215-662-5501
E-mail: info@msche.org Web: www.msche.org

New England Association of Schools and Colleges
Commission on Institutions of Higher Education (NEASC-CIHE)
209 Burlington Rd.
Bedford, Massachusetts 01730
Phone 781-271-0022 Fax 781-271-0950
E-mail: CIHE@neasc.org Web: www.neasc.org

North Central Association of Colleges and Schools
The Higher Learning Commission (NCA-HLC)
30 North LaSalle St., Suite 2400
Chicago, Illinois 60602
Phone: 312-263-0456 Fax: 312-263-7462
E-mail: info@hlcommission.org Web: www.ncahigherlearningcommission.org

Northwest Commission of Colleges and Universities (NWCCU)
8060 165th Avenue, NE, Suite 100
Redmond, WA 98052
Phone: 425-558-4224 Fax: 425-376-0596
E-mail: selman@nwccu.org Web: www.nwccu.org

Southern Association of Colleges and Schools (SACS)
Commission on Colleges
1866 Southern Lane
Decatur, GA 30033

6

Internal Frame Factors

Sarah B. Keating

OBJECTIVES

Upon completion of Chapter 6, the reader will be able to:

1. Evaluate the essential internal frame factors that impact a nursing education program for the need to either develop a new program or revise an existing one.
2. Compile resources for the collection of data related to internal frame factors for comparing the data to desired outcomes for program development.
3. Analyze a case study that illustrates a needs assessment of internal frame factors for a curriculum development project.
4. Apply the "Guidelines for Assessing Internal Frame Factors" in a simulated or real curriculum development situation.

OVERVIEW

Section III introduced the reader to the frame factors model, and Chapter 5 discussed the external frame factors that nurse educators should review when conducting a needs assessment for program planning and curriculum development purposes. The data collected from a review of the external frame factors provide information related to the external environment of the educational program and feed into the decision-making process for developing new programs and revising existing ones. These factors can have a major impact on the program's existence and decisions regarding changes. Chapter 5 initiated a case study as an example of a needs assessment, using the frame factors model that is continued in Chapter 6 with the internal frame factors to consider (Johnson, 1977). See Figure 6.1 for a conceptual model of the internal frame factors that impact the curriculum. Chapter 7 discusses the components of the curriculum and continues the case study with a proposed outreach program and its curriculum plan based on the needs assessment.

Faculty continues to be responsible for curriculum development and evaluation and is part of the process for collecting information about the internal frame factors that impact the educational program. The internal frame factors include a description and organizational structure of the parent academic institution: mission and purpose, philosophy, and goals; internal economic situation and its influence on the curriculum; resources within the institution (laboratories, classrooms, library, academic services, instructional technology support, student services, etc.); and potential faculty and student characteristics. The information related to these factors is analyzed for its relevance to the program, and the findings are weighed as to their importance to the quality of the program, its existence, and possible changes.

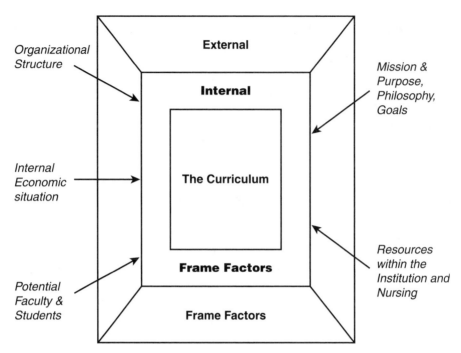

FIGURE 6.1 Internal Frame Factors for A Needs Assessment for Curriculum Development. Adapted from Johnson (1977).

Chapter 6 provides detailed information about each of these internal frame factors and there is a table with guidelines for collecting information about the factors and assessing the need according to the desired outcomes. The chapter ends by continuing the case study of a fictional nursing school that is conducting a needs assessment for an outreach program.

DISCUSSION

Description and Organizational Structure of the Parent Academic Institution

When looking at the environment that surrounds a nursing education program, the parent institution in which it resides is examined in light of the scenario it sets for the program. The physical campus and its buildings create the milieu in which the program exists with the nursing program, a reflection of its place within the institution. The nature of the institution influences the structure of the total campus, and, for nursing education programs, that institution can be health care agencies, academic medical centers, liberal arts colleges, large research universities, land grant universities, multipurpose state-supported or private universities, or community colleges. The history of the institution, such as its growth or change over the years and the role the nursing program had in its political fortunes or misfortunes, is important to know. In small private institutions, the school of nursing can be one of the largest and most influential constituents, whereas in statewide university systems, nursing can be a small department within a health-related college that is within the greater university. To appreciate the vast number of types of institutions within the United States, go to the University of Utah Web site (2010), which provides links to various U.S. higher education systems such as boards of regents, boards of governors, coordinating boards, and university systemwide administrations: http://www.utahsbr.edu/boards.htm.

All educational institutions and health care agencies have organizational structures, usually of a hierarchal nature. Faculty should analyze the structure of the parent institution as well as that of the nursing program to describe the hierarchal and formal lines of communication that guide the faculty to develop and revise programs. For example, as described in Chapter 2 on the roles and responsibilities of faculty, curriculum proposals and changes must be approved first on the local level (the nursing curriculum committee and faculty), moved to the next level of organization such as a college curriculum committee and dean, and finally, to an all-college or university-wide curriculum committee with its recommendations going to the faculty senate (or its like) for final approval. There can be administrative approval along the way from department heads, deans, and perhaps academic vice presidents or provosts, especially in regard to economic and administrative feasibility. Nevertheless, the major approval bodies are those that are composed of faculty and within-faculty governance prerogatives.

Furthermore, it is useful to know who the major players within the faculty and administrative structures are to discuss with them the plans and rationale for the proposed new programs or curriculum revisions. Prior consultation with these key people can help to smooth the way when the proposals are ready to enter the formal arena, and they can give advice related to changes that might enhance approval or advice on the best presentation formats that facilitate an understanding of the proposal. These contacts can be on a formal or informal nature; to give a word of caution, however, never blindside an administrator or decision maker, to avoid disastrous results. It is wise to keep them informed of new proposals or possible changes that place them in the advocate role as the approval process wends its way through the system.

Mission, Philosophy, and Goals of the Parent Institution

The mission/vision and purpose, philosophy, and goals of the parent institution determine the character of the nursing program. Most institutions of higher education focus their missions and philosophies on three endeavors: education, service, and scholarship/research. Nursing must examine the mission and philosophy of its parent institution to determine its place within these three basic endeavors. For example, a state-supported university may have as part of its mission and philosophy the education of the people of the state for professional, leadership, and service roles. Thus, the nursing program could focus its mission and philosophy on the preparation of nurses for leadership roles and provision of health care services to the people of the state. If the statewide system is the predominant preparer of nurses within the state as compared to independent colleges, then the additional mission or purpose might be to provide an adequate nursing workforce for the state. As nursing experienced its workforce shortages during the mid-1980s and into the early 21st century, there is evidence of federal and statewide programs for increased nursing scholarship support and in some cases, a mandate for state-supported schools to admit more students to nursing programs (Health Resources and Services Administration, 2010).

In contrast, independent or private colleges and universities may have missions and philosophies that have a sectarian flavor such as preparing individuals with strong liberal arts foundations for public service or roles in the helping professions. Again, a nursing program's mission can be very compatible with this mission. Academic medical centers are yet another example of nursing's match to health disciplines housed in one institution whose mission is to prepare individuals for the health professions. Community college or junior college missions usually focus on technical education or on prerequisite preparation for entering into upper division level colleges and universities. Although the debate still rages about the role of nursing programs in these institutions, there is no question that they fit the mission of the 2-year college as most expect that their graduates will function as registered nurses (RNs) and continue with their education at the baccalaureate and higher degree levels (Graf, 2006).

Internal Economic Situation and Influence on the Curriculum

As stated in Chapter 5, the economic health of the institution has a significant impact on the nursing program and curriculum. How much of the share of resources, income, and expenditures that the nursing program has can affect program stability and room for expansion. For example, nurse-managed clinics must be self-supporting or economic recessions can cause their demise. For state-sponsored programs, the parent institution is subject to the state economy during periods of recession and prosperity. Independent colleges, unless heavily endowed, depend on tuition, student fees, or other income generating operations.

All institutions depend on endowments, financial aid programs for students including scholarships, loans, and grants. Nursing programs are eligible for many federal grants and have a history of securing other types of grants from private foundations, state-supported programs, and private contributions including those from alumni associations. These income-generating programs illustrate to the parent institution that the nursing program is viable and at the same time, the institution's reputation and ability to garner external financial resources helps the nursing program to secure funding.

Institutions usually have support systems for assisting faculty to write grants and to seek outside financial support. Nursing programs should have close relationships with these support systems and have a plan in place for securing additional funds. Faculty plays a major role in writing grants with the perks related to them if funded of released time for program development and research activities. Two sources for funding to support program development on the national level are the Health Resources and Services Administration (http://bhpr.hrsa.gov/nursing; 2010) and the National Institutes of Health (http://www.nih.gov/ninr; 2010). The latter focuses on research; however, it is possible that faculty may wish to conduct curriculum and educational program research. A list of private foundations with funding opportunities for program development is located at http://www.research.ucla.edu/ocga/sr2/Private.htm (University of California–Los Angeles, 2010).

Assessment of the economic status of the parent institution and the nursing program provides a realistic picture of the potential for program expansion and curriculum revision. When developing curriculum, the first demand for financial support comes with the need for resources to conduct a needs assessment such as the costs of released time for those who are conducting the assessment, review of the literature, and surveys of key stakeholders. A cost analysis for revising a curriculum or mounting a new one requires a business plan to justify the costs and to forecast its financial viability. Unless there is a nursing program financial officer, the nursing program administrator and faculty should work closely with the parent institution's business office or chief financial officer in developing the business plan.

Resources Within the Institution and Nursing Program

An analysis of the existing resources within the institution and the nursing program supplies information related to possible program expansion and curriculum revisions. First, there should be adequate classrooms, learning laboratories, computer facilities, clinical practice simulations, and instructional technology and distance education support systems for the current program. When planning for revisions of the curriculum or for new programs, the need for expansion of these facilities should be identified. If expansion is not possible, then creative approaches to scheduling for the maximum use of these facilities can be examined (e.g., evening classes, weekend learning experiences, and online delivery of courses).

Academic support services such as the library, academic advisement, teaching–learning resources, and instructional technology contribute to the maintenance of a quality education program and are internal frame factors that should be assessed when developing new programs or revising existing ones. If there are to be new programs or expansion of current curricula, the library resources must be adequate. Library resources include not only those resources on campus but also services for off-campus programs and students. There should be Internet and Web-based library access for students and faculty, and this is especially true when the campus has a large commuter student population, offers distance education programs, or proposes new programs. Library and instructional-technology support staffing must be large enough and knowledgeable about nursing education needs. Thus, faculty should have strong relationships with librarians and the instructional-technology staff in order to build the resources needed to revise the curriculum or develop new programs.

Academic advisement services play an important role in program planning as new programs can require additional staffing. If the curriculum is revised, updates for academic advising are necessary so that the faculty and its support staff who provide the services have current information to impart to the students. Teaching–learning resources need to be available to keep faculty current in instructional strategies, particularly if the revisions to the curriculum have an effect on instructional design. For example, a baccalaureate program may decide to convert its RN program to a Web-based delivery system. In this case, faculty needs training in preparing and implementing Web-based courses.

Instructional support systems are part of planning as well because the nature of the proposed program or the revised curriculum may call for additional resources. These resources include programmed instruction units, audiovisual aids, hardware and software, computer technologies, simulated clinical situations, and so forth. They can generate large costs to the program and should be calculated into the business plan and the costs associated with their maintenance and replacement expenses over time. Some instructional support systems include monthly or annual fees as well. For new programs or revisions, these costs are often included in requests for external funding and because many times, these are one-time-only costs, they are funded more easily.

Student support services are equally important to nursing education programs and are an integral part of the curriculum development process. Major student services include enrollment (recruitment, admissions, registrar activities, and graduation records), maintenance of student records, advising and counseling, disciplinary matters, remediation and study skills, work study programs, career counseling, job placement, and financial aid. These services can be congregated into one department or subdivided into several, depending on the size of the university or college. Their role in curriculum development is important because expanding or changing educational programs require their support. For example, if a new program is proposed, then the recruitment and admissions staff will need to be apprised of the program to best serve the needs of the new program in recruitment and admission activities.

Financial aid programs are crucial to the recruitment, admission, and retention of students, and if the proposal brings in new revenues through grants or other financial support structures, the financial aid staff must be cognizant of the proposal. They can provide useful information to program planners and thus, a partnership between the student services staff and the nursing program staff is beneficial.

Work–study programs and job placement information can supplement the curriculum if these programs are in concert with the educational plan and not in conflict with the program of study. An example of a conflict is a revised curriculum that calls for accelerated study and clinical experiences that disallow student employment and therefore, prohibits enrollment in the work–study program. Another aspect is the potential influence of students' part-time employment on the curriculum and its role in intended and unintended outcomes on the educational experience.

The informal curriculum often takes place through the planned activities of the student services department. Again, partnerships between the staff and the nursing faculty can increase the effectiveness of the formal curriculum. Students who can benefit from remediation or learning skills workshops can be referred to student services. Faculty can help student services staff identify the learning needs of nursing students, and this is especially relevant when curriculum changes are taking place. Additionally, student services staff can educate faculty about the special needs of students with learning disabilities and the special accommodations they require without imperiling the safety of the clients for whom the students provide care. Support from the support services staff results in increased provision of accommodations for students with learning disabilities. (McCleary-Jones, 2007, 2008).

Potential Faculty and Student Characteristics

When proposing new educational programs or revising existing curricula, thought needs to go into the characteristics of the existing faculty and the student body who will participate in the educational program. If a new program is proposed, the faculty composition should be reviewed. There should be enough faculty members to reach the desired faculty to student ratio. Depending on the nature of the program, clinical supervision of students requires a low student to faculty ratio but can differ according to program. For example, master's and doctoral students are usually RNs and therefore, may not need the close supervision required of entry-level students. Although, for some advanced practice roles, there is a need for closer faculty supervision. However, in these latter cases, preceptor-ships or internships are the usual format and a faculty member can supervise more students. In entry-level programs, the student to faculty ratio is usually 8:10; however, in the senior year, it is possible to have preceptorships with approximately 12–15 students, depending on the nature of the clinical experiences. Lecture can accommodate many students to one teacher, whereas, seminars and learning laboratories demand fewer numbers of students and additional faculty. Enrollments in online courses can vary with as few at 10–12 in graduate level and seminar-type courses, whereas some didactic online courses can accommodate as many as 30 or more students. In the case of the latter, the format for the course is modified to adjust to the larger number of students and the resultant teaching load for the instructor. These are very practical issues that must be addressed owing to the quality perspectives and cost factors that they present when developing curricula.

Yet another consideration related to faculty is the match of knowledge to the subject matter, clinical expertise, and pedagogical skills. Numbers and types of faculty are pieces of information that feed into decisions about curriculum development because they are critical to the delivery of the curriculum. As with faculty considerations, the characteristics of the student body and the types of students the faculty hopes to attract to the new program or the revised curriculum are important. If it is a new program, the potential applicant pool should be identified according to interest, numbers, availability, and competition with other nursing programs. If a new program is contemplated, its type dictates the kind of applicant pool that the program and the admission department need to target. If it is a curriculum revision to update the program and plan for future demands, the applicant pool might be the same as the current one. The characteristics of the students in the program help to tailor the curriculum according to their learning needs. For example, if it is an entry-level associate degree or baccalaureate program, the applicants may be a mix of new high school graduates, transfer students with some college preparation, and adult learners with some work experience. The curriculum is then planned to meet a diversity of learning needs from traditional pedagogical learning theories to adult learning theories. Diverse racial, ethnic, and cultural characteristics are other factors to consider, and the educational program must plan to be culturally responsive as well as preparing professionals with cultural competence.

SUMMARY

Chapter 6 reviewed the internal frame factors to consider when conducting a needs assessment for developing new educational programs or revising curricula. These factors follow the assessment of external frame factors that influence the educational program and are equally important to the decision for changing a curriculum or developing a new program. While the external frame factors examined the macro environment surrounding the program, the internal frame factors looked at those factors that are closer to the program and include the parent institution as well as the nursing program itself.

Factors that were examined include the characteristics of the parent institution and its organizational structure. How the nursing program fits into this structure can determine the economic, political, and resource support for program changes, and it sets the stage for the processes that the nursing faculty must undergo to gain approval for the proposed changes. The mission and purpose, philosophy, and goals of the parent institution influence the nature of the nursing program, and to ensure success, the nursing program must be in congruence with those of the parent institution. The internal economic status and the available resources of both the parent institution and the nursing program are assessed for the financial viability as well as the necessary additional resources and support services for any proposed revisions to the curriculum or proposed new programs. Finally, the characteristics of the faculty and the potential student body are reviewed to determine their match to the proposed change. See Table 6.1 for guidelines to assess the internal frame factors when conducting a needs assessment for curriculum revision or new program proposals.

TABLE 6.1 Guidelines for Assessing Internal Frame Factors

Frame factor	Questions for data collection	Desired outcomes
Description and organizational structure of the parent academic institution	In what type of educational institution is the nursing program located? What is the milieu of the parent institution in regard to the nursing program? What is the organizational structure of the parent institution? What place in the institution does the nursing program hold? What influence does it have? What are the layers of approval processes for program approval and curriculum revisions? In what order must a program go through the approval process? Who are the major players in the various levels of approval processes?	A supportive organizational system for program planning and curriculum revision. The nursing program is recognized in the institution for its place in education, scholarship, and service to the community. A fair and comprehensive review process that results in economically sound and high quality educational programs. The approval process benefits the nursing program though the education of other entities in the home institution about the nursing program and their support for it.
Mission and purpose, philosophy, and goals of the parent institution	What are the mission, philosophy, and goals of the parent institution? Are they congruent and supportive of the nursing program?	The mission and purpose, philosophy, and goals of the parent institution are congruent with and supportive of the nursing program.
Internal economic situation and its influence on the curriculum	What is the operating budget of the nursing program? Is it adequate for the support of the existing program? Are there resources for program or curriculum development activities? Does the program have a financial officer or administrative assistant who can develop a business plan for the proposed program or curriculum revision? If not, are there resources available from the parent institution for this activity?	The nursing program has adequate resources for supporting its educational program from the parent institution. The nursing program has the resources for program or curriculum development activities. The nursing program has a business plan, the resources, and administrative support for mounting a new program or revising the existing curriculum.
Resources within the institution and nursing program	How many classrooms, laboratories, and computer laboratories does the nursing program have, and are they under the control of the nursing program? Can they accommodate additional students or newer technologies in the proposed program or curriculum revisions? Are the plans for these facilities included in the proposal and are their costs calculated in the business plan? What are the available resources for program planning and curriculum revision? Is there released time available for those involved? Is there staff support available? Are there teaching–learning continuing education programs available to faculty?	The current physical facilities such as classrooms, offices, learning laboratories, computer facilities, are adequate and can accommodate curriculum revisions or new programs, or there are plans for expansion in place that are part of the business plan and have the support of the financial bodies of the institution. There are teaching and learning support systems for faculty that facilitate program planning and curriculum revisions.

(Continued)

TABLE 6.1 Guidelines for Assessing Internal Frame Factors *Continued*

Frame factor	Questions for data collection	Desired outcomes
	What instructional support systems are in place in the institution and the nursing program? Are they adequate and what plans are there for increasing and updating them according to the revised or new program needs? How many texts and journal holdings does the library have and will they meet the needs of students and faculty in the future, especially in light of new programs or revised curricula? Is there access to the library and other electronic communications for commuter students and faculty and for distance education programs?	There are adequate instructional support systems available for the current program and for proposed future programs. The current and proposed library holdings are adequate to meet the needs of the nursing program and proposed curricular revisions. There is access to the library for commuter students and for students and faculty participating in distance education programs.
Resources within the institution and nursing program	Is the current academic advising system working to students' and faculty's satisfaction? Are there appropriate faculty to student ratios for academic advising? Will a revised curriculum or new program require additional faculty or staff for academic advising purposes? What are the current relationships of the nursing program's administration, faculty, and staff with those of student services? Is the student services department aware of the proposed revisions or proposed new programs, and have they been consulted regarding future students services needs that may be impacted by the changes?	The academic advising system can accommodate appropriate faculty–student ratios and there are support systems in it to assure the quality of advisement. The student services system (recruitment, enrollment, registrar, financial aid, remediation, student counseling, and other services) works in partnership with nursing faculty to enhance the formal curriculum.
Resources within the institution and nursing program	What are the current facilities and services related to classrooms, laboratories, computer facilities, clinical experience laboratories, the library, instructional support systems, teaching–learning support, academic advising, and student services? Are they adequate for the current program and for future program planning and/or curriculum revisions?	The parent institution and the nursing program can currently, and in the future, support the curriculum with adequate facilities and services.
Potential faculty and student characteristics	What are the number and types of faculty currently on staff? Do they meet the requirements for the current program? Identify any gaps or redundancies that exist. Based on this assessment is the faculty adequate in numbers and qualifications to meet the needs of the proposed program or revised curriculum? If it is not, what are the plans to meet the needs?	The nursing program has an adequate number and types of faculty with the required knowledge and clinical expertise to meet the requirements for the proposed new program or revised curriculum.
Potential faculty and student characteristics	Describe the characteristics of the current student body and the history of the applicant pool to the nursing program. Has the program been able to meet its enrollment targets in the past 5 years? If not, what strategies have taken place to meet the target? What are the characteristics of the student body for the proposed program or revised curriculum? Is there an adequate applicant pool to fulfill enrollment targets? Are there plans in place for their recruitment? Has the nursing program staff formed a partnership with the admissions department for recruiting and retaining students?	The parent institution and the nursing program have the resources to recruit, educate, and graduate the type of student body that the new program or curriculum revision requires.
Analysis of the data and decision making	Summarize the conclusions by generating a list of positive, negative, and neutral findings that can influence the curriculum and program planning.	Develop a final decision statement as to the feasibility for developing a new program or revising the curriculum based on the needs assessment of the external and internal frame factors.

CASE STUDY

The case study initiated in Chapter 5 presented a fictional baccalaureate and higher degree school of nursing seeking to expand its offerings in order to meet the region's increasing nursing shortage. The faculty was divided into teams and each team gathered data related to the external frame factors that influence program and curriculum development. Thus far, the information they gathered indicate a positive milieu for expanding the program for either entry-level baccalaureate or higher degree students, an accelerated track for RN to Master of Science in Nursing (MSN) students, and the possibility for a Doctor of Nursing Practice (DNP) program for advanced practice nurses. The next step is to assess the internal frame factors that can further impact the decision to revise the existing programs and/or to develop new ones.

Description and Organizational Structure of the Parent Academic Institution

The School of Nursing dean and the coordinators of the undergraduate and graduate programs put together a description of the parent institution (the college) and the School of Nursing. The most recent accreditation reports for the Commission on Collegiate Nursing Education (CCNE) and the State Board of Nursing provide the description including the organizational structure of both. With a few minor edits of the documents to update them, they have the report ready to analyze for information related to the proposed expansion.

The home campus of the college is located on the outskirts of a large metropolitan area with the campus, which is a self-contained unit in a pleasant pastoral setting. The School of Nursing shares offices, classrooms, and several laboratories with the Science Department. However, it has two clinical skills laboratories that are under its control. There is an easy access to public transportation to travel into the metropolitan area where many learning and leisure time experiences for the students take place.

The School of Nursing represents about 6% (230 undergraduates and 90 master's) of the student body and was founded within the 100-year-old institution almost 60 years ago, being the first professional school in the college. The institution averages 4,500 undergraduate students each year with the graduate enrollment at 500. It has six schools including: Arts and Sciences (46% of the enrollment), Business Administration and Economics (26% of the enrollment), Computer Science (6% of the enrollment), Education (8% of the enrollment), Extended Education (8% of the enrollment) and Nursing. All but the School of Arts and Sciences have graduate programs, and the School of Education is a graduate school only. The highest degree that the institution awards is the doctoral degree (EDD and DBA), and it awards both the Bachelor of Arts and Bachelor of Science degrees. It has an excellent reputation in the community for its dedication to community service and high quality programs, all of which hold regional and national accreditations.

Although the original purpose of the college had a strong liberal arts focus, the institution has become multipurpose with the addition of the professional schools including Business, Education, and Nursing with Computer Sciences, a relatively young school, having started 10 years ago. The School of Extended Education offers distance education programs in Business Administration, Computer Sciences, and Education from the home campus, and its outreach program in the metropolitan area is under study for a needs assessment. Each school has a dean and the School of Nursing dean has been in his position for 9 years and therefore, has a strong voice in the Council of Deans owing to his history within the college. There is an academic provost to whom the deans report, and the president, who is an ordained minister within the religious sect that sponsors the college, administers the college. There is a comptroller, a dean of Student Affairs, a dean of Enrollment Services, a director of Human Resources, and a director of Library and Instructional Support Services.

The faculty full time equivalent totals about 210 with almost 100 part-time lecturers. There is an academic senate composed of two representatives from each school's faculty, three members-at-large, undergraduate, and graduate student representatives, a presidential appointee, and the academic provost. There are three major committees of the senate: the curriculum, graduate, and faculty affairs committees. The faculty elects the chair of the senate, chair-elect, and secretary. The faculty votes for members of the three committees from the senate membership. The committee members elect committee chairs to their positions. There is one nursing faculty member on the graduate committee, one nursing member is chair of the faculty affairs committee, and another is a member-at-large of the senate. The School of Nursing faculty and the senate curriculum committee must approve new academic programs and curriculum revisions. If the proposals emanate from graduate programs, the graduate committee recommends approval after review and sends them to the senate with recommendations.

The School of Nursing faculty numbers 30 full-time, tenure-track faculty and 15 part-time clinical faculty, not including the dean and 3 administrative support staff. There are 2 coordinators, 1 for the graduate program and 1 for the undergraduate program. They have 25% released time for coordination duties. The five tracks in the nursing program have coordinators who have 15% released time for these functions. The part-time faculty's teaching role occurs primarily in supervising students during their clinical experiences. The faculty members teach in both undergraduate and graduate programs, although some are predominantly assigned to one or the other depending on their clinical expertise and academic preparation. Sixty-five percent of the full-time, tenure-track faculty members have doctorates, and there are currently three enrolled in doctoral programs. The School of Nursing faculty meets once a month during the academic year and there are three major committees: curriculum, graduate, and peer evaluation. All program and curriculum revisions must be approved through the appropriate nursing committee structure and then approved by the faculty as a whole with final administrative review and approval by the Dean. Approved proposals are forwarded to the appropriate senate committee who makes recommendations to the senate who vote for approval or disapproval. Upon approval of the senate, the provost completes a final review and makes recommendations to the president.

Preliminary Conclusions

The college has a strong reputation for high quality liberal arts and professional educa-
tion program within the region, and the School of Nursing has a significant role within
the college. The dean of nursing is an active and respected member of the college's admin-
istrative structure with a sense of the history of the college and School of Nursing.

There are clear hierarchal lines of communication for administrative decisions
and for gaining curriculum and program approval. The School had three senators with
two on senate committees, but none on the curriculum or graduate committee. Thus,
some political maneuvering will be necessary to educate the senate about the proposed
changes to solicit their support. The president, provost, and comptroller have been
aware of the proposal and are supportive owing to their awareness of the community's
demand to prepare more nurses for the health care system.

Mission and Purpose, Philosophy, and Goals of the Parent Institution

Owing to the institution's religious base, nursing's mission is congruent with
the institution's mission and goals that focus on the preparation of compassionate and responsible citizens for society and professionals who provide services to the community. While the School of Nursing sometimes finds itself in
conflict with the large School of Arts and Sciences that emphasizes strong liberal arts and science foundations for all undergraduate students, nursing often
allies itself with the other professional schools and thus, can forestall additional prerequisites by the School of Arts and Sciences that can overburden the
student load for the undergraduate degree in nursing.

Preliminary Conclusions

The School of Nursing's mission and purpose, philosophy, and goals are in congruence
with those of the college. It recognizes the need to educate other schools about the nurs-
ing shortage and the need to increase enrollments. At the same time, it must collaborate
with them in regard to the impact the new program might have on the other schools.

Internal Economic Situation and Its Influence on the Curriculum

The same team who examined the organizational structure of the college meet
with the comptroller of the college to discuss some additional issues related to
the economic situation and its effect on the proposed new outreach program.
When conducting the assessment of the external frame factors, faculty found
that both the college and School of Nursing are financially stable, the comptroller is willing to help develop a business case for the proposed program and
there are potential external funding resources for the program should it start
up. Recently, the nursing faculty identified several state and federal programs
that might fund a new program; especially if it included strategies to reduce
the current nursing shortage. However, this requires released time for faculty
to write the grants. It is calculated that two faculty members each need 5%

released time for the next semester to write these grants. The comptroller refers the dean and faculty to the provost who may have some faculty development funds that could cover the costs for this released time. The provost agrees to provide a total of $2,000 as released time for the next semester for faculty to write grant proposals for program development.

Thus far, there has been no financial support for the needs assessment and as it progresses, the dean and faculty feel the need for some support to continue to develop the proposal. Of special concern is the need to provide released time for curriculum development when and if expansion is approved. This would involve at least three faculty members and would take about 5% of their workload in assigned time activities to develop or revise the existing curriculum to fit the outreach program. This released time needs to be built into the next year's budget for the School of Nursing. The comptroller suggests that the dean of the School of Nursing bring up this need when the Council of Deans and the provost develop next year's proposed budgets. The dean discussed this with the provost who is willing to place the item into next year's budget request.

Preliminary Conclusions

The college and the School of Nursing are economically stable. The college administration indicated support for developing a business case for the proposed program. This plan will calculate estimated start-up costs and program maintenance funds for 3 years when the program should become self-sufficient. The provost will provide $2000 next semester for faculty released time to write grants for program development funds. The dean will write in the cost for faculty released time for curriculum development for the next year's budget with the approval of the provost.

Resources Within the Institution and Nursing Program

A team of faculty including representatives from faculty who teach in the nursing laboratory, the library and instructional support liaison, the school's curriculum committee chair, and the undergraduate and graduate coordinators assess the resources within the college and the School of Nursing. Because the proposed outreach changes or new programs must match the resources of the existing program and yet, meet the needs of students who may be at a distance from the school, the team assesses resources needed for possible distance outreach.

The on-campus classrooms, learning laboratories, and computer classrooms, although not under the school's control, are adequate in size and number for the on-campus student enrollment. The library has one of the largest holdings in the region for nursing journals and texts as well as for other disciplines. Recently, the library upgraded its off-campus access so that students are able to log into databases with full text journal articles including Cumulative Index to Nursing and Allied Health Literature (CINAHL), Education Resources Information Center (ERIC), and Medical Literature Analysis and Retrieval System (MEDLAR). The Instructional Support Services Department and the School of Extended Education have distance education programs including videoconferencing with a dedicated broadcasting suite and there is a contract with a Web-based delivery system for computer-based courses. These facilities were developed for the School of Business Administration and School of Education graduate programs as well as the RN to Bachelor of Science in Nursing (BSN) program. The director of Library and Instructional Support Services meets with the team and indicates that Nursing has access to these technologies, although videoconferencing services dictate scheduling of classes to avoid conflict with the School of Extended Education programs. The director indicates that monthly in-service workshops are held for faculty to improve teaching effectiveness as well as to learn new technologies such as developing Web-based courses and designing videoconference classes. Many nursing faculty attend these workshops and are always welcome as new programs and technologies are developed.

As for off-campus facilities, the team knows from the assessment of the external frame factors that the dean of Extended Education indicated that the classrooms he or she rents in the proposed off-campus outreach program site are available for rental by the nursing program as well. These rooms include an office space for faculty, one office for the coordinator of the program, a traditional classroom, and a dedicated high technology computer and videoconferencing room that can be shared with other Extended Education students. Special clinical learning laboratories are available to the program, rent free, from the religious-based health maintenance organization.

The academic advisement system in the School of Nursing requires that each faculty member carries an average of 20 advisees. Advisees are matched to faculty members' expertise and interests. In the graduate program, advisors are usually the students' thesis or research project chairs and therefore, they have fewer student advisees.

The team assesses student services needs for the expanded program. They meet with the director of Enrollment Services and discuss recruitment, student records, counseling services, financial aid programs, and work–study options for nursing students. The proposed program calls for at least one additional staff member in Enrollment Services for all of the services previously mentioned, although it is possible that such a person could work with the Extended Education program staff located in the proposed site for the program should the program decide to offer classes off-site. This needs to be included in the business plan and is duly noted for bringing to the attention of the comptroller.

Preliminary Conclusions

Current facilities and services for the School of Nursing are adequate for the on-campus program. However, the following is a list of the needs if an outreach program is decided upon. Possible resources to fill the needs are included:

Classrooms	*One room is shared with Extended Education. There is a rental fee.*
Office space	*There are two rooms in the Extended Education facility. There is a rental fee.*

Computer and videoconferencing classroom.	*One room is shared with Extended Education. There is a rental fee.*
Learning and clinical lab facilities	*There is one room with equipment donated by the health care system.*
Library and instructional support systems	*Current facilities are adequate and accessible.*
Academic counseling	*Additional faculty and staff*
Student services	*Services are in place; however additional staff may be necessary.*

Potential Faculty and Student Characteristics

Four faculty members representing the undergraduate and graduate programs are charged with identifying potential faculty and student characteristics and needs for an outreach program. They agree that a full-time coordinator for the outreach program is necessary during the planning stages as well as for managing the program when it commences. At that time, depending on the size of the student enrollment, that person could assume some teaching responsibilities in addition to coordinating the program. Faculty characteristics and needs must match those of the current faculty with tenure track and clinical positions available to the program. The size of the faculty will be determined by the choice of program, especially if it is not a prelicensure program, and the delivery mode of the program. For example, some lecture courses might be developed and delivered through videoconferencing or Web-based courses that are already part of the on-campus program and the faculty's repertoire, while new faculty will be needed for clinical supervision of students and some theory and learning laboratory courses. Although precise numbers of teachers cannot be calculated until the final decision is made to offer the program and what kind of program it will be, the faculty set the parameters for the characteristics of the faculty and its size.

Like the faculty, the characteristics and size of the student body depends on the decision to expand or offer new programs and the types of program. Based on the needs assessment of the external frame factors, the decision appears to be going toward an expansion of the RN to BSN program to the MSN program, a possible entry-level MSN program for college graduates, and the development of a post-master's DNP program, and the initiation of an outreach program. If an expansion of the undergraduate program is initiated for college graduates, the numbers of students are likely to be larger than for an entry-level master's program. However, because either program is a prelicensure program, the faculty to student ratio for clinical supervision must be calculated into the costs for mounting the program. A critical mass for the number of students needed to meet the cost of mounting the program must be calculated as well. The same prerequisites and other admission criteria for students on the home campus program must be applied to a potential outreach program.

With these factors in mind, the faculty team members look at the enrollment and retention patterns of the School of Nursing's home campus. The undergraduate program enrollments have been stable for the past 5 years; however, the applicant pool decreased in the past 4 years by 8% with a slight increase this past year. The team attributed the slight increase in the applicant pool to the lay public's increasing awareness of the nursing shortage. Although enrollment targets were met for the past 5 years, the result was that students that were admitted to the program had lower overall high school GPAs and scores on the SAT. Although they met the prerequisites and admission criteria, the average overall GPA and SAT scores fell by 3 percentage points. Thus, the students required more academic counseling and remediation programs than in the past for retention purposes and the attrition rate increased slightly from 6% to 8%. The National Council Licensure Examination (NCLEX) passing score for first-time takers averaged around 85% over the past 5 years.

Faculty informally survey entry-level MSN programs across the country and learn that the NCLEX pass rates are more than 90% and graduates are gainfully employed in nursing positions. Although formal studies were not conducted, anecdotal information indicates high satisfaction with the graduates on the part of faculty, the graduates' employers, and the graduates. The majority of faculty members reported that they enjoyed working with these students and found them challenging owing to their adult-learner needs, previous work experience, and new perspectives on nursing as a profession.

The nursing faculty learns from the admissions department that there are many college graduates in the nursing applicant pool based on the news of the nursing shortage in the public media. Based on their experiences, the admissions staff believes that recruitment for both types of students into the undergraduate or graduate programs should be fairly easy; although, owing to the other existing nursing programs, the entry-level master's program is more attractive because there is no competition for those types of students. They report that they have many inquiries for a DNP program and estimate they receive about 10 calls per week. The inquiries come from nurses who are in advanced practice roles. However, establishing a DNP program will require meetings of the staff with regional college and university advising centers' staff, public media advertisements and spot announcements, and on-site information meetings. These activities would have to be included in the business case.

Preliminary Conclusions

While the current overall nursing faculty to student ratio is 1:13, which is lower than the other schools in the college, any new programs will require a coordinator, additional faculty, and staff. A full-time coordinator is necessary to build relationships with Extended Education for an outreach program, the community, and to help admissions staff recruit students. Eventually, the coordinator role could include some teaching activities. Current faculty may be able to deliver their lecture and theory-type courses via distance education; however, skills, laboratory, and clinical experiences must take place on-site, requiring part-time clinical faculty services at the very least.

The coordinator and faculty will need to work closely with Enrollment Services in the recruitment of students into the program. A marketing and recruitment plan including a timetable needs to be developed. See Table 6.2 for a summary and analysis of the internal frame factors needs assessment and the conclusions based on the findings.

TABLE 6.2 Analysis of the Internal Frame Factors

Frame factor	Findings	Negative	Neutral	Positive	Conclusions
Description and organizational structure of the parent academic institution	The college and School of Nursing have positive reputations. Organization and hierarchal communication lines are clear for program and curriculum development processes and approvals. The dean has influence in the college. The college administrators are aware of the proposed program and supportive thus far.	There are no nursing senators on the senate curriculum or graduate committees.		The school has three senators on the academic senate. Organization lines are clear. There is administrative support. The dean has influence. The school has a positive reputation.	Positive. The college organizational structure and administrators are supportive. The dean has influence. Neutral. There is a need to educate key members of the senate about the program.
Mission and purpose, philosophy, and goals of the parent institution	The School of Nursing matches the college mission, purpose, philosophy, and goals. It has good relationships with the professional schools.	A few of the other schools may present roadblocks to the development of an expanded program if it impacts their programs.		Mission is congruent. Relationships with professional schools are good.	Positive. Nursing is congruent with the college mission, purpose, philosophy, and goals. Nursing has the support of the professional schools. Neutral. A campuswide education effort about the nursing shortage is indicated.
Internal economic situation and its influence on the curriculum	The college and the School of Nursing are financially secure. The college administrators favor the proposed program and will develop a business case for it. There is $2000 released time for writing grants.	There is no support for the needs assessment and program or curriculum development.		The college and the School of Nursing are financially secure. The costs for released time to develop the curriculum will be included in next year's proposed budget.	Positive. The college and the School of Nursing are financially secure. The comptroller will develop a business case for the proposal. There is money for faculty to write grants. Negative. Plans for released time for curriculum development must be included in next year's budget.

(Continued)

TABLE 6.2 Analysis of the Internal Frame Factors *Continued*

Frame factor	Findings	Negative	Neutral	Positive	Conclusions
Resources within the institution and nursing program	The current on-campus program has adequate resources and services. The costs for some facilities may be offset by donated space.	An outreach program will require rental fees for classrooms, labs, offices, a coordinator, support staff, and faculty. Student services may need to increase staff for marketing and recruitment purposes.		Some support staff and instructional support services can be covered by existing services. Current resources on campus are adequate.	Positive. The college and school have adequate resources for the on-campus program, some of which can be shared with the outreach program. Negative. The business case must include the costs for a coordinator, increases to faculty and support staff, physical facilities, and student services.
Potential faculty and student characteristics	The current faculty is well qualified. Inquiries from college graduates are increasing. Entry-level master's graduates and employers are satisfied. NCLEX pass rates are excellent.	A coordinator for new programs and support staff for start-up is necessary. Part-time faculty at the very least will be necessary for learning lab and clinical supervision purposes. Recently, the quality of the undergraduate applicant pool decreased. Additional marketing and recruitment services are indicated for recruiting students.		Faculty is qualified. The applicant pool to the baccalaureate had a slight increase in the past year. There have been increased inquiries from college graduates and from advanced practice nurses for a DNP. Entry-level MSN programs are successful.	Positive. Faculty is well qualified. Negative. Selecting coordinators for new programs are of priority. Neutral. Faculty and staff needs can be identified when the program starts. Positive. There is an increased interest in entry-level master's program. Survey indicates high NCLEX pass rates and employers are satisfied. Negative. Support for marketing and recruitment purposes are of highest priority.
Overall decision internal frame factors		9 negative entries	0 neutral entries	15 positive entries	11 positive conclusions. 4 negative conclusions. 3 neutral

Conclusion

The needs assessment of the internal frame factors clarified some of the issues raised by the assessment of the external frame factors. Overall, the college and School of Nursing has the experience and knowledge to expand its programs. Other schools in the college, particularly the professional schools and Extended Education are supportive of nursing. The nursing faculty is well prepared and the library and instructional support systems of the college can facilitate the development of new programs within certain financial limitations. Released time for faculty ($2,000) to write grants for external funding for program development is available. However, released time for program planning and curriculum development is of highest priority. The dean, provost, and comptroller plan to develop a business case and request for support of these activities into next year's budget. Student services works closely with the school and with a small increase in staffing can provide marketing and recruitment support. Applications and enrollment patterns have been stable for the School of Nursing; although, the RN to BSN and master's programs have been more stable than the undergraduate program.

Specific items for the business case have been iterated. The recommendations from the needs assessment of the external factors and the conclusions reached from the assessment of the internal factors led to the decision to decrease the basic baccalaureate enrollments by 10 new admissions each year and expand the RN to BSN program into an accelerated master's program with the majority of the courses online, as there is no other program in the region that accelerates RNs to the MSN. Interest from college graduates supports the initiation of an entry-level master's program that provides college graduates with the equivalent of a baccalaureate in nursing to move into the master's program. In addition, a post-master's DNP program will be initiated to accommodate advanced practice nurses and to provide a pathway for graduates of the entry-level masters, the RN to BSN to MSN, and the MSN graduates to continue into the doctoral program. Because the state-supported school prepares nurse practitioners, it was decided that the Family Nurse Practitioner (FNP) program limit its enrollment to 20 per year in light of the other program in the region. The clinical specialty tracks will remain steady at 20 per year. The plans call for a decrease of 30 students in the MSN specialty track to accommodate 30 new entry-level students and 10 RN students. However, as the curricula are revised and new ones developed, it is anticipated that enrollments will grow each year except for the basic undergraduate program that will decrease slightly. Eventually, graduates of the BSN program could move into the DNP program, while the MSN programs are phased out. The program would follow the national trend to offer advanced practice education at the doctoral level.

It was determined by the faculty and administrators that there is an adequate applicant pool for graduates of the programs, there are no other programs like them in the region, and the school meets the demand for preparing additional nurses prepared at the baccalaureate and higher degree levels for the workforce. The first order of business is to identify program coordinators for the DNP and entry-level MSN to lead curriculum development, marketing of the programs, and recruitment of students. (The existing RN to BSN coordinator can continue with the RN to BSN to MSN program.) A new coordinator will be appointed for the entry-level MSN and the FNP Coordinator will assume coordination of the DNP Program. The following are the recommendations for initiation of the program and plans for their follow-up:

1. Develop an entry-level MSN curriculum to meet the needs of college graduates (baccalaureates or higher *not* in nursing)
2. Appoint a coordinator for the program and support staff.
3. Develop the curriculum for the entry-level MSN that is congruent with upper division level BSN courses and provide a segue into the existing MSN tracks.
4. Initiate information meetings about the program to the college community and the public.
5. Expand the RN to BSN program into an accelerated RN to BSN to MSN program.
6. Work with the coordinator of the RN to BSN program and the coordinators of the MSN clinical specialty tracks to expand the curriculum.
7. Appoint faculty to revise the existing RN to BSN curriculum to accelerate students into the MSN program.
8. Work with faculty to revise the format of courses to an online delivery.
9. Work with the coordinator of the FNP track to develop a post-master's DNP program.
10. Appoint a task force to develop the curriculum for the DNP.
11. Initiate information meetings about the program to the college community and the public.
12. Establish an infrastructure for program development, planning, and implementation, for the expanded RN program and the initiation of the entry-level MSN and DNP programs.
13. Develop a business case for the proposed plans in collaboration with the comptroller for presentation to the college community.
14. Work with the comptroller to develop a business plan for a start-up year and implementation of the program for the following 3 years leading to self-sufficiency.
15. Identify all costs for management and planning for the program, support staff, faculty, facilities, resources, and services.
16. Balance the costs with income from start-up grants, tuition, and fees.
17. Initiate start-up activities for the program including the following plans.
18. Meet with key stakeholders about the program, (e.g., the provost, body politic, other nursing program directors and faculty, focus groups of potential students, health care facilities administrators and educators, potential funding agencies, and feeder educational institutions).
19. Hold information and planning meetings with the dean and other deans of schools within the college, the provost and the president, the director of the

Library and Instructional Support Services, the dean of Enrollment Services, nursing faculty, the nursing graduate committee, current enrolled entry-level master's students and graduates of that program, and members of the senate.

20. Establish curriculum development task forces for the RN to BSN to MSN, the entry-level MSN, and the DNP programs to develop curricula.
21. Begin a written record for the program to incorporate into grant proposals, accreditation reports, and proposals for approval by the School of Nursing and the academic senate.
22. Develop a program evaluation and review technique (PERT) chart.
23. Develop an evaluation plan for each program that is congruent with the Nursing Master Plan of Evaluation.

DISCUSSION QUESTIONS

1. To what extent do you believe an assessment of the internal frame factors that affect a nursing education program influences a decision to revise a program or propose a new one?
2. Of the five major internal frame factors, how would you prioritize findings from their assessment in terms of the potential success for a proposed education program or revision of the curriculum?

LEARNING ACTIVITIES

Student Project

As a student group, continue your needs assessment for a potential nursing program that you started in Chapter 5. Use Table 6.1 "Guidelines for Assessing Internal Frame Factors" to collect data on the frame factors that you need to consider. After you collect the data, summarize your findings and compare them to the "Desired Outcomes" listed in the table. Based on the findings, justify why or why not a new nursing program is needed.

Faculty Project

Using Table 6.1. "Guidelines for Assessing Internal Frame Factors", continue your work on the existing nursing curriculum that you identified in Chapter 5. Collect data for each internal frame factor as it applies to the curriculum. Summarize your findings and compare them to the "Desired Outcomes" listed in the table. In light of your summary, is a curriculum revision indicated? Explain your reasons for the decision to revise or not to revise.

REFERENCES

Graf, C. M. (2006). ADN to BSN: Lessons learned from human capital theory. *Nursing Economics. 24*(3), 135–141.

Health Resources and Services Administration, Bureau of Health Professions, Division of Nursing. (2010). *Nurse Education and Practice Grant Programs.* Retrieved from http://bhpr.hrsa.gov/nursing

Johnson, M. (1977). *Intentionality in Education.* (Distributed by the Center for Curriculum Research and Services, Albany, NY). Troy, NY: Walter Snyder, Printer.

McCleary-Jones, V. (2007). Learning disabilities in the community college and the role of disability services departments. *Journal of Cultural Diversity. 14*(1), 43–47.

McCleary-Jones, V. (2008). Strategies to facilitate learning among nursing students with learning disabilities. *Nurse Educator. 33*(3), 105–106.

National Institutes of Health. National Institute of Nursing Research. (2010). Retrieved from http://www.nih.gov/ninr/

University of California–Los Angeles (UCLA), Office of Contract and Grant Administration. (2010). *Private Foundations and Organizations.* Retrieved from http://www.research.ucla.edu/sr2/Private.htm

University of Utah. USA Higher Education Systems. (2010). Retrieved from http://www.utahsbr.edu/boards.htm

IV Curriculum Development Applied to Nursing Education and the Practice Setting

Sarah B. Keating

OVERVIEW OF CURRICULUM DEVELOPMENT

Prior to discussing curriculum development, it is useful to review the definition of curriculum. According to this text, "a curriculum is the formal plan of study that provides the philosophical underpinnings, goals, and guidelines for the delivery of a specific educational program." Chapter 7 introduces the components of the curriculum and the process for its development followed by specific chapters on associate, baccalaureate, master's, advanced practice doctorates, and research-focused doctoral degrees. The last chapter in this section discusses application of the components of the curriculum to the development of education programs in the practice setting.

Experienced educators will testify to the fact that as a curriculum ages, changes that were unintended in the original curriculum plan occur. These changes occur in response to feedback from students, faculty, and consumers; faculty's individual interpretations of the objectives and course content; changes in faculty personnel who are not familiar with the curriculum; changes in the practice setting; and the expansion of nursing knowledge. Unless there is continuous evaluation of the curriculum, the plan will eventually become so corrupted that it is barely recognizable.

Section 5 that follows these chapters describes in detail the value of evaluation activities as they apply to approval, review, and accreditation of the nursing program. However, it is wise in this section on curriculum development to recognize the need for continually monitoring the program, at least annually, to ensure that it is meeting the original mission, framework, goals, and objectives of the curriculum. The data collected from evaluation reviews and the recommendations issuing from them indicate to faculty the need for revising the curriculum, discontinuing certain programs within it, or initiating new tracks. If this exercise is conducted every year, maintaining the integrity of the curriculum becomes easy and there are fewer hoops to go through in seeking approval for major or minor changes. Annual review and minor revisions contribute to a curriculum that is current and is a living, vibrant organism that prepares nursing professionals for current and future markets.

Purpose of Curriculum Development

The overall purpose of curriculum development is to meet the learners' needs by ensuring that it meets educational and professional standards and that it is responsive to the current and future demands of the health care system. To accomplish this long-term goal, the curriculum serves as the template for faculty to express its vision, mission, philosophy, framework, goals, and objectives of the nursing program. Although curriculum development is the prerogative of the faculty, consumers of the program need to be involved in the process. Consumers include the students, their families, the health care system that utilizes its graduates, nurse educators, and staff in the practice setting, and lastly, the patients that receive nursing care from students and graduates.

Components of Curriculum Development

The classic components of a school of nursing curriculum include (a) the mission of the program; (b) the philosophy of the faculty that usually contains beliefs about teaching and learning processes, diversity, the metaparadigm of nursing (i.e., nursing, person, health, and environment); critical thinking and evidence-based practice; and other selected concepts or theories that define the specific nursing education program; (c) the purpose or overall goal of the program; (d) a framework by which to organize the curriculum plan; (e) the end-of-program objectives or student learning outcomes; and (f) an overall implementation plan (program of study). The components should be congruent with the parent institution's mission and philosophy. Chapter 7 discusses the components in detail and the pros-and-cons of frameworks to organize the curriculum plan including the use of nursing and other disciplines' theories and concepts and professionally defined standards or essentials of education.

Levels of Nursing Education

Chapters 8 through 12 apply the components of the curriculum to the various levels of nursing education including the associate degree, the baccalaureate, master's, Doctor of Nursing Practice (DNP), and research-based doctorates (e.g., the PhD, DNSc, and DNS). Each chapter provides a summary of the role that each level of education plays in the mission, philosophy, organizational framework, goals, and end-of-program objectives for its parent institution. Issues that apply to each such as entry into practice, opportunities for further education, advanced practice, contributions to nursing education, evidence-based practice, and research are discussed.

Curriculum Development Applied to the Practice Setting

Chapter 13 assists staff developers and patient and family educators to adapt the information in the text to their arena of nursing practice. Although the major focus of the text is on curriculum development and evaluation in schools

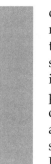

of nursing, many of the same components and activities for curriculum planning apply to staff development and patient and family education, even though the target audiences differ. The processes of conducting a needs assessment, setting the mission, philosophy, purpose, and goals for an education program in the practice setting must be in line with the health agency's mission and purpose. This applies to all types of staff development programs including orientation, specialty and cross training, maintenance of skills competency, and continuing education. The current role of educators in nursing practice settings, their qualifications, and desired educational levels are discussed. Issues and trends that apply to staff development are reviewed.

7 # The Components of the Curriculum

Sarah B. Keating

OBJECTIVES

Upon completion of Chapter 7, the reader will be able to:

1. Compare curriculum development activities among various types of educational institutions and levels of nursing education.
2. Distinguish the formal curriculum from the informal curriculum.
3. Analyze the components of curriculum development according to their role in producing a curriculum plan.
4. Analyze a case study that illustrates the adaptation of an existing curriculum to a distance education program.
5. Assess an existing curriculum or educational program by using the "Guidelines for Assessing the Key Components of a Curriculum or Educational Program."

OVERVIEW

Chapter 7 provides an overview of types of educational institutions in higher education and how the various levels of nursing education fit into them. It continues with a discussion of the classic components of the curriculum, which include the following:

- Mission/Vision
- Philosophy
  - Beliefs about teaching and learning processes
  - Critical thinking
  - Diversity and cultural competence
  - Genetics
  - Social justice
  - Research and evidence-based practice
  - Informatics and technology
  - Quality health care and patient safety
  - Nursing paradigm
- Organizational framework and concept mapping
- Overall program goal and purpose
- Implementation plan
  - Student learning outcomes (SLOs; end-of-program objectives)
  - Level objectives
  - Course objectives

- Course prerequisites
- Course descriptions
- Content outlines
- Course schedule
- Learning activities
- Evaluation methods

The chapter provides a sample nursing curriculum developed from the fictional case study in Section III, the needs assessment. Table 7.1 provides guidelines for assessing the key components of a curriculum or educational program. Chapters 8 through 13 discuss in detail levels of nursing education from the associate degree through the PhD with Chapter 13 applying the components of the curriculum to staff development and health education. The last chapter (17) of the text responds to the issues that arise from the myriad of levels of nursing education for entry into practice. Chapter 17 proposes several plans that promote a unified approach to nursing education for the readers' consideration and debate.

TYPES OF INSTITUTIONS

Types of educational institutions are classified as **private** or **public, undergraduate** or **graduate**, and **research-intensive** or **research-extensive**. The types of nursing education programs addressed in this text range from the associate degree to the doctorate level. Many nursing curricula include step-in and step-out educational programs that provide career ladder opportunities for nurses. Most institutions of higher education identify themselves according to classifications found in the Carnegie Foundation for Advancement of Teaching Classification (2009). The Carnegie classification was first published in 1970 with the most recent classification occurring in 2005 and an update planned for 2010. The 2005 designations are according to what institutions teach (undergraduate and graduate programs), to whom they teach (student profiles), and the size and setting of the institution. The original classifications continue to be used and appear at the end of the new list identified as "Basic Classifications" (Carnegie Foundation for Advancement of Teaching Classification). A listing with a detailed description of each type of classification is available at: http://www.carnegiefoundation.org/classifications.

McCormick and Zhao (2007) describe the recent changes in the Carnegie Classifications, the reasons for the changes, and the rationale behind the reorganized classifications. McCormick (2009) has an interesting perspective on the utilization of the Carnegie Classification system compared to that of the annual U.S. News & World Report that ranks institutions according to region, specific disciplines, and national recognition. McCormick raises the issue of how to differentiate between types of higher education institutions and brings into question the methodology for rating schools according to quality within various classifications.

For this text, the discussion about types of higher education institutions includes private (nonprofit and for-profit) and public institutions (federal, state, or regionally supported) as well as community colleges, small liberal arts colleges, large multipurpose or comprehensive colleges and universities, research-intensive and research-extensive universities, and academic health science/medical centers. **Sectarian** and **nonsectarian**

institutions are yet another classification with sectarian institutions reflecting a religious affiliation, for example, Catholic University, Southwest Baptist University, Brigham Young, and so forth. Although curriculum development activities are quite the same across types of institutions, the differences arise when examining the overall purpose of the institution and the financial and human resources that are available for revising or initiating new programs.

LEVELS OF NURSING EDUCATION

The levels of nursing education discussed in this text include associate degree programs that are usually housed in community colleges. These colleges are regional, public-supported institutions; although, there are some privately funded 2-year colleges that include nursing programs. Baccalaureate, master's, and doctorate nursing programs are found in both state-supported and privately funded institutions. There are a few **"single-purpose," nursing-only schools**. Many of these schools are or were former diploma, hospital-based programs with the latter converting to associate degree or baccalaureates in nursing. There are relatively few diploma program left because of the financial constraints they face as well as the need for providing the liberal education and basic sciences that undergird nursing programs (Raines & Taglaireni, 2008).

For all types of programs, administrators and faculty should plan in advance for financial support of curriculum development and evaluation activities and should investigate external resources such as grants that support curriculum changes and program development. A very visible program that has been available over the years for nursing program development or expansion is the Division of Nursing Title VIII grants for basic nurse education, diversifying the workforce through education programs, advanced nurse education, advanced nurse training grants, scholarships, and nurse faculty loans and development (Health Resources and Services Administration, Bureau of Health Professions, Division of Nursing, 2010). Detailed information is available at the following Web site: http://bhpr.hrsa.gov/nursing.

THE FORMAL AND INFORMAL CURRICULA

The **formal curriculum** is the planned program of studies for an academic degree or discipline. It includes the components of the curriculum that are discussed in this chapter and the curriculum plan is visible to the public through its publication in catalogs, recruitment materials, and on Web sites. The **informal curriculum** is sometimes termed as the hidden curriculum, cocurriculum, or as extracurricular activities. These planned and unplanned influences on students' learning should be kept in mind as faculty assesses and develops the curriculum. Examples include special convocations with invited speakers, student organization activities that parallel course work, and outside-of-class meetings with students and faculty to enrich learning experiences. The cocurriculum incorporates planned activities such as collaboration with other academic units, student affairs meetings (information meetings, orientation, counseling sessions, etc.), field trips, and planned volunteer services in the community. Examples of extracurricular activities are athletics, social gatherings, and student organization events.

The Informal Curriculum in Nursing

Some examples of the informal curriculum's influence in nursing are student services activities and counseling, special convocations, graduations, honor society meetings, study groups, student nursing association meetings, student invited attendance at faculty meetings, participation in academic committees, and so forth. Many schools of nursing schedule informal student–faculty meetings, holiday parties, and special events such as pinning ceremonies, honors convocation, and so forth. These activities provide opportunities for student–faculty interchanges to enrich and supplement the formal classroom setting as well as facilitate leadership opportunities for the students.

Examples of the Cocurriculum

An example of student affairs working with the academic side of the institution was illustrated by Thornburg, Uline, and Wilson (2006). They describe an orientation program for upper division level and master's students transferring into a teacher education program. Although it applies to teacher education, the same principles apply to students transferring into nursing programs from other higher education institutions. The orientation was held in seminar style with faculty and students establishing relationships that helped them to plan for study and for the practica that are part of professional education programs. Information in the seminar included admission requirements, expectations for the practicum, the conceptual framework of the program, and orientation to online education strategies.

Another article described the orientation needs of international students. Many nursing programs have students from other countries and students whose primary language is not English. Personal needs of these students were part of the orientation including on- and off-campus living, health care needs, insurance, transportation, and discrimination issues. These same needs apply to high school students and transfer students entering nursing programs (Poyrazli & Grahame, 2007).

Registered nurse (RN) students are a rather unique group of adult learners who, in essence, are transfer students. They require responsive educational programs that recognize their needs and their strengths as adult learners in both bachelor's completion and graduate programs. Some of the strategies for meeting the needs of RN students include distance and online education (especially attractive to working RNs), clinical experiences in which teachers respect the RNs' competence and facilitate advancement of their competencies, learning contracts, alternative validation approaches for previous learning, and classroom teaching tailored to the preferences of the adult learner.

Effects of Student–Faculty Interactions on the Curriculum

Student–faculty relationships are important factors to consider and influence the unplanned curriculum. Clark (2008) interviewed seven nursing students including several who graduated or left the nursing program. The participants represented baccalaureate, master's, and doctoral levels. She asked participants for instances in their educational program of uncivil behavior on the part of faculty toward them. Types of reported behaviors included demeaning students, gender bias, unfairness, and pushing students to conform to faculty demands. Students in turn felt anger, hopelessness, and powerlessness. Clark and Springer (2007) looked at incivility on the part of faculty to students and students to faculty. They list common uncivil behaviors exhibited by students and faculty and call for additional research to identify the problem and find solutions to prevent the behaviors that lead to negative psychological and sociological consequences.

Federizo (2009), in an unpublished thesis, surveyed freshman and senior students in a baccalaureate nursing program for their reported instances of horizontal violence in classroom and clinical settings. Sixty-nine percent of the respondents reported experiencing horizontal violence from peers, faculty, and staff nurses in the clinical setting. She identified major reported themes such as humiliation, powerlessness, lack of respect, and concern for the decline in the image of nursing. These studies point out the need to assess and determine the extent of incivility among students, faculty, and the staff with whom they work and to take measures to prevent them.

Longo and Sherman (2007) offer strategies for tackling horizontal violence in the workplace that also apply to the educational setting. They report that it is a common phenomenon occurring in oppressed groups and urge nurses to understand the nature of horizontal violence in the workplace and its effects on the staff. Victims of horizontal violence experience psychological, sociological, and physical stress because of it. The authors suggest setting cultural expectations with a zero-tolerance policy for aggression and to develop approaches that support and empower staff.

Sitzman and Leners (2006) conducted a study on facilitating and encouraging caring behaviors in an online classroom. They surveyed students in an RN to Bachelor of Science in Nursing (BSN) program and asked them to report their impressions of caring behaviors exhibited by the instructor and students in the class. Eight themes emerged from the data including frequent feedback, timeliness, reciprocity of caring online, personal connection and empathy, clarity, multiple contact opportunities, second-fiddle worries, and the teacher's commitment to learning. Although the study was limited in size to only 11 students, the findings help to illuminate the influence of student–faculty interactions in online education and should lead to additional studies on the topic.

The Campus Environment

The physical environment for the delivery of the educational program is important to the image of the home institution and plays a major role in building a sense of belonging for students and alumni alike. Broussard (2009) talks about the influence of the architecture and landscape of the home campus that creates lasting relationships among students, alumni, faculty, staff, and the community. He talks about "transformational places" on campus where the college community has time to congregate and share ideas and experiences. He makes a point about commuter students and the need for campuses to build into the landscape, places where they too can experience a feeling of community.

Although the physical environment plays a small role in programs that are delivered in cyberspace, some colleges and universities require periodic on-campus academic program meetings or residencies and special events for distance education students to experience the on-site campus. Another strategy is to provide program information materials that include pictures of the campus and campus life. This helps students to identify with the physical plant and landscape to form images unique to the home campus. Other strategies for delivering the informal curriculum and an academic environment online include virtual faculty office hours and student and faculty meeting rooms.

The Doctoral Online Community for Students (DOCS) is an example of an extracurricular meeting place for students in the PhD online nursing program offered by the University of Nevada Las Vegas (UNLV). The DOCS site was established as an informal, online community with tips for students progressing through the program and a meeting place to share ideas and for social networking. Although faculty and students developed the site, a portion of the site is a student-only place and faculty only meet there when invited by students (University of Nevada Las Vegas, 2009).

The following discussion examines each of the major components of the curriculum from the vision or mission statements to the philosophy statement that embraces faculty beliefs and values about teaching and learning, critical thinking, diversity and cultural competence, genetics, social justice, research and evidence-based practice, informatics and technology, quality health care and patient safety, and the nursing metaparadigm. A description follows on how the organizational framework, overall goal or purpose, SLOs (end-of-program objectives), and level objectives constitute the implementation plan that flows from the mission and philosophy statements.

COMPONENTS OF THE CURRICULUM

The Mission or Vision Statement

Traditionally, higher education institutions in the United States have three major components in their mission, (i.e., teaching, service, and research [scholarship]). The mission statement for each institution depends on the nature of the institution and the three major components are often divided into separate permutations of the components. In more recent times, some organizations either replace or supplement the mission statement with a vision statement. For this discussion, the **mission statement** is the institution's beliefs about its responsibility for the delivery of programs through teaching, service, and scholarship. A **vision statement** is outlook oriented and reflects the institution's plans and dreams about its direction for the future. It is possible that a mission statement includes a vision statement and that the vision statement includes the mission. With this in mind, the following discussion emphasizes the development of the traditional mission statement, but also recognizes the more recent utilization of vision statements.

Morphew and Hartley (2006) reviewed more than 300 mission statements from the worldwide Web from universities and colleges that represented the Carnegie Classification of Baccalaureate Institutions, Master's Institutions, and Doctoral/Research Intensive and Extensive Institutions. They further divided the programs into public and private institutions. Major elements in the mission statements were categorized to identify similarities and differences among them. The authors hypothesized that the missions would or would not reflect classification differences and that consistent use of certain elements would communicate their differences to the public they served. They also hypothesized that normative or aspirational elements would be used to legitimize their purpose. It was found that the designation of public or private had more influence on the mission statements than the Carnegie Classifications. In addition, commitment to diversity and liberal arts appeared frequently across all programs. Although service appeared frequently, the definition of service varied.

An overall theme was the primary message the institutions hoped to convey to their constituents. For example, public institutions talked about service to the local or regional area (state-supported), whereas private institutions appealed to a wider population. They found few aspirational statements such as "to be the best," which as the authors state, is difficult to measure as an outcome. They concluded that the analysis of mission statements is complex and recommended further study to break down the classifications into subsets such as urban, women's, religious, and so forth.

Meacham (2008) conducted another analysis of mission statements in higher education. He studied more than 300 missions of universities identified by The Princeton Review (2001) as the 331 best colleges across the United States. Findings were similar to those of Morphew and Hartley (2006) with most missions emphasizing liberal arts, service, and social responsibility. Meachem discusses the utility of mission statements for orientation of new faculty and administrators to the history and purpose of the institution, assessment of the program and its relevance to current goals, utilization for campuswide discussions on current issues confronting the institution, and visualization of the future direction of the university/college.

Chief administrators (presidents) of institutions of higher learning assume much of the responsibility for ensuring that the mission is current and reflects the purpose of the college or university. They provide the leadership for administrators, staff, faculty, and students to implement the mission, to maintain its relevancy in the community, and to meet future education needs. Developing or revising a mission statement is usually a part of a strategic planning process that involves all of the constituents within the institution. Again, administration provides the leadership and resources for these activities. The purpose of the institution is examined and a vision statement is developed that looks into the future for the next decade or two. These activities foster creativity and a movement toward the future that provide the framework for planning. After consensus is reached for the vision, the mission is developed into a statement of purpose or mission of the college or university. This statement serves as the guiding document for developing long-range goals and implementing them. Another consideration related to the mission is the congruence of the statement with its actual implementation. Measures to determine if the mission is realized throughout the educational process and according to the expectations of graduates' performance in the real world, give feedback as to how well the mission is met. For example, if the mission has a strong research emphasis, there should be adequate support and funding for faculty to write grants to sponsor research and released time and facilities to conduct their studies.

Another aspect to the implementation of the mission is a cost analysis of the budget to relate the amount of monies allocated to the various functions of the program that support the mission. Academic and infrastructure support systems are analyzed for congruency with the mission. An example from nursing is an institution's support and commitment to a nurse-managed primary care clinic that serves the underserved and unserved populations of the community in which the institution is located. In this example, the clinic meets the institution's mission to serve the community.

Unless the school or department of nursing is a stand-alone academic entity, the mission of the major academic division (e.g., college or school, in which it resides) is examined in addition to that of the parent institution. Both the missions of the parent institution and its academic subdivision should be congruent with each other and provide guidelines for the mission statement of the nursing program. These statements depend on the nature of the institution and the nursing program. Smaller institutions may focus on liberal arts as a basis for all disciplines and professional programs to meet societal needs, whereas large research-oriented universities or academic health sciences centers might espouse new knowledge breakthroughs by its faculty and graduate students' research. In the case of the former, nursing's mission statement would reflect the graduation of well-prepared nurses to meet current and future health care demands; the latter would have an emphasis on nursing research and leadership in the profession. As mentioned previously, mission statements focus on the three elements of higher education (i.e., teaching, service, and research) thus, nursing's mission statement will reflect all three with emphasis on certain ones according to the nature of the parent institution and its divisions.

In the past, nursing and other health care disciplines recognized the need for interprofessional education, and with the complexity of the U.S. health care system, this is an important consideration for nursing programs to include in their mission statements and philosophies. Several examples from the literature serve as models for developing curricular experiences that are interdisciplinary in nature.

Rossen, Bartlett, and Herrick (2008) describe clinical experiences for nursing students that took place in a mental health care setting with other health-related disciplines such as social work, psychology, clients, and the clients' families. They found that students developed collaborative skills in working with other disciplines and improved their communication skills in the delivery of care. Lennon-Dearing, Florence, Garrett, Click, and Abercrombie (2008) describe a rural learning experience that put together nursing, medicine, social work, nutrition, and public health students. They found that the experience improved patient outcomes and the attitudes of the students toward interprofessional collaboration.

As with the presidents of universities and colleges, deans and directors of nursing education programs have a leadership role in developing program missions that are not only congruent with the parent institutions, but look to the future. Additionally, the mission needs to be examined frequently for its relevance to the rapidly changing health care system and the needs of society.

Philosophy

One definition for **philosophy** listed in the *American Heritage Dictionary* (2005) that applies to building a philosophy for a school of nursing curriculum is "the critical analysis of fundamental assumptions or beliefs." Such an analysis should flow from the mission and give faculty members the opportunity to discuss their beliefs, values, and attitudes about nursing and an education that imparts a body of knowledge and skills for the next generation of care providers. When building or revising a philosophy, faculty members discuss their beliefs about their specific school of nursing and its role in preparing nurses for the future, including statements on teaching and learning theories, the development of critical thinking, beliefs about diversity and cultural competence, social justice, research and evidence-based practice, patient safety and quality health care, and the nursing paradigm. Each individual member holds his/her own personal philosophy of education and nursing and thus, the development of a philosophical statement can become an arduous task for reaching consensus. Nevertheless, the resulting statement reflects the faculty's (as an entity) rationale for the school of nursing's existence and it serves to flavor the remainder of the curriculum components, their implementation, and their outcomes.

The first task related to developing the philosophy statement is to look at those of the parent institution and the subdivision of the parent in which nursing is housed. The ideal nursing philosophy incorporates all of the components of the other two philosophies; although, at times there are mismatches to some of the specific components. In those instances, a rationale as to why that incongruence exists and how the nursing program meets other components of the philosophy should be discussed. Eventually, this rationale is documented so that members of the school and external reviewers understand the fit of the nursing program into its parent institution and subdivision.

Some examples of incongruence of a nursing program's philosophy with its parent institution's philosophy occur when the program is within a traditional, liberal arts college that has no other professional programs. In this case, the nursing program's philosophy speaks to the importance of a strong liberal arts foundation for its graduates and the role of the nursing program to produce graduates who provide health care for the community. Another example is a nursing program housed within a school of engineering, along with several other professional programs such as computer science and journalism. In this case, nursing emphasizes the professional education aspects and preparation of professionals who serve the community.

The majority of nursing education programs' philosophies includes basic theories, concepts, beliefs, and values of faculty. The statement can be brief and succinct or lengthy; however, it should offer guiding principles for the remainder of the curriculum and should be evident in the organizational framework(s), goals, objectives, and implementation plan. The following discussion reviews many of the concepts found in nursing education program philosophies and is offered as a way for faculty to share ideas and beliefs and find consensus for developing or revising the program's philosophy.

Beliefs About Teaching and Learning and the Roles of Faculty and Students

Beliefs about teaching and learning form the premise for the delivery of the nursing curriculum. In the past, courses were traditionally delivered through classroom lecture, clinical laboratory sessions, and clinical experiences in the reality setting. The emphasis was on teaching and the curriculum reflected that modality. In the more recent past, with the focus on program outcomes and the advent of technology, the emphasis changed to learner-centered education. The role of the teacher, instead of transmitter of knowledge, became a role of mentor and coach. Teaching strategies fostered student participation in learning activities instead of acting as passive receivers of knowledge. With the change in focus to the learner, theories and principles of teaching and learning served as guides for assessing the characteristics of the learners and adapting those theories and principles to the needs of the learner.

Candela, Dalley, and Benzel-Lindley (2006) make a strong case for learner-centered education in nursing. They offer several helpful suggestions for faculty to make the change from a teaching-centered modality for delivering the educational program to one that centers on student learning. Ideas on best practice and strategies for teaching in nursing programs may be found at the Carnegie's Study of Nursing Education (2009): http://www.carnegiefoundation.org/programs/sub.asp?key=1829&subkey=2309&top key=1829. The Carnegie study's findings provide information gathered from case studies of schools of nursing related to theory and clinical teaching, which serve as exemplars for professional education

Chapters 3 and 4 of this text include in-depth discussions regarding learning theories and teaching principles, critical thinking, and educational taxonomies. They provide an overview of current ideas on these topics and foster faculty's sharing of ideas and beliefs regarding the application of learning theories to specific student populations. The educational taxonomies and strategies for developing critical thinking give faculty members ideas on how these theories and concepts apply to their specific nursing program. The resultant sharing and discussions are summarized and become part of the philosophy statement.

Critical Thinking

Chapter 4 of this text discusses critical thinking, definitions of it, and its application to nursing education. Development of critical thinking is essential to the preparation of nurses for clinical decision making and judgment. Most philosophies for nursing curricula contain some mention of it and thus, it is useful for faculty to discuss its place in the curriculum and how it applies to its specific nursing program. The following discussion presents thoughts from the literature that apply to the development of critical thinking skills and some ideas for faculty as they philosophize about the integration of critical thinking into the education program.

Faculty members need to discuss definitions of critical thinking and agree on one that fits their nursing program. Ways to measure achievement or an increase in critical thinking skills are important considerations when developing a philosophical statement. Lunney (2008) discusses critical thinking and metacognition as they apply to the education of nursing students. She contends that they require a blend of the two, (i.e., thinking about thinking (metacognition) and carrying out the processes for critical thinking). The critical thinking processes that Lunney identifies include the ability to use metacognition, interact with empirical knowledge in nursing, and have repeated experiences in applying the knowledge to the clinical setting. Points are made that each person is an individual and has varying levels of cognitive abilities and that critical thinking can be taught. A method for developing these skills that Lunney supports is the use of the written case study. She proposes that case studies offer situations that promote critical thinking based on actual health care situations. At the same time, she recognizes that they are not reality; however, they provide opportunities for students to practice metacognition and critical thinking in a controlled, safe environment.

Kennison (2008) describes a nursing-specific Critical Thinking Scale (CTS) to measure the development of critical thinking skills in baccalaureate nursing program seniors. She compared the scale to the California Critical Thinking Skills Test (a standard measurement for critical thinking). Three faculty members familiar with the critical thinking test evaluated reflective writings by the senior students based on a significant clinical experience that they identified. Interrater reliability was found among the three faculty members and the construct validity between the CTS and the CCTS was also affirmed. Although her sample was limited to one school and cannot be generalized, the findings indicate that the CTS is a tool that can be used to measure the development of critical thinking skills in nursing students and can be used over time from entry level to time of graduation.

Zygmont and Shaefer (2006) studied the critical thinking skills of faculty and students in a baccalaureate program. They interviewed the participants to identify their use of the steps of critical thinking. They listed these steps as analysis, evaluation, inference, and inductive and deductive reasoning. Although the findings from those measures indicated low levels of critical thinking on the part of faculty for some of the steps, they found that faculty used the skills when evaluating students' performance. Faculty gave examples of students' clinical experiences that demonstrated the use of these critical thinking for making clinical decisions. However, they could not provide examples from the classroom experience that helped to develop critical thinking for students. The authors linked this to the lecture and instructional-centered style of education common to nursing curricula and recommended that the strategies used in clinical experiences be applied to classroom settings as well.

Carter and Rukholm (2008) considered the development of RN students' critical thinking skills through discipline-specific writing opportunities in online education. They describe an online health assessment course that included asynchronous writing assignments to demonstrate the students' use of empirical knowledge from the discipline as well as critical thinking skills. Her definition of critical thinking included aesthetic, personal, ethical, and empirical thinking processes. Throughout the course, students received thought-provoking comments from the instructor to encourage additional seeking of knowledge and the application of critical thinking skills to client situations. Based on an analysis of the students' postings, she was able to demonstrate their use of empirical knowledge, clinical experience, and critical thinking skills when assessing clients. Her study illustrates the occurrence of positive learning outcomes with the use of teacher interactions and the posting of writing assignments on discussion boards in online classrooms. She encourages additional studies related to the use of writing assignments to assess the development of critical thinking skills.

The literature is rich in discussions about critical thinking and its relationship to problem solving and clinical decision making. Faculty members are urged to review current literature on the theories and concepts related to critical thinking and metacognition and their application to the nursing process. They should state their beliefs about these processes and how they define them; its role in nursing knowledge and practice, and how faculty can mentor students as nursing competencies are developed and increased through the educational experiences.

Diversity

Diversity can be considered in its broadest sense, not only in terms of race, ethnicity, culture, language, and gender, but also in terms of the diversity of opportunities in nursing. For example, although the majority of the nursing workforce (56.2%; Health Resources and Services Administration, Bureau of Health Professions, Division of Nursing, 2010) remains in the acute care delivery system, there are many opportunities in community-based settings such as primary care, public health, industry, schools, home care, skilled nursing facilities, rehabilitation hospitals, and so forth. Although the core of nursing knowledge and practice remains the same for all settings, community-based settings call for different interests, values, educational preparation, and skills sets. Thus, when faculty develops the curriculum philosophy, it must consider these factors and how the curriculum will meet society's diverse health care needs from entry-level graduates who function in all settings to those in advanced nursing roles in selected specialty settings.

Diversity of the Nursing Workforce

As discussed in this chapter's "Overview," the nursing profession and its education system must commit itself to diversifying the workforce to more closely resemble that of the populace. Although many gains were realized in the latter part of the 20th century, the profession needs to continue to build its diversity. The characteristics of the population whom the graduates serve should be taken into account so that student character-istics match the population as closely as possible and at the same time, graduates are culturally competent.

According to the U.S. Census Bureau (2005), one third of the nation's population is part of a group other than White, non-Hispanic. Hispanics are the largest minority group and the fastest growing. The second largest minority group was Blacks followed by Asians, American Indians and Alaska Natives, and Native Hawaiians and other Pacific Islanders. In contrast, the employed nursing population in 2004 was composed of White, 81.2%; Black, 4.4%; Asian, 3.1%; Native Hawaiian/Pacific Islander, 0.2%; American Indian/Alaska Native, 0.3%; Hispanic/Latino (any race), 1.7%, two or more races, 1.5%; and not known, 7.5% (Health Resources and Services Administration, 2009). The Nursing Data Review 2004–2005 reports that the total percentage of minority nursing students slipped from 20% in 2002 to 18% in 2004–2005. Graduate numbers for diversity are somewhat better than student enrollments but still worrisome according to the 2007 National League for Nursing (NLN) survey data of schools of nursing. The survey found that 23.6% of new graduates were from minority groups compared to 24.5% in the previous year (Kaufman, 2009).

According to these statistics, not only must schools of nursing increase their minority recruitment, they also need to retain and graduate them and ensure that all students are culturally competent when they graduate. The discussion thus far talks about increasing the diversity of the nursing workforce to prepare a more representative nursing workforce. Another major issue is the need to increase the diversity of nursing faculty who serve as role models for students. Milone-Nuzzo (2007) reinforces this statement by pointing out a modest (4%) increase in nurses from minority groups seeking advanced degrees. Although this has promise for increasing their representation in faculty ranks, nursing must con-tinue to increase the diversity in its pipeline for advanced degrees and faculty roles.

Cultural Competence

"**Cultural and linguistic competence** is a set of congruent behaviors, attitudes, and poli-cies that come together in a system, agency, or among professionals that enables effec-tive work in cross-cultural situations" (Health Resources and Services Administration, 2001). Calvillo et al. (2009) reports on the work by the American Association of Colleges of Nursing (AACN; 2010c) to identify standards for baccalaureate nursing curricula for developing cultural competence. These standards can be adapted to other levels of nursing education. The group identified five standards for graduates to:

- Apply knowledge of social and cultural factors that affect nursing and health care across multiple contexts;
- Use relevant data sources and best evidence in providing culturally competent care;
- Promote achievement of safe and quality outcomes of care for diverse populations;
- Participate in continuous cultural competence development; and
- Advocate for social justice, including commitment to the health of vulnerable populations and the elimination of health disparities.

The guidelines for integrating these standards into the curriculum may be found at the following Web site http://www.aacn.nche.edu/Education/pdf/toolkit.pdf.

Language as a major part of culture is an important component in examining beliefs about graduates' communication skills and cultural competence. Many nursing programs are considering proficiency in another language other than the native language as a competency expected of their graduates. Carter and Xu (2007) discuss building cultural sensitivity and competence into the nursing curriculum for international students and students whose primary language is not English. Surveys of the students' experiences in one nursing program with people from different cultures indicated that students, for the most part, had positive experiences in relating to culturally diverse patients, their families, and staff. Faculty reported that language barriers for students with English as a Second Language (ESL) presented major challenges to the educational process and clinical experiences. They indicated that working with ESL students required additional amounts of faculty time. A workshop for faculty on the issues proved successful and it was believed that the integration of cultural awareness and cultural competence into the curriculum was positive. Ideas for integrating these concepts into the curriculum are offered by Carter and Xu.

Faculty serve as role models and mentors in the development of cultural competence in nursing students. Kardon-Edgren (2007) surveyed nursing faculty across the country for their cultural competence as measured by Campinha-Bacote's Inventory for Assessing the Process of Cultural Competency among Health Care Professionals-Revised (IPCC-R; 2003). She found that the faculty scores demonstrated cultural competence with faculty from regions with more culturally diverse populations scoring a bit higher. Her findings were positive and indicated awareness on the part of nursing faculty for the importance of cultural competence in nursing education and for practice. Faculty should discuss beliefs, values, and issues surrounding diversity and include a final statement in the philosophy that posits beliefs about the preparation of graduates who will serve multicultural and ethnic clients. In addition, the implementation plan and master plan of evaluation should assess to what extent this philosophical statement is realized in the educational process and its outcomes.

Genetics and the Genome Project

According to the Human Genome Project Information (2010), **genetics** is the study of inheritance patterns of specific traits. The definition for **genome** is: all the genetic material in the chromosomes of a particular organism; its size is generally given as its total number of base pairs. The **Genome project** is the research and technology development effort aimed at mapping and sequencing the genome of human beings and certain model organisms (http://www.ornl.gov/sci/techresources/Human_Genome/project/about.shtml). The Genome project was a major breakthrough in the science of genetics and its application to the management of human diseases. Prior to the breakthrough, nursing education did not include knowledge related to the topic except for very basic information in human biology courses and in nursing courses as it relates to major genetic/inherited diseases such as certain birth defects, diabetes, sickle cell disease, hemophilia, and so forth.

With the growing recognition of the role of genetics in major health disease such as cardiovascular disease, mental health disorders, certain cancers, and so forth, the need for the incorporation of genetics and the importance of the genome project's findings into nursing curricula has been recognized by nurse educators. The AACN in its *Essentials* documents for baccalaureate, master's, and the doctorate of advanced nursing practice (AACN, 2010a) lists genetics as one of the essential concepts to be included in nursing education. In an editorial, Cashion (2009) urges nurse educators to integrate genetics into the curriculum by citing several examples of nurses in practice who felt they were not prepared with basic education in genetics that provide the foundation for more advanced concepts in genetics and their influence on diseases and health care management.

Maradiegue (2008) has an especially useful article on integrating genetics into the nursing curriculum. She reviews the history of the human genome project and genetics and their impact on health care. Especially useful in the article are common terms and definitions used in genetics and resources for nurse educators as they incorporate genetics into the curriculum. Jenkins and Calzone (2007) review the processes used for developing competencies and curricula guidelines for the incorporation of genetics into the curriculum. The competencies were developed through a nationwide initiative of nurse leaders, educators, and scholars and endorsed by many professional nursing organizations including those with considerable influence in nursing education. The article includes a table of the competencies that should be useful to nurse educators as they integrate genetics into the curriculum.

Social Justice

Cultural diversity segues into the complexities of concepts related to social justice. Many of the standards for accreditation of nursing programs and requests for proposals for educational funding refer to the notion of inequality, health disparities, and access to health care. Certain populations and oppressed groups suffer the consequences of discrimination and unfair treatment in the health care system. Nursing as a prime caring profession must be cognizant of these injustices and have the power and strategies to advocate for their clients and themselves to provide quality health care for all. Social justice is an important concept often found in the missions and philosophies of educational programs; however, it is sometimes difficult to find evidence of its integration into the curriculum plan and its implementation.

Boutain (2005) discusses the concept of social justice and presents an example of how it is integrated into a Professional Nursing course for entry-level students. Vickers (2008) discusses social justice and the need for its integration into baccalaureate education. She discusses the profession and its behavior as an oppressed group, its emphasis in the past on clinical/apprentice-type learning, and its more recent move away from behaviorist-styled curricula to student-centered education. She is a proponent for assuring that students have opportunities for reflective and critical thinking in social justice venues to develop nurses who act on behalf of themselves, the profession, and the clients they care for when confronted with social justice issues.

Fahrenwald, Taylor, Kneip, and Canales (2007) present several definitions of social justice from a nursing perspective and the importance of it to nursing education and practice. They review the complexities of social justice and the need to analyze it from many perspectives and its role in the discipline of nursing. It has been a tradition for teaching social justice in public health courses; however, they point out that it transcends all specialties in nursing and needs to be integrated throughout the curriculum. In addition to analyzing the characteristics and concepts related to social justice, they advocate for its presentation in the nursing program through transformative learning activities. They believe that learners must participate in confronting issues related to social justice to become leaders in the health care system and advocates for the people who suffer health disparities and limited access to quality care. This idea applies to all concepts related to the philosophy that guides the curriculum and goes back to the theories related to teaching and learning. Each concept discussed and integrated into the philosophy and program of study must be considered by faculty for how it will be presented to students and how students will interact with it to assimilate and practice what the program defines as expectations for its graduates.

Research and Evidence-Based Practice

RESEARCH. Research provides the foundation for evidence-based practice. Both concepts appear in nursing curricula and should be addressed by faculty when developing or revising the philosophy of the educational program. Research concepts begin at the associate degree level and continue in complexity to the PhD where new knowledge is tested and added to the body of scientific knowledge for the discipline. Faculties identify the research competencies they expect of their graduates according to the level of the educational program and the practice areas or role functions that they expect their graduates to achieve. For example, associate degree programs expect their graduates to use evidence-based practice based upon credible, research-based nursing interventions and to challenge practices that lack data to support their use and do not result in quality patient outcomes.

Baccalaureate programs usually require a basic statistics course to support a separate nursing research course in the curriculum with expectations that graduates will understand the research process so that they can be discerning consumers of the research literature and use it to provide evidence-based practice. In an editorial on the critique of research, Morse (2006) describes research-related competencies for baccalaureate students. She advocates the development of an appreciation for research and its processes for its dissemination. She states that finding flaws and limitations in research is useful for baccalaureate students in reviewing research, the art of critiquing it for its significance and application to practice has a more practical purpose.

Most master's programs require a graduate level statistics course and at least one course in research, either as the sole topic or integrated with other related concepts such as nursing theory. They usually have options for theses, scholarly projects, or professional papers. Many include comprehensive examinations in addition to the thesis or project or as the only capstone requirement. The thesis can serve as a pathway to doctoral studies and uses extensive reviews and analysis of the literature in addition to utilization of research processes to investigate a problem. Projects or other scholarly works and professional papers at the master's level include extensive reviews of the literature and its integration to support the project or paper.

At the doctoral level, both research intensive and applied research projects require supporting research and statistical analyses courses. The number and depth of knowledge contained in these courses depend upon the type of doctoral program. Applied practice or professional doctoral projects and dissertations translate existing knowledge on a selected topic to develop new evidence-based strategies for advanced practice and/or application to leadership roles. Research-based PhD or DNSc dissertations synthesize knowledge of nursing science on a selected topic and generate new knowledge through quantitative, qualitative, or triangulation processes. Cowling (2005) offers advice to faculty in PhD programs. He states "A school that develops or has an existing PhD program should articulate a clear philosophical statement about the substance of the discipline of nursing and what constitutes advancement of nursing science. From my perspective, nursing's territory of knowledge encompasses the wide array of phenomena and concerns that are related to the health/illness experience of humans expressed individually and collectively by families, groups, communities, and societies" (p. 14).

EVIDENCE-BASED PRACTICE. Research is the base for evidence-based practice. Therefore, it is important for all levels of nursing education to graduate students who understand this concept and can discern between valid and reliable evidence-based nursing interventions and interventions that have no supportive data or rationale for their use. Evidence-based practice applies to all health care disciplines and its utilization has a major role in patient outcomes and quality care. As with the research process, evidence-based practice is leveled according to the type of nursing education program. Associate degree students should have theory and clinical experiences that demonstrate the use of evidence-based practice. Baccalaureate students further this knowledge by raising questions related to practice and seeking answers through literature review.

Spizale and Jacobson (2005) replicated a 2002 study of nursing programs across the country to learn what essential concepts in nursing commonly appeared in nursing curricula. Evidence-based practice was one of four items that demonstrated greater current emphasis or plans to develop greater emphasis in curricula for the future. BSN and diploma programs reported greater emphasis on evidence-based practice in 2003 than in 1998 and expected this trend to continue through 2008. Associate Degree in Nursing (ADN) programs did not have as great an emphasis but they expected it to have greater importance in the future.

An exemplar for integrating evidence-based practice into the undergraduate curriculum is offered by Aronson, Rebeschi, and Killion (2007). They describe a course on evidence-based practice for beginning level students in a baccalaureate program. Concepts related to the topic and instructional strategies in the laboratory and clinical settings were included. Aronson et al. surveyed students and faculty who participated in the course and found that students and faculty were satisfied with the course and both believed students were better prepared for evidence-based practice in the reality setting.

Another exemplar for integrating evidence-based practice into the curriculum, this time for senior baccalaureate students, is described by Kim, Brown, Fields, and Stichler (2009). They studied the outcomes related to an interactive teaching strategy used in two schools of nursing for students in evidence-based practice. The interactive strategy included lecture-style sessions to present concepts related to the topic followed by group projects and clinical opportunities with preceptors in the practice setting. Control groups received standard teaching. The authors reported statistically significant differences between the groups in knowledge gain with the interactive style demonstrating higher scores on a posttest than those of the control groups. However, there were no differences between the two groups in attitude toward evidence-based practice. The authors recommend replication studies to demonstrate the efficacy of the strategy and to delve into methods for changing attitudes toward evidence-based practice.

Master's students apply evidence-based practice in advanced roles, raise questions, and investigate current research to inform their practice. Students in applied practice or professional doctoral program synthesize this knowledge and generate new interventions for evidence-based practice. Theory-based doctoral students study the domain of evidence-based practice and develop new knowledge related to its use and value.

Research- and evidence-based practices are important concepts to include in philosophical statements for nursing curricula. The concepts can be leveled according to type of program and the statements provide guidelines for how the concepts will be delivered in the instructional program.

Informatics and Technology

Informatics and technology are crucial components of nursing education in order to meet their expanding development and impact on communications, research and scholarly activities, the delivery of health care, and teaching and learning modalities. As with many other concepts in nursing education that are discussed, technological advances are mentioned in the NLNAC Standards and Criteria for Associate Degree Programs in Nursing (NLNAC, 2010). Informatics and technology are listed in the essentials documents for the baccalaureate, master's, and the doctorate of advanced nursing practice (AACN, 2010d). Technology and informatics serve as platforms for the delivery of nursing education programs such as Web-based, hybrid, and Web-enhanced courses, and they apply to the practice setting as students gain nursing competencies in the care of clients.

In the clinical setting, students use personal digital assistants (PDAs), patient information systems, computerized medical records, telemedicine/nursing, and the high-tech devices for patient monitoring and care. It is important for faculty to be competent in these skills and knowledge for students to develop the necessary knowledge and skills in informatics and technology.

Thompson and Skiba (2008) conducted a survey of various levels of nursing programs (licensed practical nurse [LPN], ADN, Bachelor of Science in Nursing (BSN), and master's) on the integration of informatics into the curriculum. Although most programs reported integration of informatics into the curriculum, there remains confusion on the part of administrators and faculty as to what constitutes information literacy, computer literacy, and informatics competencies. The authors identified major gaps in all programs for using informatics to communicate with patients and care providers, manage care, and make clinical decisions.

To illustrate the findings of Thompson and Skiba, Fetter (2009) surveyed graduating baccalaureate nurses for their perceptions on their competencies in the application of information technology to their practice. The graduates reported confidence in computer skills such as word processing, Internet communications, and Web searching. However, they were not as confident in using informatics and technology in the patient care setting such as documentation and care planning. They indicated that integrating health information into practice is a priority. Fetter summarized by stating, "to facilitate current and future skills attainment and innovation, nursing informatics education and evaluation must keep pace" (p. 86).

Coyle, Duffy, and Martin (2007) report on a community health nursing experience for community college nursing students to provide health promotion services in a senior health center. Students maintained contact with the seniors through telephone calls to monitor their health status and to provide health counseling. Students were surveyed after the experience for their perceptions on the experience and the majority reported that the experience proved to be above average. The authors recommend follow-up of the seniors to gain their views on the experience with students through telehealth strategies. Although the follow-up study was not done, an anecdotal note from one of the seniors reported that she was an undiagnosed hypertensive prior to the contact with the program and with a year of the services from a nursing student lost 30 pounds to help control her hypertension. Although this is a low-tech strategy in today's high-tech world, it illustrates one way that technology can serve clients and provide students with clinical experiences in remote places.

Tilghman, Raley, and Conway (2006) reported on the use of PDAs in a family nurse practitioner (FNP) program. Students used the PDAs as a resource in the clinical setting and to record clinical findings for later documentation and case study analysis. The authors found that it is essential that faculty and students be trained in the use of the PDA and faculty needs to be supportive of its use. The authors also surveyed preceptors for their observations on the utility of the PDAs in the clinical setting. Preceptors were supportive of the use of PDAs because it gave students rapid access to information and helped them to gain confidence in differential diagnoses.

Quality Health Care and Patient Safety

Quality health care and patient safety concepts are embedded in nursing knowledge and clinical practice. However, they are receiving increased emphasis in the delivery of health care as the system becomes more complex. Increased acuity levels and patients with complex physiological and psychosocial challenges add to the challenges for providing safe and quality care. In addition, all of these factors call for interdisciplinary collaboration to assure a safe and compassionate health care environment. Therefore, these concepts need to be discussed when assessing and updating the philosophy of the educational program.

The Agency for Healthcare Research and Quality (2010) lists quality indicators and prevention strategies for patient safety. A useful Web site for finding the latest information on quality health care and patient safety is http://www.ahrq.gov. Hall, Moore, and Barnsteiner (2008) reviewed quality improvement strategies and linked them to the six quality indicators listed by the Institute of Medicine (IOM), that is, Patient-Centered Care, Teamwork and Collaboration, Evidence-Based Practice, Quality

Improvement, Safety, and Informatics (IOM, 2003). Hall et al. provide strategies for nurses in the practice setting to carry out these core competencies and present several examples of how nurses use these competencies. Their contribution provides ideas for nurse educators to include in the curriculum for the educational program.

Smith, Cronenwett, and Sherwood (2007) reported on a survey of faculty in prelicensure nursing programs for their perception of content experiences in the six core competencies for quality of health care and patient safety. Faculty indicated that the content was in the curriculum. However, later studies involving separate focus groups of faculty and new graduates found varying beliefs about the presence of the content in the curriculum. The faculty participants could not identify pedagogical methods for teaching quality and patient safety and the new graduates reported that they did not have experiences in their curricula and it was their belief that faculty did not have the expertise to teach it.

Cherot (2007) developed six research questions regarding content on patient safety in prelicensure programs. She surveyed nursing students from seven schools regarding their perceptions of patient safety defined by nurse experts as comfort, error reporting, denial, and culture factors. Cherot found differences among the students according to their racial/ethnic groups and type of prelicensure nursing program. All seven of the schools had content relating to at least three of the core competencies on patient safety and one school had evidence of all six. These findings identify the need for patient safety content in nursing curricula with appropriate learning strategies to assure the graduation of competent nurses. The competencies should be included in the assessment of the curriculum and their integration into it. A useful Web site for educators can be found at the Quality and Safety Education for Nursing home page (2010): http://www.qsen.org

Nursing's Metaparadigm

Although the debate continues about nursing as a science and a discipline, in most nursing education circles, a **metaparadigm for the nursing** discipline is recognized and included in the philosophy and organizing framework of the curriculum. Although there are numerous terms for the four domains of the nursing metaparadigm, the most commonly accepted terms are nursing (practice), environment, health, and the client (Fawcett, 1996).

Plummer and Molzahn (2009) conducted a concept analysis of "quality of life" as a possible replacement for one of the major concepts contained in the metaparadigm (i.e., health). They analyzed the concept of quality of life in its broader context and its application to nursing theorists' discussions about health. They found similarities in five theorists' discussions of quality of life that included Peplau (1952), Leininger (1997), Rogers (1970), King (1972), and Parse (1992). Plummer and Molzahn argue that quality of life encompasses psychological, sociological, and cultural aspects in addition to physical health and add that the consumer of health care is more apt to think of health as physical health.

The work of Plummer and Molzahn (2009) points out the need for the discipline to reflect on the usefulness of the metaparadigm to define itself and the possibility for conducting similar concept analyses to examine the other three components (i.e., nursing, environment, and person). The metaparadigm is a useful tool for organizing the numerous other concepts discussed under the curriculum components of the philosophy. It can serve the faculty as it begins to synthesize the various concepts into one overall statement of philosophy. Many of these same concepts are listed as critical for nursing education in the Commission on Collegiate Nursing Education (CCNE; 2010) and the National League for Nursing Accreditation Commission, Inc. (NLNAC; 2010) accreditation standards.

Organizational Frameworks and Concept Mapping

ORGANIZATIONAL FRAMEWORKS. Although accreditation is voluntary, most schools of nursing in the United States are accredited by a national organization, either the CCNE or the NLNAC (CCNE, 2010; NLNAC, 2010). At one time, both accrediting bodies required or implied that organizational frameworks were necessary to design the educational program's objectives, content and instructional design. It was common for schools of nursing to use theoretical or conceptual models from nursing or other related disciplines as organizational frameworks. These frameworks served a useful purpose to place certain theories, concepts, content, and clinical learning experiences into the curriculum. Although they are no longer explicitly required in the standards for accreditation, both CCNE (2010) and NLNAC (2010) make reference to an organizational structure for the curriculum. Many of the concepts listed under the discussion of the philosophy in this text are included in the accreditation standards for the curriculum (e.g., social justice, cultural diversity, patient safety, quality health care). The accreditation standards/competencies for CCNE and NLNAC may be found at their Web sites: http://www.aacn.nche.edu.Accreditation/pdf/standards09.pdf and http://www.nlnac.org

A word of caution: Faculty should check the regulations of the governing body in which the school of nursing is located such as state boards of nursing, when developing or revising the curriculum. Some of these agencies may require a conceptual or theoretic framework for the curriculum.

The organizational framework serves to logically order the delivery of the body of knowledge in the curriculum and provides a checklist of sorts that assures that no concepts are omitted. CCNE (2010) states in its standards for accreditation that baccalaureate and graduate programs including the Doctor of Nursing Practice (DNP) should demonstrate evidence for integrating the essentials and competencies developed by the American Association of Colleges of Nursing (AACN) for each level of education. Information on how to access these documents may be found at AACN's Web site (2010): http://www.aacn.nche.edu/Publications/PubsCatalog.htm. Likewise, the National League for Nursing (2010), in collaboration with the National Organization for Associate Degree Nursing Programs (NOADN), developed *Educational Competencies for Graduates of Associate Degree Nursing Programs* that provides guidelines for ADN programs. Information on how to access the document may be found at: http://www.nln.org/publications/ADN/index.htm. NLNAC lists competencies for other levels of nursing education including LPN, diploma, baccalaureate, master's, and the practice doctorate.

Scott Tilley (2008) analyzed the literature for a definition and measurement of competency in nursing students and how nurses who are in practice maintain competency. She found numerous articles from nursing including educational programs and state boards of nursing that describe the concept of competency. She pointed out that all health disciplines must find ways to demonstrate competencies for their professionals. Scott Tilley reports on several strategies to measure nursing competencies such as portfolios and measurements of skills and competencies as students move through a program. However, the major findings from her analysis were the continuing need to find ways in which to measure competencies and to analyze the concept of competencies. Because both of the major accrediting bodies for nursing education list competencies as part of their standards for accreditation, this is imperative and is a fertile ground for research on the topic.

CONCEPT MAPPING. The process of concept mapping is useful for assuring that essential knowledge and skills are integrated into the curriculum. Concept mapping is a detailed analysis of a concept and its relationships. As Novak and Canas (2008) advise, a concept analysis begins with a focus question. For example, nursing faculty could pose the question, "Where should the concept and skills for the nursing process occur in the curriculum and in what depth"? To answer the question, the major concept is placed on the top of the map with the related and subconcepts under it. Directional symbols are used to explain the relationships among them. The map can be composed of simple linear steps or complex with multiple pathways to illustrate integration of the concept into cognitive understanding and related behaviors or psychomotor skills.

Conceição and Taylor (2007) related concept mapping to constructivist learning theories and it is similar to systems theory. Giddens, Brady, Brown, Wright, Smith, and Harris (2008) describe a revised baccalaureate curriculum that was concept driven and based on the AACN Essentials document (AACN, 2010c). Although it is not a concept map per se, it illustrates an initial analysis for concept mapping by identifying the key concepts to be integrated into the curriculum. A sample of a concept map is found in the case study at the end of this chapter.

Once the mission and philosophy for the program are finalized, faculty identifies the major theories, concepts, and skills it believes should be in the curriculum. As the implementation plan for the curriculum is developed or as faculty assesses the curriculum, the process of concept mapping helps to identify where these elements occur. A useful Web site that discusses in detail the process of concept mapping is found at http://cmap.ihmc.us/ Publications/ResearchPapers/TheoryCmaps/TheoryUnderlyingConceptMaps.htm.

An example of how concept mapping applies to the development of critical thinking in the implementation of the curriculum is described in the article by Kinchin, Cabot, and Hay (2008) who analyzed the literature on professional knowledge and clinical practice. They discuss the terms of intuitive reasoning and tacit knowledge and compare them to the use of concept mapping to promote the development of expertise in clinical practice. They argue that both tacit knowledge and intuitive behaviors exhibited by experts in the discipline can be described through concept mapping. Their model for concept mapping includes the linear model of reasoning, which is a lock-step process, and a network model that maps out the relationship between the knowledge pieces and the processes that link them. The authors believe that using concept mapping for instructional design can lead to the development of critical thinking and clinical competence.

Implementation of the Curriculum

Overall Purpose and Goal of the Program

After the philosophy, mission, and organizing framework are chosen; the next logical step in curriculum development is to state the overall purpose or goal of the program. There are arguments against behavioral statements for goals as postmodernistic and humanistic philosophies take hold in the 21st century. The arguments against them relate to the lack of freedom they provide for the learner and for the teacher whose role is to empower the learner. At the same time, there are accountability issues that relate to graduates' competencies in meeting the health care systems' demands and the health care needs of the people they serve. Faculty must grapple with these issues as it develops statements of the purpose of the nursing program and the overall long-term goal for graduates. Whether the statement becomes global and idealistic or specific and stated in measurable terms depends upon the faculty's philosophy, values, and beliefs and subsequent statements and objectives that specify the graduates' learning outcomes.

In addition to a choice of the format of the statement of purpose or goal for a nursing program (i.e., global or behavioral), there are certain components belonging to professional nursing education that faculty may wish to consider and include, if not explicitly, implicitly. Examples of concepts that might be emphasized include statements on caring, health promotion, and other types of nursing interventions, client systems, professional behaviors and competencies, the health care system, and so forth. Characteristics of the graduate that are unique to the specific school of nursing can be included. For example, "a caring, compassionate health care provider."

The type of nursing education program influences the overall program purpose or goal statement. Levels of clinical competence and knowledge acquisition will differ among licensed vocational nursing, associate degree, baccalaureate, master's, and doctoral programs. Programs with multiple layers of preparation including undergraduate and graduate education usually have a global statement of purpose and then, each program, adapts that statement to meet its own level of education. Although the statement of purpose and overall goal can be succinct, it acts as the guide for end-of-program objectives. The statement must also reflect the faculty's mission statement, philosophy, and organizational framework.

Tanner, Gubrud-Howe, and Shores (2008) describe in detail the process for developing a statewide curriculum for nursing in Oregon that includes an overall goal and the objectives and outcomes that follow it. Swearington (2009) provides an example of an overall goal to develop nursing leadership in the practice setting. She describes the overall goal for the program and how it was leveled into learning outcomes throughout the curriculum.

Student Learning Outcomes or End-of-Program and Level Objectives

As reiterated throughout this chapter, nursing programs must demonstrate that they meet the overall program mission, purpose, and goal. SLOs or end-of-program objectives reflect the organizing framework and define the specific expectations or competencies of graduates upon completion of the nursing program. To reach these objectives, intermediate level or semester objectives are developed in sequential order. For example, in a 2-year associate degree program, there are end-of-first-year expectations and end-of-second-year expectations all of which lead to the end-of-program objectives. In a baccalaureate program, there may be freshman, sophomore, junior, and senior level objectives. Some programs prefer to divide the objectives into semesters and could be titled in that fashion (i.e., first semester, second semester, third semester, etc.). Graduate programs may indicate junior or senior levels, semester levels, first year and second year, doctorate candidate, and so forth.

Chapter 4 of the text presents educational taxonomies such as the classics developed by Bloom et al. (1956). These taxonomies categorize domains of learning and provide guidelines for writing objectives related to the domains. The major domains are cognitive, affective, psychomotor, and behavioral. Furthermore, these domains are divided into levels of development and difficulty. For example, in nursing, the psychomotor skill of measuring blood pressure moves from recognition of the blood pressure measurement tools to mastery of the skill. At the same time, the student is using the cognitive domain by first recalling the physiology of blood pressure and identifying the norms for blood pressure. The student continues to comprehend, apply, analyze, synthesize, and evaluate knowledge that results in nursing diagnosis and actions such as referral of clients for management of abnormal findings, teaching clients how to manage hypertension or hypotension, or in the case of the advanced practitioner, prescribing interventions to control hypertension.

The classic taxonomies assist in the development of end-of-program, level (intermediate), and course objectives. To develop or assess end-of-program objectives, the first task is to look at the program mission, purpose, and overall goal. Faculty members discuss what they expect of their graduates at the end of the program to meet the overall goal. A list of these expectations is developed into end-of-program objectives, which are analyzed for their specificity to meet the overall goal and the selected organizing framework of the curriculum. For example, if the NLNAC core competencies for associate degree nursing are used for the curriculum's organizational framework, the end-of-program objectives should include statements on nationally established patient health and safety goals as applied to nursing practice (Standard 4.8.1., NLNAC, 2010).

Level or semester objectives follow the end-of-program objectives and each of these steps may be viewed deductively or inductively to ensure that the total body of knowledge and skills expected at the end of the program are included in the curriculum plan. All levels of objectives provide the guidelines for planning and implementing the curriculum.

When developing objectives, there are basic components in them that provide ways in which to meet their expectations and to determine to what extent they are attained. The cardinal rule is that objectives must be learner focused. Additional components include the content as it relates to the outcome, expected learner behavior and at what level, feasibility, and the time frame. The content of the objective is what knowledge and/or skills that students are expected to learn. An example of an end-of-program objective is "the graduate will provide competent, compassionate nursing care based on assessment of clients and families across the life span." In this example, the content is nursing care, assessment, and clients and families. The behavior expected of the graduate is to "provide, competent, compassionate nursing care." This statement implies that the graduate will provide this care 100% of the time competently and also, compassionately. Objectives like these require definitions of competence and compassion and how to measure consistency in these behaviors (100% of the time). Thus, faculty agrees on definitions for these terms and prepares statements that describe them, usually in the philosophy and/or organizational framework. Based on these definitions, the faculty assesses the feasibility for accomplishing the objectives that includes the time frame (end of the program) and expected levels of performance and consistency. These are defined according to the type of program (i.e., associate degree, baccalaureate, advanced practice, or other graduate level tracks). Additional considerations relate to the resources available for implementing the objectives, the abilities of the graduates to accomplish them, and at what level.

Level or semester objectives follow the same pattern as the SLOs. Faculty reviews each level for the progression of objectives toward the end-of-program objectives. Some programs start from basic knowledge and skills at the first level or semester to the complex knowledge and skills expected at the senior level of the program. Other programs expect mastery of specific knowledge and skills earlier in the program that are reinforced throughout the program and practiced after graduation. Still other programs use a combination of both. Decisions on the patterns of progression will depend on the philosophy and organizational framework, including the developmental stage of the learner. These decisions should be documented with a rationale for their placement in the curriculum to aid in evaluation of the curriculum and total quality management of the program.

Program of Study

The overall goal, SLOs, level objectives, and organizing framework serve as a master plan for placing content into the curriculum and developing a program of study. Faculty is responsible for developing the curriculum plan and revising it periodically as needed. The prerequisites for the program are examined for their logical location in the curriculum. Prerequisites for prelicensure nursing programs include the liberal arts; social, physical, and biological sciences; communications; mathematics; and other general education (GE) requirements.

Graduate nursing programs usually require a baccalaureate in nursing; although students with associate degrees in nursing and a baccalaureate in another discipline can sometimes be admitted conditionally subject to completing prescribed courses in nursing that the faculty designates as requirements for meeting the equivalent of a baccalaureate in nursing. The same principles apply to nursing or other disciplines' doctorate programs. Each doctoral program will prescribe the courses or degree work necessary to meet the equivalent of their lower degree requirements.

Once the prerequisites are completed, the nursing curriculum plan has a progressive order for sequencing nursing courses. For example, a Nursing 101 (Fundamentals of Nursing) course is a prerequisite for Nursing 102 (Nursing Care of the Older Adult), and Nursing 501 (Nursing Research) is the prerequisite for Nursing 502 (Master's Thesis). Corequisites are courses that can be taught simultaneously and are complementary; for example Nursing 301 (Health Promotion of Children and Adolescents) and Nursing 303 (Nursing Care of Children and Adolescents). Again, the placement of courses depends on the organizing framework with the course objectives and content leading toward the achievement of level objectives and eventually, the program outcomes.

The numbers of units or credits are assigned to each course keeping in mind the total allotted to the major. For associate degree in nursing programs, nursing credits average 30 semester credits with total degree requirements averaging 60 to 70 semester credits. It should be noted that some programs operate on quarter credits or units that are usually 10 weeks in length as contrasted to the usual semester length of 15 weeks. In that case, 1-quarter credit or unit is equivalent to two thirds of a semester credit or unit.

Baccalaureate programs average 60 nursing credits with 120 to 130 credits for the degree. The master's in nursing program ranges from 30 to 60 or more total credits depending on the nature of the program, with advanced practice roles requiring the higher number of credits. Because of the wide range of nursing credits at the master's level, the profession is moving toward advanced practice degrees at the doctoral level. The AACN issued a position paper recommending that the preparation of advanced practice nurses move to the doctorate level by 2015 (AACN, 2009). The majority of master's and doctorate degree credits are in the nursing major with only a few from other disciplines or electives.

Content experts serve as guides for nursing course placements and once the courses have been placed in logical sequence, the course descriptions are written, usually by the content expert or the person who will serve as "faculty of record" (in charge of the course). For example, the content expert of the course "Nursing Care of Children and Adolescents" would probably be a faculty member certified as a clinical specialist or nurse practitioner in pediatrics. Course descriptions are brief paragraphs with several comprehensive statements that provide an overview of the content of the course. They do not contain student-centered objectives.

Course objectives follow the course description, are learner centered, based on the content of the course, their place in the curriculum plan, relationship to the level and end-of-program objectives, and relevance to the organizational framework. Finally, an outline of the course content is listed and should be tied to the objectives of the course. A course schedule is usually included and tied to the content outline. See Exhibit 7.1 for a classic outline for a course syllabus.

All of these components are subject to faculty approval as well as the parent institution. Once established, faculty members who are assigned to courses have the freedom to rearrange or update the content and to teach the courses in their preferred method. However, changes to the course title, credits, objectives, or descriptions must undergo the same approval processes as the original courses. Although this may appear stifling to academic freedom, it ensures the integrity of the curriculum.

Usually, new or revised course descriptions, objectives, and content outlines are presented to the program's curriculum committee for recommendations and approval, are submitted to the total faculty for approval, and continue through the appropriate channels of the parent institution for final formal approval. Because of the many layers of approval, faculty must be mindful of the initial proposals so that they will not need frequent revision as any changes to course titles, credits, descriptions, number of credits, and objectives are subject to the same review processes.

EXHIBIT 7.1 The Major Components of a Syllabus

Parent Institution Logo School of Nursing

Type of Program

Course Number and Title

Course Description:

Credits:

Prerequisite or Corequisites:

Class Type: (Lecture, Seminar, Laboratory, Practicum)

Faculty Information:

Required and Recommended Texts:

Course Objectives:

Teaching and Learning Strategies: (include teacher and student expectations)

Attendance and Participation Requirements:

Evaluation Methods:

Assignments:

Course Content and Schedule:

Academic Dishonesty Statement:

Disability Statement:

SUMMARY

This chapter reviewed the components of the curriculum and the processes faculty undergo in developing or revising curricula. Assessing and revising (if necessary) each component of the curriculum in logical sequence helps to maintain its integrity and assure its quality. Faculty members are experts in their discipline and are therefore, responsible for ensuring that essential knowledge as well as the latest breakthroughs in its science is in the curriculum. Curriculum development and revision processes must be based on information from evaluation activities; the latest changes in the profession, health care, and society; and forecasts for the future. Table 7.1 provides guidelines for assessing the key components of a curriculum or educational program.

TABLE 7.1 Guidelines for Assessing the Key Components of a Curriculum or Educational Program

Component	Questions for data collection	Desired outcomes
Mission	What are the major elements of the parent institution and subdivision (if applicable) missions? Are these major elements in the nursing mission? If not, give a rationale as to why. How does the nursing mission speak to its teaching, service, and research/scholarship roles?	The nursing mission is congruent with that of its parent institution and if applicable, the academic subdivision in which it is located. The mission reflects nursing's teaching, service, and research/scholarship role.
Philosophy	Is the nursing philosophy congruent with that of the parent institution philosophy and subdivision (if applicable)? If not, give the rationale as to why they are not. What statements in the philosophy relate to the faculty's beliefs and values about, teaching and learning, critical thinking, diversity and cultural competence, social justice, research and evidence-based practice, quality health care and patient safety, and nursing's metaparadigm?	The philosophy statement is congruent with that of the parent institution and academic subdivision (if applicable). The philosophy reflects the faculty's beliefs and values on teaching and learning, critical thinking, diversity, and cultural competence, genetics, social justice, research and evidence-based practice, informatics and technology, quality health care and patient safety, and nursing's metaparadigm.
Organizing framework	What is the organizing framework for the curriculum and how does it reflect the mission and philosophy statements? To what extent does the framework appear throughout the implementation of the curriculum? Are its concepts readily identified in all of the tracks of the programs?	The curriculum has an organizing framework that reflects its mission and philosophy. The concepts of the organizing framework are readily identified in all tracks of the nursing education program.

(Continued)

TABLE 7.1 Guidelines for Assessing the Key Components of a Curriculum or Educational Program *Continued*

Component	Questions for data collection	Desired outcomes
Overall Purpose and Goal of the Program	To what extent does the overall goal or purpose statement reflect the mission, philosophy, and organizing framework?	The overall goal or purpose statement reflects that of the mission, philosophy, and organizing framework.
	Is the statement broad enough to encompass all tracks of the nursing program?	The overall goal or purpose includes all tracks of the nursing program.
	To what extent does the statement lead to the measurement of program outcomes?	The overall goal or purpose is stated in such a way that it is a guide for measuring outcomes of the program (program review).
Student Learning Outcomes (SLOs) **End-of-Program and Level Objectives**	To that extent are the mission, overall goal or purpose, and organizational framework reflected in the objectives?	The objectives reflect the mission, overall purpose or goal, and organizing framework.
	How are the objectives arranged in logical and sequential order?	The objectives are sequential and logical.
	Is each objective learner centered and does it include the content, expected level of behavior of the learner, feasibility, and time frame?	The objective statements are learner centered and include the content, expected learner behavior and at what level, feasibility, and time frame.
Implementation plan	To what extent does the curriculum plan reflect the organizing framework, overall goal, end-of-program, and level objectives?	The implementation plan for the curriculum reflects the organizing framework, overall goal or purpose, end-of-program, and level objectives.
	Is there documentation of approval of the curriculum plan in the permanent records?	The curriculum plan and its prerequisites and courses have the approval of the appropriate governing bodies.
	Does each track in the program have a curriculum plan that includes course descriptions, credits, prerequisite and corequisites, objectives, and content outlines?	The implementation plan for each track includes all courses and credits, prerequisite or corequisites, descriptions, objectives, and content outlines.
Summary	Has each component of the curriculum been addressed?	Each component is addressed based on an analysis of the curriculum.
	To what extent is each component congruent with those of the parent institution? If not congruent, has the rationale for incongruence been addressed?	The curriculum components are congruent with the parent institution and with each other.
	Are the components of the curriculum listed, and do they flow in a logical and sequential order?	The components flow in a logical and sequential order.
	To what extent does the implementation plan flow from the overall goal, SLOs or end-of-program objectives, and level objectives?	The implementation plan flows from the overall goal, SLOs, and level objectives.
	To what extent is the implementation plan congruent with the organizing framework?	The implementation plan is congruent with the organizing framework.
	To what extent is the curriculum relevant to current and future nursing practice demands and needs for nurses?	The curriculum reflects relevance to current nursing practice demands and the need for nurses and projected future changes in the health care system.

CASE STUDY

*T*he Case Study from Chapters 5 and 6 continue with a description of the processes faculty used in a fictional school of nursing to revise its RN to BSN program that accelerates into the MSN and to develop an Entry-Level Master of Science Nursing (EL-MSN) program and a post-master's DNP curriculum. The EL-MSN will produce new RNs into the workforce, whereas the RN to BSN to MSN and the DNP program will produce advanced practice nurses for the evolving health care system. The decision to revise the curriculum and develop new programs was agreed upon by the faculty. Administrative units in the College were advised of the proposals and approved them and the State Board of Nursing approved the EL-MSN tentatively, while awaiting the final proposal. The accrediting agencies were made aware of the proposed programs and are standing by for review and approval of the program proposals.

Because the school of nursing has an RN to BSN program and there are three tracks in the MSN program, it is anticipated that it will take 1 academic year to develop the program. The EL-MSN program accelerates college graduates through baccalaureate level nursing courses into the MSN program. It is anticipated that it will be developed in tandem with the RN to BSN to MSN program. The school plans to admit the first classes for both tracks in the spring semester following completion of the curricula and approval of the state board of nursing and accrediting bodies. The post-master's DNP program will be developed over 1.5 academic years with the first class admitted in the fall of the second year.

Mission

The faculty reviews the existing College and School of Nursing mission statements that are found in the most recent accreditation reports as well as the College catalogue and recruiting materials. The College mission states: "The mission of the College is to educate students in the traditions of the liberal arts, sciences, and spiritual beliefs of its founding fathers to become intellectually and socially responsible, compassionate citizens and leaders in their communities and society." The School of Nursing mission statement states: "The mission of the School of Nursing is to prepare intellectually and socially aware, competent, and compassionate nurses and nurse leaders to meet the health care needs of their communities and society."

The faculty agrees that both missions are similar and contain elements of teaching, service, and research. Specifically, the School of Nursing mission implies teaching and learning by the verb *prepare* and all that it entails including acquisition of knowledge and skills. The service element specifies that the graduates will provide competent and compassionate care to communities and society and the allusions to intellectual and social awareness imply research or in this case, scholarly activities and evidence-based practice. Because the RN to BSN to MSN program is an adaptation of the existing RN to BSN program and operates within the mission, it is determined that it is not in conflict with the current College and School of Nursing mission statements that, in turn, are congruent. The same is true for both the EL-MSN and the DNP programs and in addition, both prepare nurse leaders.

Philosophy

The Philosophy statement of the College is as follows: "The College fosters the liberal study of the arts and sciences of humanity in its diverse historical and cultural forms and of the insight derived from spiritual and religious study. Students and faculty interact in critical and creative thinking processes and effective communication to acquire the skills needed for active participation and leadership in transforming their communities and the world. Through faculty's research and scholarly activities and collaborative teaching and learning processes, students cultivate a global perspective that embodies the values of social justice and compassion and results in the responsible valuing and sharing of knowledge and skills as articulate and responsible citizens and leaders in their communities."

The School of Nursing Philosophy states: Students and faculty of the School of Nursing interact in teaching and learning processes that empower students to build upon a strong liberal arts and sciences foundation and assimilate the nursing knowledge and skills that lead to the provision of competent and compassionate nursing care and leadership for multicultural and ethnic persons, families, aggregates, and communities. The nursing paradigm guides the students and faculty in the teaching and learning processes to foster creative thought, critical thinking, clinical decision making, and ethical and professional judgments. The faculty defines the metaparadigm as follows:

Nursing: A science and profession that provides evidence-based practice for client systems in various health care settings. Nursing uses research, informatics, and technology to inform practice and coordinate care. Nursing uses effective communication and collaboration with other professions to assure safe and quality health care.

Client system: It is composed of multicultural, racial, and ethnic individuals, families, aggregates, and communities and is the focus of nursing care. The individual, as a recipient of nursing and health care services, is a spiritual, biopsychosocial being. The family is composed of persons with close biological or psychosocial ties that bind them together as a subsystem of the community in which they are members. The aggregate is a group of persons with at-risk health needs within the community in which they are members. The community is composed of individuals, groups, and aggregates with social, geographical, functional, or political ties.

Health: The optimum state of well-being along a continuum of wellness and illness throughout the life span from conception to death. Nursing has a key role in providing health promotion and prevention of disease services for client systems.

Environment: The milieu and external factors that surround the caregiving phenomenon and the interactions of the client system and care provider with these factors. The profession has a major role in analyzing the health care system and its financial structure to recognize social justice issues and shape public policies that affect the health of the local, regional, and world communities.

An analysis of the philosophies of the College and School of Nursing reveals that they are congruent. Although the nursing philosophy does not speak specifically to that of the College's statement on religious study, it incorporates the notion of spirituality and designates the study of the liberal arts and sciences including religious studies as the foundation for nursing knowledge and skills. The nursing statement includes teaching and learning, ethnic diversity, and critical thinking, clinical decision making, and professional and ethical judgments. The philosophy is broad enough to incorporate all levels of the nursing program and its definitions of the components of the nursing paradigm include concepts from the AACN Essentials documents.

Organizing Framework

The School of Nursing uses the "Essentials" documents for the undergraduate and graduate programs published by the AACN (AACN, 2010a) serving as the organizing framework for the programs. Thus, the generic BSN and the RN to BSN programs are organized according to the *Essentials for Baccalaureate Education for Professional Nursing Practice* (AACN, 2010c). The graduate program uses the *Essentials of Master's Education for Advanced Practice Nursing* (AACN, 2010e) and AACN's (2010d) the *Essentials of Doctoral Education for Advanced Nursing Practice* for the new DNP program. Faculty members analyze the Essentials documents for their relationship to the mission and philosophy statements and find them to be congruent. For example, the baccalaureate Essentials (AACN, 2010c) have most of the same concepts discussed in the school's philosophy and states that it: "emphasizes such concepts as patient centered care, interprofessional teams, evidence-based practice, quality improvement, patient safety, informatics, clinical reasoning/critical thinking, genetics and genomics, cultural sensitivity, professionalism, and practice across the life span in an ever-changing and complex health care environment" (p. 3). The DNP builds upon the undergraduate and master's programs and as stated by AACN (2010d): "One constant is true for all of these models. The DNP is a graduate degree and is built upon the generalist foundation acquired through a baccalaureate or advanced generalist master's in nursing" (p. 6).

Overall Purpose and Goal of the Program

The School of Nursing's overall goal is: The School of Nursing prepares highly competent and compassionate nurses and nurse leaders to deliver professional nursing care and interprofessional health care for multicultural and ethnic people, families, aggregates, and communities in all settings.

The faculty agrees that the goal is broad enough to encompass the undergraduate and graduate programs. Some members raise the question about the term *nurse leaders* as it applies to the baccalaureate program; however, they agree that leadership in its broadest terms apply to those graduates as well as the graduates of the master's program. They point to the baccalaureate senior level Nursing Management course as well as the Health Policy course as foundations for preparing nurse leaders. The overall goal provides guidelines for the end-of-program objectives for all of the tracks and for evaluation of the outcomes of the program. By analyzing the mission and philosophy of the school, terms in the goal statement can be traced back to terms in those statements.

Student Learning Outcomes (End-of-Program) and Level Objectives

Both the accelerated RN to BSN to MSN program and the entry-level master's program are adaptations of the existing baccalaureate and master's programs. Therefore, the SLOs (end-of-program objectives) are the same as the existing master's program SLOs. Please see Table 7.2 for a listing of the SLOs and the level objectives to reach these SLOs for each of the programs (i.e., BSN, RN to BSN to MSN, EL-MSN, and the DNP). Note the increasing depth in the SLOs from the BSN to the DNP and the alignment with the AACN Essentials documents. An analysis of the SLOs for all of these programs demonstrates that the they are congruent with the mission, philosophy, conceptual framework, and overall goal.

BSN Program

The BSN program is an upper division level program, thus students begin nursing courses in the junior year. There are two levels of objectives, Level 1 and Level 2, with the latter identical to the SLOs (end-of-program objectives). See Table 7.2 for a list of SLOs and level objectives. A sample syllabus from the BSN program appears at the end of the case study.

RN to BSN to MSN Program

To move into graduate level courses, RNs complete the equivalent of upper division level BSN courses having completed lower division courses in their entry-level nursing programs (ADN or Diploma). It is planned that the accelerated RN to BSN to MSN program will take 3 years to complete. The first year is 1 calendar year (3 semesters) and students complete the equivalent of upper division nursing courses in the BSN program. Therefore, the level objectives for Year 1 of the RN program are the same as the SLOs for the basic BSN. The RNs take many of the same courses that junior and senior students in the BSN program take (i.e., Pathophysiology, Genetics, Health Assessment, Interprofessional Health Care Practice: Communication and Collaboration, Introduction to Nursing Research, Nursing Leadership, Community Health Nursing Theory and Practice, Analysis of the Health Care System, and two upper division

TABLE 7.2 Student Learning Outcomes and Level Objectives for the BSN, RN to BSN to MSN, MSN, and DNP Program

Objectives	Basic BSN	RN to BSN to MSN
Level 1	1. Relate knowledge from other disciplines to the evidence-based nursing care of multicultural and ethnic individuals and families across the life span. (Junior level) 2. Build nursing knowledge and skills to provide competent and compassionate care for multicultural and ethnic individuals and families in select health care settings. 3. Discuss the professional role of nursing and its collaborative role with other health care disciplines. 4. Examine the organization of the health care system, its financial structure, and the role of nursing in health-related issues, ethics, and public policy. 5. Relate current and relevant informatics, technology, and nursing research to the generalist practice of nursing. 6. Discuss social justice issues related to the health care delivery system and the role of nursing. 7. Discuss continuing education, lifelong learning, and graduate study in nursing.	1. Analyze knowledge from other disciplines to evidence-based nursing care of multicultural and ethnic individuals and families across the life span. 2. Apply nursing knowledge and skills with competency and compassion for multicultural and ethnic individuals, families, and communities in select health care settings. 3. Analyze the professional role of nursing and its collaborative role with other health care disciplines. 4. Discuss the organization of the health care system, its financial structure, and the role of nursing in health-related issues, ethics, and public policy. 5. Apply current and relevant informatics, technology, and nursing research to the generalist practice of nursing. 6. Identify social justice issues by participating in nursing and community action groups that seek to improve the health care delivery system. 7. Build a foundation for lifelong learning and graduate study.
Level 2	*This is senior level See SLOs for Basic BSN.*	1. Synthesize knowledge from other disciplines to develop intellectual and social knowledge and skills that apply to advanced nursing practice and responsibilities as citizens and leaders in the community and society. 2. Apply nursing knowledge and skills with competency and compassion for multicultural and ethnic individuals, families, and communities in select health care settings. 3. Analyze the professional role of nursing and inter-professional collaboration through community service and scholarly activities. 4. Analyze the organization of the health care system, its financial structure, and the role of nursing in health-related issues, ethics, and public policy. 5. Analyze the development of nursing as a science through the review of theory, scientific processes, research, informatics and technology. 6. Analyze social justice issues as they apply to nursing and health policy actions for improving the health care delivery system. 7. Analyze professional nursing as it pertains to advanced practice nursing and doctoral studies.

MSN	Entry-Level MSN	DNP
1. Synthesize knowledge from other disciplines to develop intellectual and social knowledge and skills that apply to advanced nursing practice and responsibilities as citizens and leaders in the community and society.	1. Relate knowledge from other disciplines to the evidence-based nursing care of multicultural and ethnic individuals and families across the life span.	Level objectives to be developed
2. Build advanced nursing knowledge and skills to provide evidence-based, competent and compassionate nursing care for multicultural and ethnic people, families, aggregates, and communities across the life span in various health care settings.	2. Build nursing knowledge and skills to provide competent and compassionate care for multicultural and ethnic individuals and families in select health care settings.	
3. Analyze the professional role of nursing and interprofessional collaboration through community service and scholarly activities.	3. Discuss the professional role of nursing and its collaborative role with other health care disciplines.	
4. Analyze the organization of the health care system, its financial structure, and the role of nursing in health-related issues, ethics, and public policy.	4. Examine the organization of the health care system, its financial structure, and the role of nursing in health-related issues, ethics, and public policy.	
5. Analyze the development of nursing as a science through the review of theory, scientific processes, research, informatics and technology.	5. Relate current and relevant informatics, technology, and nursing research to the generalist practice of nursing.	
6. Analyze social justice issues as they apply to nursing and health policy actions for improving the health care delivery system.	6. Discuss social justice issues related to the health care delivery system and the role of nursing.	
7. Analyze professional nursing as it pertains to advanced practice nursing and doctoral studies.	7. Discuss continuing education, lifelong learning, and graduate study in nursing.	
This is final year See SLOs for MSN.	1. Analyze knowledge from other disciplines to evidence-based nursing care of multicultural and ethnic individuals and families across the life span.	See SLOs
	2. Build nursing knowledge and skills to provide competent and compassionate care for multicultural and ethnic individuals and families in select health care settings.	
	3. Analyze the professional role of nursing and its collaborative role with other health care disciplines.	
	4. Analyze the organization of the health care system, its financial structure, and the role of nursing in health-related issues, ethics, and public policy.	
	5. Apply current and relevant informatics, technology, and nursing research to the generalist practice of nursing.	
	6. Identify social justice issues by participating in nursing and community action groups that seek to improve the health care delivery system.	
	7. Build a foundation for lifelong learning and graduate study.	

(Continued)

TABLE 7.2 Student Learning Outcomes and Level Objectives for the BSN, RN to BSN to MSN, MSN, and DNP Program *Continued*

Objectives	Basic BSN	RN to BSN to MSN
Level 3	*There is no Level 3 in Nursing for the Basic BSN*	*There is no Level 3 in Nursing for the RN to BSN to MSN*
Student learning outcomes (SLOs) (End-of-program objectives)	1. Analyze knowledge from other disciplines to the evidence-based nursing care of multicultural and ethnic individuals and families across the life span. 2. Apply nursing knowledge and skills with competency and compassion for multicultural and ethnic individuals, families, and communities in select health care settings. 3. Analyze the professional role of nursing and its collaborative role with other health care disciplines. 4. Analyze the organization of the health care system, its financial structure and the role of nursing in health-related issues, ethics, and public policy. 5. Apply current and relevant informatics, technology, and nursing research to the generalist practice of nursing. 6. Identify social justice issues by participating in nursing and community action groups that seek to improve the health care delivery system. 7. Build a foundation for lifelong learning and graduate study.	1. Evaluate knowledge from other disciplines to develop intellectual, social, and political knowledge and skills that apply to nursing and responsibilities as citizens and leaders in the community and society. 2. Apply advanced nursing knowledge and skills to provide evidence-based, competent and compassionate advanced practice nursing care for multicultural and ethnic people, individuals, families, aggregates, and communities across the life span and in various health care settings. 3. Value the professional role of nursing and interprofessional collaboration in the delivery of health care through community service and scholarly activities. 4. Evaluate the organization of the health care system, its financial structure, and the role of nursing in health-related issues, ethics, and public policy. 5. Contribute to the development of nursing as a science through the use of theory, scientific processes, research, informatics, and technology. 6. Using a broad understanding of social justice issues, participate in nursing and health care policy actions to improve the health care delivery system. 7. Gain the foundation for advanced practice nursing and doctoral studies.

MSN	Entry-Level MSN	DNP
There is no Level 3 in Nursing for the MSN	1. Synthesize knowledge from other disciplines to develop intellectual and social knowledge and skills that apply to advanced nursing practice and responsibilities as citizens and leaders in the community and society.	See SLOs
	2. Build advanced nursing knowledge and skills to provide competent and compassionate care for multicultural and ethnic individuals and families in select health care settings.	
	3. Analyze the professional role of nursing and interprofessional collaboration through community service and scholarly activities.	
	4. Analyze the organization of the health care system, its financial structure, and the role of nursing in health related issues, ethics, and public policy.	
	5. Analyze the development of nursing as a science through the review of theory, scientific processes, research, informatics, and technology.	
	6. Analyze social justice issues as they apply to nursing and health policy to improve health care delivery.	
	7. Analyze nursing as it relates to advanced practice and doctoral studies.	
1. Evaluate knowledge from other disciplines to develop intellectual, social, and political knowledge and skills that apply to nursing and responsibilities as citizens and leaders in the community and society.	1. Evaluate knowledge from other disciplines to develop intellectual, social, and political knowledge and skills that apply to nursing and responsibilities as citizens and leaders in the community and society.	1. Apply knowledge from other disciplines to assume leadership in nursing, the health care system, and as citizens in the community and society.
2. Apply advanced nursing knowledge and skills to provide evidence-based, competent and compassionate advanced practice nursing care for multicultural and ethnic people, individuals, families, aggregates, and communities across the life span and various health care settings.	2. Apply advanced nursing knowledge and skills to provide evidence-based, competent and compassionate advanced practice nursing care for multicultural and ethnic people, individuals, families, aggregates, and communities across the life span and in various health care settings.	2. Provide evidence-based practice to improve nursing and health care for multicultural and ethnic client systems in various health care settings.
3. Value the professional role of nursing and interprofessional collaboration in the delivery of health care through community service and scholarly activities.	3. Value the professional role of nursing and interprofessional collaboration in the delivery of health care through community service and scholarly activities.	3. Assume leadership in health care systems through nursing and interprofessional collaboration in the delivery of health care through advanced practice, community service, and scholarly activities.
4. Evaluate the organization of the health care system, its financial structure, and the role of nursing in health-related issues, ethics, and public policy.	4. Evaluate the organization of the health care system, its financial structure, and the role of nursing in health-related issues, ethics, and public policy.	4. Participate in professional and ethical nursing activities that relate to issues and changes in the organization of the health care system, its financial structure, and public policy.
5. Contribute to the development of nursing as a science through the use of theory, scientific processes, research, informatics, and technology.	5. Contribute to the development of nursing as a science through the use of theory, scientific processes, research, informatics, and technology.	5. Apply nursing theories, analytical processes, clinical research, informatics, and technology to the provision of evidence-based advanced nursing practice.
6. Using a broad understanding of social justice issues, participate in nursing and health care policy actions to improve the health care delivery system.	6. Using a broad understanding of social justice issues, participate in nursing and health care policy actions to improve the health care delivery system.	6. Address social justice issues by evaluating nursing and health care policies to act as a change agent and client advocate in the health care delivery system.
7. Gain the foundation for advanced practice nursing and doctoral studies.	7. Gain the foundation for advanced practice nursing and doctoral studies.	7. Use research and evidence for lifelong learning and to bring about change in health care.

GE required core courses. A Professional Nursing course is the first course that RNs take to bridge concepts from lower division courses to upper division. A sample syllabus for this course appears at the end of the case study.

After completing Level 1 courses, the RNs spend 2 semesters in the first level of the MSN program. They select the advanced practice option they wish to major in (i.e., Family Nurse Practitioner (FNP), Adult Health Clinical Specialty, or Family Health Care Specialty. The objectives for Level 2 of the RN to BSN to MSN program are the same as Level 1 of the MSN program. The Level 3 objectives for the RN to BSN to MSN program are the same as the SLOs of the MSN program (see Table 7.2).

MSN Program

The existing MSN program has three tracks (i.e., FNP, and two Clinical Specialties in Adult and Family Health Care). The full time program is 2 calendar years long with 2 summer terms. All students have core courses in nursing theory, research, health care policy, and advanced pathophysiology, pharmacology, and health assessment. Their specialty courses consist of three didactic courses with clinical preceptorships for each. Students complete 600 hours of supervised clinical practice by the end of the program. In addition, students complete either a thesis or project as a capstone experience. Like the BSN program, it has two levels, Level 1 with intermediate objectives and Level 2, which have objectives identical to the SLOs of the MSN program (see Table 7.2). A sample syllabus from the MSN program appears at the end of the case study.

Entry-Level MSN Program

The entry-level master's program consists of three levels. The first level is the prelicensure content and is 4 semesters in length (including a summer session) ending with the SLOs of the BSN program. The second level is at the graduate level, meets graduate Level 1 objectives, and is another 3 semesters including summer. The third level is 3 semesters including summer. The level objectives for that year are the same as those of the MSN student learning outcomes. The total program is 8 semesters full time for a total of 3.5 calendar years (see Table 7.2). A sample syllabus from the Entry-Level MSN program that is the same as a Level 2 SLO course in the MSN appears at the end of the case study.

The DNP Program

To guide the Task Force of faculty members who are developing the DNP program, the Curriculum Committee develops SLOs for the program. As with the other programs in the school, the organizational framework used for the DNP program is the AACN's (2010d) *Essentials of Doctoral Education for Advanced Nursing Practice*. Upon completion, the committee brings the objectives to the faculty as a whole for approval. Once approved, they go to the DNP Task Force for developing level objectives and the courses needed for students to meet the objectives (see Table 7.2 for the list of the DNP SLOs).

A sample syllabus from the DNP program appears at the end of the case study. It is a course that occurs in the last semester of the DNP program.

Summary

The faculty agrees that the level objectives for the RN to BSN to MSN, the entry-level MSN, and the DNP programs come from the SLOs (end-of-program objectives); are learner focused; contain the content of what is to be learned; and specify when they are to be completed and to what extent. The level objectives imply mastery of the content, they must be met by the end of course-work for each level, and are arranged in sequential order. All of the objectives are measurable and serve as guides for collecting data for formative (course and level reviews) and summative (program review) evaluation.

Sample Courses for the BSN, RN to BSN to MSN, the MSN, the entry-level MSN, and the DNP program follow. A concept map for one theme (inter-professional collaboration) that runs throughout the nursing program is presented.

Sample Courses

BSN Level 1

Overarching Objective for Level 1 of the BSN Program

Discuss the professional role of nursing and its collaborative role with other health care disciplines.

Course title: Nursing and Health Care
Credits: 3 units (theory)
Prerequisite courses: Completion of lower division level GE requirements, Anatomy, Physiology, Chemistry, Genetics, Microbiology, Nutrition, Human Development.
Description: Introduces the nursing profession, its history, the science of nursing, current issues, and ethics. Discusses the role of the interprofessional health care team. Reviews the definitions of health and the health and illness continuum across the life span.
Objectives: At the end of the course, the student will:

1. Analyze the history of nursing and its impact on its status as a profession and a discipline.
2. Compare the definitions of a profession and an academic discipline to nursing.

3. Review the major health disciplines and their role in providing health care.
4. Formulate a definition of health and illness across a continuum and the life span for multicultural and ethnic people.
5. Examine selected issues in health care and nursing that have an impact on health care and the ethics for providing nursing care.

Content outline:

1. Nursing History
2. Nursing as a Profession
3. Nursing as a Science and an Academic Discipline
4. The Interprofessional Health Care Team
5. Health and Illness Definitions
6. Diversity and the Delivery of Competent and Compassionate Nursing Care
7. Health Care Issues and the Ethics of Nursing Care

RN to BSN to MSN Level 1 (bridge course between levels 1 and 2 of the BSN)

Overarching Objective from the SLOs BSN Program

Analyze the professional role of nursing and its collaborative role with other health care disciplines.

Course title: The Nursing Profession
Credits: 3 units (theory)
Prerequisite courses: Graduation with a GPA of 3.0 from an associate degree program in nursing. Diploma graduates must have an overall 3.0 GPA from the Diploma program *and* complete a portfolio to demonstrate equivalency to the ADN.
Course description: Reviews nursing education and the profession, the science of nursing, current issues, and ethics. Discusses the role of nursing and collaboration with the interprofessional health care team. Analyzes health and the health and illness continuum across the life span as it applies to the nursing role.
Objectives: At the end of the course, the student will:

1. Analyze nursing education and its impact on its status as a profession and a discipline.
2. Analyze the nursing profession as an academic discipline.
3. Identify the major health disciplines and their relationships to nursing in providing health care.
4. Discuss nursing's role in health and illness across its continuum and across the life span for multicultural and ethnic people.
5. Analyze selected issues in health care and nursing that have an impact on health care and the ethics for providing nursing care.

Content outline:

1. Nursing Education
2. Nursing as a Profession
3. Nursing as a Science and an Academic Discipline
4. Interprofessional Collaboration
5. Health and Illness
6. Diversity and the Delivery of Competent and Compassionate Nursing Care
7. Health Care Issues and the Ethics of Nursing Care

MSN Level 1

Overarching objective from Level 1 of the MSN Program

Analyze the professional role of nursing and interprofessional collaboration in the delivery of health care through community service and scholarly activities.

Course title: Advanced Practice and Leadership Roles in Nursing
Credits: 3 units (theory)
Prerequisite courses: Admission into the MSN program *or* completion of Level 1 courses for RN to BSN to MSN program *or* completion of Level 1 and 2 of the Entry-Level MSN program.
Course description: Reviews the evolution of advanced practice and leadership in nursing and their impact on issues facing the nursing profession and health care. Reviews evidence-based advanced practice and leadership in nursing and their place in interprofessional collaboration and quality care in health care delivery system.
Objectives: At the end of the course, the student will:

1. Analyze advanced practice roles in nursing according to their history, regulating issues, ethics, and contributions to the health care system.
2. Differentiate among the various levels of leadership roles in nursing and their influence on the delivery of health care.
3. Debate evidence-based practice and how advanced practice nurses and the leadership of nursing can bring about change in the health care delivery system.
4. Analyze communication and interpersonal relationships for effective collaborative interprofessional strategies.
5. Analyze quality assurance methodologies and the role of advanced practice nurses to deliver safe and quality care to multicultural and ethnic clients.

Content outline:

1. The History of Advanced Practice Nursing
2. Regulation, Certification, and Licensure Issues for Advanced Practice Nursing
3. Ethics for Advanced Practice Nurses
4. Leadership Concepts Roles in Nursing from the Beginning to Executive Levels

5. Evidence-based Practice for Advanced Practice Nurses and Nurse Leaders
6. Delivery of Culturally Competent Advanced Practice Nursing
7. What It Takes for Interprofessional Collaboration
8. Advanced Practice Nurses and Quality Care and Patient Safety

Entry-Level MSN (same end-of-program course for all tracks of the MSN program)

Overarching objective from SLOs of the MSN Program

Value the professional role of nursing and interprofessional collaboration in the delivery of health care through community service and scholarly activities.

Course title: Role Development for Advanced Practice
Credits: 2 units (seminar)
Prerequisite courses: Completion of Level 1 courses for the MSN program or its equivalent.
Course description: Develops the role for ethical, advanced practice nursing and leadership in nursing. Analyzes experiences from the clinical setting in evidence-based advanced practice and their effect on interprofessional collaboration, quality of care and patient safety, and changes in the health care delivery system. Discusses current issues in advanced practice roles in nursing.
Objectives: At the end of the course, the student will:

1. Analyze the phases of development to become an advanced practice nurse from novice to expert and the expectations placed upon self and the health care system for the novice advanced practice nurse.
2. Analyze ethical dilemmas in advanced practice nursing.
3. Analyze clinical experiences in the delivery of evidence-based advanced practice for multicultural and ethnic clients.
4. Analyze clinical experiences in the role of the advanced practice nurse and effective strategies for interprofessional collaboration in the delivery of safe and quality health care.
5. Present a persuasive case for a current issue in advanced practice nursing and how professional nursing can bring about change in the health care system.

Content outline:

1. Theories and Concepts Related to Professional Socialization in Advanced Practice Roles
2. Ethical Issues Confronting Advanced Practice Nurses in the Health Care System
3. Leadership and Change Theories
4. Evidence-based Advanced Practice Nursing for Multicultural and Ethnic Clients

5. Safe and Quality Care Through Effective Interprofessional Collaboration
6. Current Issues in Advanced Practice Nursing
7. The Art of Persuasion

DNP (one of the end-of-program courses)

Overarching objective from the SLOs of the DNP program

Assume leadership in health care systems through nursing and interprofessional collaboration in the delivery of health care through advanced practice, community service, and scholarly activities.

Course title: Forum on the DNP Role
Credits: 2 units (seminar)
Prerequisites: Completion of previous 4 semesters of course work in the DNP program.
Course description: Evaluates the role of advanced practice and leadership in nursing to bring about change in the health care delivery system.
Objectives: At the end of the course, the student will:

1. Analyze the health care system and nursing profession for needed changes to deliver safe and quality health care to multicultural and ethnic clients.
2. Synthesize evidence-based advanced-practice strategies and interprofessional collaboration to demonstrate examples of their impact on changes in the health care delivery system.
3. Evaluate leadership strategies that bring about change in the health care delivery system.

Content outline:

1. Current State of the Health Care Delivery System Related to the DNP Role
2. Current State of the Nursing Profession and Its Educational System and the DNP Role
3. Current State of Interprofessional Collaboration and the DNP Role
4. Strategies for the Application of Change Theories to the Health Care System and Nursing Practice
5. Leadership Strategies for Macrosystems and the DNP Role

Concept Map for Interprofessional Theme

The following model is an example of the beginning of a concept map for the theme of interprofessional collaboration that is threaded through the various levels of curriculum in the case study curriculum. Note the listing or learning activities directed by the course objectives on the right side of the figure. To complete the concept map, faculty would list the relevant course objectives and the learning activities that contribute to the objectives that lead to the level objectives or the SLOs.

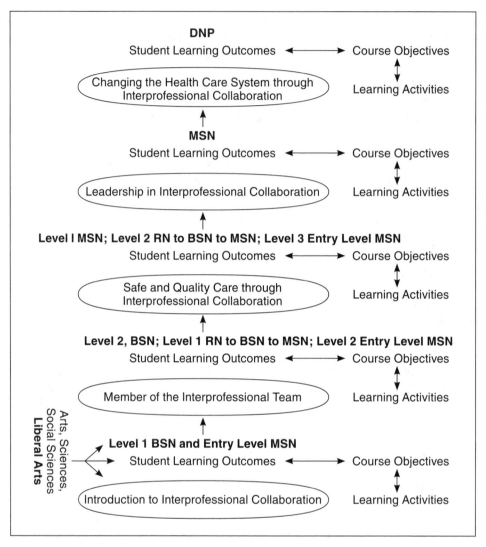

FIGURE 7.1 Concept Map for Interprofessional Theme

DISCUSSION QUESTIONS

1. Which component(s) of the curriculum do you believe has/have the most impact on the implementation of the curriculum?
2. In which ways do you believe organizational frameworks serve to ensure quality of the educational program? Give an example of an organizational framework that illustrates your belief.
3. Why do you agree or disagree with the principle of faculty control of the curriculum?

LEARNING ACTIVITIES

Student Learning Activities

1. Using the "Guidelines for Assessing the Key Components of a Curriculum or Educational Program," assess the educational program in which you are enrolled for the components of the curriculum. Are they easily identified? What resources do you need to locate them?

2. Attend one or more Curriculum Committee meetings and identify which of the components of the curriculum are addressed. Observe faculty members' interactions, their commitment to curriculum development and evaluation, and the role they play in developing or revising the curriculum. Note evidence of the routes of approval for any changes to the curriculum.

Faculty Development Activities

1. Using the "Guidelines for Assessing the Key Components of a Curriculum or Educational Program," assess the educational program in which you teach for the components of the curriculum. Are they easily identified? What resources do you need to locate them?

2. When you attend the next curriculum committee meeting, identify which of the components of the curriculum are addressed. Observe faculty members' interactions, their commitment to curriculum development and evaluation, and the role they play in developing or revising the curriculum. Note evidence of the routes of approval for any changes to the curriculum.

REFERENCES, RESOURCES, AND WEB SITES

Agency for Healthcare Research and Quality. (2010). *Home page. Department of Health and Human Services.* Retrieved from http://www.ahrq.gov

American Association of Colleges of Nursing. (2010a). *Curriculum standards. AACN. "Essentials" Series.* Retrieved from http://www.aacn.nche.edu/Education/curriculum.htm

American Association of Colleges of Nursing. (2010b). *Fact sheet: The doctor of nursing practice.* Retrieved from http://www.aacn.nche.edu/Media/pdf/FS_dnp.pdf

American Association of Colleges of Nursing. (2010c). *The essentials of baccalaureate education for professional nursing practice.* Retrieved from http://www.aacn.nche.edu/Education/bacessn.htm

American Association of Colleges of Nursing. (2010d). *Essentials of doctoral education for advanced nursing practice.* Retrieved from http://www.aacn.nche.edu/DNP/pdf/Essentials.pdf

American Association of Colleges of Nursing. (2010e). *Essentials of master's education for advanced nursing practice.* Retrieved from http://www.aacn.nche.edu/Education/mastessn.htm

American Association of Colleges of Nursing. (2010f). *Standards for Accreditation of Baccalaureate and Graduate Nursing Programs.* Retrieved from http://www.aacn.nche.edu/Accreditation/pdf/standards09.pdf

The American Heritage® Dictionary of the English Language (4th ed.). (2005). Boston: Houghton Mifflin.

Aronson, B. S., Rebeschi, L. M., & Killion, S. W. (2007). Enhancing evidence bases for intervention in a baccalaureate program. *Nursing Education Perspectives, 28*(5), 257–262.

Bloom, B. S., et. al. (Eds.). (1956). *Taxonomy of educational objectives: Handbook I: Cognitive domain*. New York: D. McKay.

Boutain, D. (2005). Social justice as a framework for professional nursing. *Journal of Nursing Education*, *44*(9), 404–408.

Broussard, E. (2009). The power of place on campus. *The Chronicle of Higher Education*, *55*(34), 812–813.

Calvillo, E., Clark, L., Ballantyne, J. E., Pacquiao, D., Purnell, L. D., & Villaruel, V. M. (2009). Cultural competency in baccalaureate nursing education. *Journal of Transcultural Nursing*, *20*(2), 137–145.

Campinha-Bacote, J. (2003). The process of cultural competency in the delivery of healthcare services: A culturally competent model of care. Cincinnati, OH: Transcultural C.A.R.E. Associates.

Candela, L., Dalley, K., & Benzel-Lindley, J. (2006). A case for learning centered curricula. *Journal of Nursing Education*, *45*(2), 59–66.

Carnegie Foundation for Advancement of Teaching Classification. (2009). *Carnegie Study of Nursing Education*. Retrieved from http://www.carnegiefoundation.org/nursing-education

Carter, L., & Rukholm E. (2008). A study of critical thinking, teacher–student interaction, and discipline-specific writing in an online educational setting for registered nurses. *Journal of Continuing Education in Nursing*, *39*(3), 133–138.

Carter, K. F., & Xu, Y. (2007). Addressing the hidden dimension in nursing education: Promoting cultural competence. *Nurse Educator*, *32*(4), 149–153.

Cashion, A. (2009). The importance of genetics education for undergraduate and graduate nursing programs. *Journal of Nursing Education*, *48*(10), 535–536.

Cherot, T. M. (2007). Frameworks for patient safety in the nursing curriculum. Retrieved September 18, 2000, from CINAHL database.

Clark, C. M. (2008). Student voices on faculty incivility in nursing education: A conceptual model. *Nursing Education Perspectives*, *29*(5), 284–289.

Clark C. M., & Springer P. J. (2007). Thoughts on incivility: Student and faculty perceptions of uncivil behavior in nursing education. *Nursing Education Perspectives*, *28*(2), 93–97.

Commission on Collegiate Nursing Education. (2010). *About CCNE*. Retrieved from http://www.aacn.nche.edu/Accreditation/AboutCCNE.htm

Conceição, S. C. O., & Taylor, L. D. (2007). Using a constructivist approach with online concept maps: Relationship between theory and nursing education. *Nursing Education Perspectives*, *28*(5), 268–275.

Cowling, W. R. (2005). Directions for doctoral dissertation research. *Nursing Science Quarterly*, *18*(1), 14–15.

Coyle, M., Duffy, J., & Martin, E. (2007). Teaching/learning health promoting behaviors through telehealth. *Nursing Education Perspectives*, *28*(1), 18–23.

Fahrenwald, N. L., Taylor, J. Y., Kneip, S. M., & Canales, M. K. (2007). Academic freedom and academic duty to teach social justice: A perspective and pedagogy for public health nursing faculty. *Public Health Nursing*, *24*(2), 190–197.

Fawcett J. (1996). On the requirements for a metaparadigm: An invitation to dialogue. *Nursing Science Quarterly*, *9*(3), 94–97.

Federizo. A. (2009). *Nursing students' perceptions of horizontal violence: Are the seeds of departure planted prior to licensure?* Master of Science in Nursing Thesis, University of Nevada–Reno.

Fetter, M. (2009). Graduating nurses' self-evaluation of information technology competencies. *Journal of Nursing Education*, *48*(2), 86–90.

Giddens, J., Brady, D., Brown, P., Wright, M., Smith, D., & Harris, J. (2008). A new curriculum for a new era of nursing education. *Nursing Education Perspectives*, *29*(4), 200–204.

Hall, L. W., Moore, S. M., & Barnsteiner, J. H. (2008). Quality and nursing: Moving from a concept to a core competency. *Urologic Nursing*, *28*(5), 417–425.

Health Resources and Services Administration. (2001). Using cultural competence to improve the quality of health care for diverse populations and add value to managed care arrangements. Retrieved from ftp://ftp.hrsa.gov/financeMC/cultural-competence.pdf

Health Resources and Services Administration, Bureau of Health Professions, Division of Nursing. (2010). *HRSA Health Professions*. Retrieved from http://bhpr.hrsa.gov/grants/nursing.htm

Health Resources and Services Administration, Bureau of Health Professions, Division of Nursing. (2010; Released 2002). *The national sample survey of registered nurses.* Washington, DC: Author.

Health Resources and Services Administration. (2009). *The registered nurse population: findings from the 2004 national survey of registered nurses.* Retrieved from http://bhpr.hrsa.gov/healthworkforce/rnsurvey04/appendixa.htm#1

Human Genome Project Information. (2010). *About the human genome project.* Retrieved from http://www.ornl.gov/sci/techresources/Human_Genome/project/about.shtml

Institute of Medicine. (2003). *Health professions education: A bridge to quality.* Washington, DC: National Academies Press.

Jenkins, J., & Calzone K. A. (2007). Establishing the essential nursing competencies for genetics and genomics. *Journal of Nursing Scholarship, 39*(1), 10–6.

Kardon-Edgren, S. (2007). Cultural competence of Baccalaureate nursing faculty. *Journal of Nursing Education, 46*(8), 360–366.

Kaufman, K. A. (2009). Headlines from the NLN. Annual survey of schools of nursing academic year 2006–2007: Executive summary. *Nursing Education Perspectives, 30*(2), 136–137.

Kennison, M. M. (2006). The evaluation of students' reflective writing for evidence of critical thinking. *Nursing Education Perspectives, 27*(5), 269–273.

Kim, S. C., Brown, C. E., Fields, W., & Stichler, J. F. (2009). Evidence-based practice-focused interactive teaching strategy: A controlled study. *Journal of Advanced Nursing, 65*(6), 1218–27.

Kinchin, I. M., Cabot, L. B., & Hay, D. B. (2008). Using concept mapping to locate the tacit dimension of clinical expertise: Toward a theoretical framework to support critical reflection on teaching. *Learning in Health and Social Care, 7*(2), 93–104.

King, I. (2009). Toward a theory of nursing [Original article published 1972.]. *Nursing, 2*(2), 29.

Leininger, M. (1997). Transcultural nursing research to transform nursing education and practice: 40 years. *Journal of Nursing Scholarship, 29*(4), 341–347.

Lennon-Dearing, R., Florence, J., Garrett, L., Click, I. A., & Abercrombie, S. (2008). A rural community-based interdisciplinary curriculum: A social work perspective. *Social Work in Health Care, 47*(2), 93–107.

Longo, J., & Sherman, R. O. (2007). Leveling horizontal violence. *Journal of Nursing Management, 38*(3), 34–7, 50–1.

Lunney, M. (2008). Current knowledge related to intelligence and thinking with implications for the use and development of case studies. *International Journal of Nursing Terminologies and Classifications, 19*(4), 158–162.

Maradiegue, A. (2008). A resource guide for learning about genetics. *Online Journal of Issues in Nursing, 13*(1), 10.

McCormick, A. C., & Zhao, C. (2007). *Inside Higher Education.* Retrieved October 8, 2009, from http://www.insidehighered.com/views/2007/05/10/mccormick

Meacham, J. (2008). What's the use of a mission statement? *Academe, 94*(1), 21–24.

Milone-Nuzzo, P. (2007). Diversity in nursing education. How well are we doing? *Journal of Nursing Education, 46*(8), 343–348.

Morphew, C. C., & Hartley, M. (2006). Mission statements: a thematic analysis of rhetoric across institutional type. *The Journal of Higher Education, 77*(3), 456–471.

Morse, J. M. (2006). The critique of research. *Qualitative Health Research, 16*(2), 171–172.

National League for Nursing Accrediting Commission, Inc. (2010). NLNAC Homepage. Retrieved from http://www.nlnac.org/home.htm

National League for Nursing Accrediting Commission. (2010). *NLNAC 2008 Standards and Criteria.* Retrieved from http://www.nlnac.org

Newman, M. S., Sime, A. M., & Corcoran-Perry, S. A. (1991). The focus of the discipline of nursing. *Advances in Nursing Science, 14*(1), 1–6.

Novak, & Canas. (2006, January) *The theory underlying concept maps and how to construct and use them* [Technical Report Florida Institute for Human and Machine Cognition, Revised 2008, January]. Retrieved from http://cmap.ihmc.us/Publications/ResearchPapers/TheoryCmaps/Theory underlyingConceptMaps.htm

Parse, R. R. (1992). Human becoming: Parse's theory of nursing. *Nursing Science Quarterly, 5*(1), 35–42.

Peplau, H. (1952). *Interpersonal relations in nursing.* New York: Putnam.

Plummer, M., & Molzahn, A. E. (2009). Quality of life in contemporary nursing theory: A concept analysis. *Nursing Science Quarterly, 22*(2), 134–140.

Poyrazli, S., & Grahame K. M. (2007). Barriers to adjustment: Needs of international students within a semi-urban campus community. *Journal of Instructional Psychology, 34*(1), 28–45.

The Princeton Review. (2001). The Best 331 Colleges (2002 ed.). New York: Princeton Review Publishing.

Quality and Safety Education for Nursing. (2010). Funded by the Robert Wood Johnson Foundation. Retrieved from http://www.qsen.org

Raines, C. F., & Taglaireni, M. E., (2008). Career pathways in nursing: Entry points and academic progression. *Online Journal of Issues in Nursing, 13*(3), (11p).

Rogers, M. E. (1970). *An introduction to the theoretical basis of nursing.* Philadelphia: F. A. Davis

Rossen, E. K., Bartlett R., & Herrick, C. A. (2008). Interdisciplinary collaboration: The need to revisit. *Issues in Mental Health Nursing, 29*(4), 387–396.

Scott Tilley, D. D. (2008). Competency in nursing: A concept analysis. *Journal of Continuing Education, 39*(2), 58–64.

Sitzman, K., & Leners, D. W. (2006). Bachelor of Science in Nursing student perceptions of caring online. *Nursing Education Perspectives, 27*(5), 254–259.

Smith, E. L., Cronenwett, L., & Sherwood, G. (2007). Current assessments of quality and safety education in nursing. *Nursing Outlook, 55*(3), 132–137.

Spizale, H. J. S., & Jacobson, L. (2005). Trends in registered nurse education programs: 1998–2008. *Nursing Education Perspectives, 26*(4), 230–235.

Swearington, S. (2009). A journey of leadership: Designing a nursing leadership development program. *The Journal of Continuing Education in Nursing, 40*(3), 107–112.

Tanner, C. A., Gubrud-Howe, L., & Shores, P. (2008). The Oregon consortium for nursing education: A response to the nursing shortage. *Policy, Politics, & Nursing Practice, 9*(3), 203–209.

Thompson, B. W., & Skiba, D. J. (2008). Headlines from the NLN. Informatics in the nursing curriculum: A national survey of nursing informatics requirements in nursing curricula. *Nursing Education Perspectives, 29*(5), 312–317.

Thornburg R. A., Uline C., & Wilson, J. D. (2006). Creating a teacher orientation seminar for certification candidates: Priming your students for success. *Journal of Instructional Psychology, 33*(1), 58–62.

Tilghman J., Raley D., & Conway, J. J. (2008). Family nurse practitioner students: Utilization of personal digital assistants (PDAs): Implications for practice. *ABNF Journal, 17*(3), 115–117.

University of Nevada Las Vegas. (2009). Doctoral Online Community. Retrieved from https://webcampus.nevada.edu/webct/urw/lc33129041.tp0/cobaltMainFrame.dowebct

U.S. Census Bureau. (2005). Nation's population one-third minority. Retrieved from http://www.census.gov/Press-Release/www/releases/archives/population/006808.html

Vickers, D. A. (2008). Social justice: A concept for undergraduate nursing curricula? *Southern Online Journal for Nursing Research, 8*(1), 1–18.

Zygmont, D. M., & Schaefer, K. M. (2006). Assessing the critical thinking skills of faculty: What do the findings mean for nursing education? *Nursing Education Perspectives, 27*(5), 260–268.

Curriculum Planning for Associate Degree Nursing Programs

Karen E. Fontaine

OBJECTIVES

1. Provide examples of the steps involved in curriculum development for associate degree nursing educational programs.
2. Analyze current regulatory, accreditation, political, and social factors affecting associate degree curriculum development.
3. Provide examples of concepts that are used in curriculum development for associate degree nursing.
4. Describe current national issues affecting associate and baccalaureate prelicensure nursing educational programs.

OVERVIEW

Chapter 8 begins with a history and describes the current status of associate degree nursing (ADN). It outlines the current pressures on this type of nursing program. A sample nursing curriculum that follows the outline in Chapter 7 is presented along with a rationale for the components that were used. Examples are provided.

INTRODUCTION

There are several different types of prelicensure programs for the education of nurses in the United States: associate, baccalaureate, entry-level master's, and diploma. Most nurses enter the profession through ADN educational programs (National League for Nursing [NLN], 2006). The development of a curriculum for all types of prelicensure programs follows a similar process, and there are many factors that must be considered. They are accreditation and regulatory standards, social and political climates, the health care industry, professional nursing, and economic factors.

This chapter defines ADN education and summarizes the process of curriculum development and revision for such programs, using a concept-based curriculum design. Issues surrounding the basic educational preparation of nurses in a rapidly changing environment are discussed. A sample program of instruction from an ADN nursing program in a community college is provided.

THE HISTORY OF ASSOCIATE DEGREE NURSING

ADN education has its genesis in a post-World War II nursing shortage. At the time, community colleges were expanding their role. At the same time, the existing educational systems for nurses, consisting of either university education or hospital-based diploma programs, were not able to address the shortage. Haase (1990) describes the sequence of events that began in 1948 with a recommendation from the Committee on the Functions of Nursing that nursing practice would consist of two tiers of nurses, one professional the other technical. Haase credits Mildred Montag with further developing the idea in her doctoral dissertation, presenting an educational model for the community college setting that was intended to create the technical worker in nursing, which would have a more limited scope than a professional nurse but broader than that of a practical nurse. Several pilot studies implemented the model and found that there was little difference in the graduates of associate degree programs than those from the existing educational systems (Haase). Implementation of the proposed model of education effectively removed the education of nurses from hospitals where an apprentice model of instruction was used and created a new model of nursing education housed in the nation's colleges and universities. However, it did not address the professional versus technical issue in practice, nor was the recommendation for prelicensure education at the baccalaureate level implemented.

The discussion regarding two tiers of nursing preparation and practice, professional versus technical, was resurrected when the American Nurses Association (ANA, 1965) recommended that all nursing education should take place at institutions of higher education and that beginning preparation for professional nursing should be at the baccalaureate level. The controversial issue of how to differentiate the practice differences between Bachelor of Science in Nursing (BSN) and ADN educational preparation has continued. Although there are increasing numbers of entry-level master's in nursing programs, today's workforce represents mainly three levels of basic nursing preparation: diploma, associate degree, and baccalaureate prelicensure programs. (American Association of Colleges of Nursing [AACN], 2008).

CURRENT STATUS OF ASSOCIATE DEGREE NURSING

According to the National League for Nursing (NLN, 2006), ADN programs currently comprise both the majority of students in nursing programs and the graduate nurses working in the profession. Fifty-nine percent of all basic registered nurse (RN) programs are associate degree, and they graduate 63% of all registered nurses (NLN).

Despite the continued efforts of nursing leadership, professional organizations, government-sponsored task forces, and educators to clarify the differences between associate and baccalaureate degree nurses, the issue continues to be divisive (Orsolini-Hain & Waters, 2009). Further complicating the issue, hospitals, traditionally the major employers of nurses, do not consistently differentiate among the educational levels of staff nurses in assigning patient care responsibilities or salary.

ADN programs have responded to demands to create a nurse who is able to take care of increasingly complex patients in a rapidly changing health care environment by continuously modifying and adding to the curriculum. This created the current problem of content saturation, which is endemic among all nursing programs. Tanner (2007) enumerates the competencies and content that nursing faculty have been asked to include in the curriculum: genetics, gerontology, community health, perioperative care, pharmacology, bioterrorism, mass casualty response, health economics, cultural competence, health policy, palliative and end-of-life care, evidence-based practice, assessment, interdisciplinary team management, leadership, and informatics. The ANA created standards of practice for generalist and specialty nurses (2004).

Accrediting and regulatory organizations, such as the National Council of State Boards of Nursing (NCSBN, 2009), individual state boards of nursing, and the National League for Nursing Accrediting Commission (NLNAC, 2008), require specific content. In addition, general education and sciences courses are corequisite and prerequisite for admission into nursing programs. Consequently, most associate degree programs are at least 3 years long. As pressure once again is exerted on nursing to define the entry into practice at the baccalaureate level, Orsolini-Hain and Waters (2009) state that "this shortened span between ADN and BSN program length may make continuing on to earn a BSN more appealing, especially if the barriers to doing so are few" (p. 5).

There are emerging trends and support within the system of nursing education that would help to reconcile the controversies surrounding associate and baccalaureate education of nurses. Manthey (2005) suggests either that associate degree programs be transformed into baccalaureate programs or that graduates of associate degree programs have a pathway to a realistic plan for obtaining a bachelor's degree within a specific period. The National Advisory Council on Nurse Education and Practice, a group that advises the federal government and Congress, recommends that there be an increased proportion of BSNs in the workforce and suggests that partnerships between ADN and BSN programs be a methodology for attaining this goal (U.S. Department of Health and Human Services, Health Resources and Services Administration, 2008). Several states now allow community colleges to confer baccalaureate degrees in nursing (Orsolini-Hain & Waters, 2009). The Oregon Consortium of Nursing Education (OCNE, 2007) provides an example of collaborative models that have been developed to promote a seamless transition between associate and baccalaureate education. A shared pathway, combined with agreements among the community colleges and universities that participate in the consortium, creates the expectation and availability for students to continue their education and receive their BS degree (OCNE).

CURRICULUM REFORM IN ASSOCIATE DEGREE EDUCATION

The NLN has called for the reform and transformation of nursing education and recommended a move to a more evidence-based curriculum that is founded in research findings (NLN 2003, 2005). The Institute of Medicine (IOM, 2003) has recommended major educational reform for all health care professions. To meet the demands of the health care system, the IOM called for a delineation of the relationship between education and quality of care and the identification of the most effective educational methods for teaching the competencies necessary for practice (IOM). These same competencies have been imbedded in the NCSBN's Model Nurse Practice Act (2009). They are as follows:

1. Using informatics to communicate, manage knowledge, mitigate error, and support decision making.
2. Employing evidence-based practice to integrate best research with clinical expertise and client values for optimal care, including skills to identify and apply best practices to nursing care.
3. Providing client-centered, culturally competent care.
   a. Respecting client differences, values, preferences, and expressed needs.
   b. Involving clients in decision making and care management.
   c. Coordinating and managing continuous client care.
   d. Promoting healthy lifestyles for clients and populations.
4. Working in interdisciplinary teams to cooperate, collaborate, communicate, and integrate client care and health promotion.
5. Participating in quality improvement processes to measure client outcomes, identify hazards and errors, and develop changes in processes of client care (p. 4).

Content saturation and overly crowded curricula are a primary challenge to reform for the current nursing curriculum and the movement toward an evidence basis for nursing education according to the NLN (2003), IOM (2003), and Giddens (2007). Giddens states that nursing education must solve the content saturation issue before it can determine the essential skills and knowledge required of graduates. Ironside (2004) concurs, stating that the current nursing education practice of relying on competency-based education and tradition creates a curriculum in which content is increasingly added, but little removed.

Changes in health care delivery, an academic-practice gap, and an information explosion are just some of the factors that have historically impacted and added to nursing educational content. Ironside (2004) further states that these are barriers to the faculty's understanding to determine which aspects of traditional nursing education should be retained and which should be discarded when revising curriculum.

A body of evidence is emerging that suggests different pedagogical approaches to nursing education. Giddens (2007) believes that concepts can be used as tools for managing content that provides an organizational framework for curriculum that allows students to apply learning to new situations and builds on previous knowledge as students move from course to course. Carrieri-Kohlman, Lindsey, and West (2003) state that concepts are a means for organizing content and that discussion of the management of phenomena, concepts, or processes can be related to different individuals, groups, and illnesses. Tanner (2007) supports this approach, and she agrees that students should be provided a foundation of knowledge in the context of a framework, thus gaining experience in comparing and contrasting practical knowledge that can then be applied to clinical situations.

An example of a conceptual approach to teaching is provided by Vacek (2009) who describes using a process for teaching students to provide care for psychotic patients by applying the concepts learned from that experience to patients across multiple settings.

Tanner (2007) suggests that case studies can be used as a method for gaining deep understanding and relating concepts. Concept mapping is a further demonstration of meaningful learning that promotes critical thinking and helps students connect new information and past learning (Abel & Freeze, 2006). Methods of teaching are being explored that help faculty show students how to discover the meaning of content and how to develop critical thinking.

COMPONENTS OF AN ASSOCIATE DEGREE CURRICULUM

Nursing programs exist within a context of regulation, accreditation, professional standards, and an educational milieu. Any nursing program that educates prelicensure candidates for registered nursing must adhere to regulations. At the national level, the NCSBN developed a model nurse practice act that offers guiding principles for state boards of nursing and applies to education and practice (NCSBN, 2009). ADN programs are offered accreditation status by the National League for Nursing Accrediting Commission (NLNAC), which maintains and updates national accreditation standards (NLNAC, 2008).

Nursing programs that exist within a public or private educational institution must meet regional accreditation standards for the parent institution, such as the Northwest Commission on Colleges and Universities. Public or privately funded programs may belong to an organization or system that has additional requirements. These may require compliance with standards generated by a statewide consortium of publicly funded community colleges or a nationwide chain of associate degree granting private colleges.

Components common to the various types of programs of nursing were described in Chapter 7. Applying a construction analogy can help explain the function, structure, and purpose of each and how the parts of a curriculum work together. For example, the foundation of a house can be seen as the mission and vision of the curriculum, providing support to the overall curriculum. Seen as the parent institution and the social and political setting, infrastructure (sewer, water, and fire and police services in our construction analogy) is based on location and resources available and must be considered when building the foundation. Next is the building frame, providing support for the roof, ceilings, and walls. This is the organizational framework of the curriculum that provides a common support and envelops the curriculum in form and structure. The rooms in the building are thus the courses and content, such as pediatric nursing, family nursing, or a pathosphysiology or diversity class. All of the disparate rooms in the structure have ceilings, floors, and a common purpose, which are the curriculum threads, or concepts that run throughout the program.

Mission or Vision and Philosophy Statements

NLNAC (2008) accreditation standards for ADN programs require that the nursing program's mission and/or philosophy reflects the governing organization's core values and is congruent with the outcomes and strategic goals and objectives. When developing or revising the mission and philosophy statements, the faculty and leaders of the nursing program should examine the program's mission in relation to those of the institution. Recommended sources of guidance are other programs within a system or programs that are similar or have good reputations. A sample mission statement is provided in Exhibit 8.1 by the Truckee Meadows Community College (TMCC) Nursing Program, which exists within a community college in Reno, Nevada, and is part of a publicly supported statewide system, the Nevada System of Higher Education. The information provided is used with permission (TMCC, 2009a). An ongoing program evaluation process ensures that the mission statement is continuously evaluated, for both congruence and currency.

The philosophy flows from the mission statement and reflects the beliefs of the program's faculty and staff about nursing, nursing education, students, and learning. The sample philosophy provided in Exhibit 8.2, used with permission from the nursing program at TMCC, is based on the nursing metaparadigm and explains and expands on the college's philosophy of associate degree education (TMCC, 2009b).

EXHIBIT 8.1 Sample Mission Statement

College Mission Statement

Vision

Truckee Meadows Community College creates the future by changing lives.

Mission

Truckee Meadows Community College promotes student success, academic excellence and access to lifelong learning by delivering high quality education and services to our diverse communities.

Values

The values upon which Truckee Meadows Community College bases its mission and vision statements are the principles, standards and qualities the college considers worthwhile and desirable. Truckee Meadows Community College is committed to:

- Student access and success
- Excellence in teaching and learning
- Evidence of student progress through assessment of student outcomes
- Nurturing a climate of innovative and creative thought
- Collaborative decision making
- Community development through partnerships and services
- Ethical practices and integrity
- Respect, compassion, and equality for all persons
- Responsible and sustainable use of resources
- Fostering attitudes that exemplify responsible participation in a democratic society

Nursing Program Mission Statement

The mission of Truckee Meadows Community College's Nursing Program is congruent with the college's mission, providing high quality associate degree nursing education in order to positively influence the health and well-being of the community and the clients our students serve. Valuing social and cultural differences, the faculty believes that students are active learners and use current nursing educational theory and practice to prepare students to be critical thinkers and competent professionals. Student success is encouraged by providing a thorough welcome and orientation to the nursing program and access to essential services, college resources and community mentors for the duration that the student is enrolled in the TMCC nursing program. The importance of lifelong learning for the graduate is emphasized.

From Truckee Meadows Community College (2009a).

EXHIBIT 8.2 Sample Associate Degree Nursing Program Philosophy

Philosophy of the A.D. Nursing Program

The philosophy of the nursing program at TMCC embraces the nursing paradigm of person, health, environment and nursing. It also incorporates the eight core components and competencies for graduates of associate degree programs as identified by the National League for Nursing (NLN) and addresses nursing education within a state supported community college.

PERSON

A unique, valued, multifaceted biopsychosocialspiritual individual seeking an optimal level of wellness that considers personal and cultural needs, choices and motivation.

HEALTH

An individualized homeostatic state that is achieved when the person and environment interact to maximize quality of life experiences.

ENVIRONMENT

Dynamic internal and external components that impact the person in pursuit of health.

NURSING

Nursing provides an essential direct service to society. The nurse collaborates with the person across the life span to achieve health and provides caring and compassion at the end of life.

Nursing is both art and science incorporating theories and concepts from the biological, physical, behavioral and social sciences. Evidence based nursing practice, nursing process and standards of nursing care are combined with legal, ethical and cultural considerations to provide collaborative holistic care to individuals, families and communities.

Nursing is an evolving profession and requires dedication to lifelong learning. The core competencies of nursing include: professional behaviors, communication, assessment, clinical decision making, caring interventions, teaching and learning, collaboration and managing care. (Coxwell, G. & Gillerman, H. (Eds). (2002). *Educational competencies for graduates of associate degree nursing programs.* Sudbury, MA: Jones and Bartlett Publishers.).

ASSOCIATE DEGREE NURSING EDUCATION

We believe that the TMCC Nursing Program Learning Outcomes with Supporting Definitions serve as the guide for nursing education. Nursing education in an institution of higher learning incorporates knowledge gained from nursing courses and those in general education, physical, behavioral and social sciences and cultural diversity.

Identification of general education courses provides a common foundation for all students in the nursing program. We recognize that individual educational and life experiences also contribute to each student's nursing education process. A balance between general education and nursing courses with early introduction of technical skills and person/student interaction facilitates development of nursing knowledge by recognizing needs of the individual adult learner.

Nursing education must address use of the nursing process across the life span at various points along the health–illness continuum and in a variety of health care settings. Nursing education at the community college must also consider the demographic and cultural needs of the community that will serve as the nursing practice environment for the graduate of the nursing program.

Integral to the education of nursing students is providing opportunities to observe and participate in both simulated and actual patient centered learning experiences. Laboratory and clinical courses are structured to allow application of concepts and principles learned from theory courses. Each semester of education builds upon previous learning and encourages the development of clinical decision making. Nursing faculty are both educators and skilled practitioners of nursing responsible for maintaining expertise and current knowledge and serve as role models for the importance of lifelong learning. Nursing faculty are responsible for identifying learning experiences that will expose the students to a variety of settings and serve as liaisons with registered nurses within those settings. Nursing faculty review and analyze current trends in nursing and health care issues that impact the role of the registered nurse.

The ultimate goal of nursing education at TMCC is to prepare a safe, competent, beginning level practitioner who possesses knowledge, skills and professionalism required by the registered nurse. The nursing education obtained by the graduate of the TMCC nursing program serves as the starting point for continued development and education as an accountable and responsible member of the nursing profession.

(Continued)

EXHIBIT 8.2 Sample Associate Degree Nursing Program Philosophy *Continued*

Philosophy of the A.D. Nursing Program

COMMUNITY COLLEGE EDUCATION

The mission of TMCC is to provide access for lifelong learning opportunities to improve quality of life for our diverse community. A variety of educational offerings and student and academic support services help individuals achieve goals and aspirations. Strategic Goals of TMCC that are of special interest to nursing are fostering academic excellence and diversity, incorporation of technology and provision of a welcoming and supportive environment.

The population utilizing TMCC as an institution of higher learning includes residents from the greater Reno-Sparks community, outlying areas of Fernley, Fallon, Dayton and Carson City. Residents of California cities and communities including Susanville, Truckee and Tahoe City enroll as part of the "good neighbor" community. Fostering flexibility and diversity through classroom, online and distance education course offerings in addition to workforce or continuing education courses provides a variety of learning opportunities to the community.

LEARNER

The adult learner in the Associate Degree Nursing Program has unique values, beliefs, needs, experiences and educational backgrounds. Each individual has personal and professional aspirations that serve as motivation to succeed. The combination of readiness, motivation, culture and life experiences of the learner will influence the learning process. It is the responsibility of the learner to take advantage of all educational opportunities, to adhere to program and course policies and requirements and to seek out academic and support services as needed.

NURSE EDUCATOR

The nurse educator facilitates learning by providing a variety of meaningful learning experiences and assisting learners to develop the core competencies of nursing. The nurse educator provides ongoing evaluation of the learner utilizing verbal and written feedback to stimulate growth. The nurse educator is a professional role model in the classroom and clinical settings, participates in continuing education and professional activities including maintaining membership in professional organizations and involvement in community service.

From Truckee Meadows Community College Nursing Program Student Handbook (2009).

Organizational Framework

Although an organizational framework is not required by the NLNAC (2008), the curriculum standards state that student learning outcomes should be used to organize the curriculum, guide the delivery of instruction, direct learning activities, and evaluate student progress. Programs should first identify the overall student learning outcomes desired from their graduates. These are behaviors, and they differ from program outcomes such as first-time National Council Licensure Examination-Registered Nurse (NCLEX-RN) graduate pass rates, retention rates, employment rates, and program satisfaction. Student learning outcomes describe desired and expected behaviors of the program's graduates and should be a result of and reflected in level and course objectives. See Chapter 7 for further discussion. Exhibit 8.3 offers sample student learning outcomes for the associate degree program that was presented previously.

Giddens et al., (2008), in proposing a new curriculum model for nursing, state that there is no longer a body of knowledge in nursing that can be learned and that students must instead be taught how to learn. They recommend that population or setting-based teaching be de-emphasized in the curriculum and suggest instead that practice, theory, and clinical activities be integrated (Giddens et al.). Carrieri-Kohlman et al. (2003) suggest the use of a conceptual basis for education, organizing content around concepts, phenomena, or processes and providing a framework for course content. In a

EXHIBIT 8.3 Sample Student Learning Outcomes

Student Learning Outcome

GRADUATES OF TMCC'S NURSING PROGRAM WILL BE ABLE TO:

1. Utilize comprehensive and accurate assessment, employing knowledge and concepts of evidence-based practice and critical thinking to provide effective care in meeting client needs and outcomes.
2. Coordinate and delegate responsibilities for those who work cooperatively in the interdisciplinary team, communicating and interacting with all to achieve the client needs, goals, and outcomes.
3. Utilize the teaching/learning processes, including informatics, to promote and maintain health and reduce risk for the client, the significant support person, and interdisciplinary health team.
4. Practice professional behaviors within the nursing standards of legal, ethical, and regulatory frameworks, as well as demonstrate behaviors to include concern for others, personal accountability, and lifelong learning.

From Truckee Meadows Community College (2009).

concept-based curriculum, the concepts are tied to all classes (Giddens & Brady, 2007). Students gain exposure to concepts before formal study, and the clinical experience provides opportunities to understand the concepts within multiple age groups along a health–illness continuum; they learn ways that the concepts are interrelated (Giddens & Brady). Concepts should cross environmental settings, the life span, and the health–illness continuum and are the foci within courses (Giddens & Brady). Recognizing content through concepts for students and freeing nursing faculty from content saturation are the goal of conceptual-based teaching and learning (Giddens, 2007).

Concepts

Concepts can be based on existing frameworks but should be faculty generated and validated through a review of the literature and definitions established (Giddens & Brady, 2007). The faculty who designed the curriculum that is used as an example in this chapter developed a concept-based curriculum. They had previous experience with using the core components that are defined within the Educational Competencies for Graduates of Associate Degree Nursing Programs developed by the Council of Associate Degree Nursing Competencies Task force for the NLN with support from the National Organization of Associate Degree Nursing (Coxwell & Gillerman, 2000). Believing that the core components were clearly defined as concepts, they requested and received permission from the NLN for their use as concepts in creating the framework for their curriculum.

Giddens (2007) suggests that one way to limit content is by the use of exemplars to represent a specific concept, thereby reducing content by using large concepts. Exemplars restrict content to that which is most prevalent or appears most frequently in practice or the literature (Giddens). In an effort to limit content, the faculty at TMCC chose to use selected exemplar diseases as a basis for pathophysiologic content in the curriculum, adding a physiologic concept within which they identify a body systems approach to the study of disease. Prevalence, incidence, and hospital discharge data were used to select exemplar diseases, which represent each body system and address the subconcepts of life span, health–illness continuum, and patient safety. All diseases are taught across the life span, as appropriate, and are taught only once. Teaching of exemplar diseases is leveled within the curriculum. Students learn about appropriate lab value alterations, medications, and the related nursing processes of assessment, diagnosis, care planning, intervention, and evaluation within the context of the exemplar disease.

An example is provided in Exhibit 8.4. Shown are two concepts: One is the physiologic concept and associated exemplar diseases, and the second concept is derived from the NLN's Educational Competencies for Graduates of Associate Degree Nursing Programs (Coxwell & Gillerman, 2002) as discussed previously and has been used with permission.

Evaluation of competency in the sample curriculum provided is also loosely derived from the NLN competencies (Coxwell & Gillerman, 2002). Faculty defined the

EXHIBIT 8.4 Sample Concepts Exemplar Diseases, and Clinical Expectations

Physiologic Concept Circulation

The circulatory system (or cardiovascular system) is an organ system that moves nutrients, gases, and wastes to and from cells, helps fight diseases and helps stabilize body temperature and pH to maintain homeostasis. Humans have a closed circulatory system (meaning that the blood never leaves the network of arteries, veins and capillaries).

The physiological concept of circulation includes the human circulatory system and its related physiology and the pathophysiology of diseases that affect clients across the life span. The care of clients with alterations in the circulatory system includes an understanding of the pathophysiology of the diseases of the circulatory system and related clinical findings. The nurse will be responsible for knowledge of the related targeted assessment, lab and diagnostic tests, medical treatment including medications, fluid and electrolyte imbalances, and acid-base issues. The nurse is also responsible for care planning for the client to include nutritional issues, family issues, and care coordination across health care settings.

Exemplar Diseases for Circulatory Body System

- Tetralogy of Fallot
- Hypertension
- Anemia
- Multiple System Organ Failure
- Acute Lymphocytic Leukemia
- Congestive Heart Failure
- Hemorrhage
- Acute Coronary Syndrome
- Disseminated Intravascular Coagulopathy

Sample Concept

Communication

Communication in nursing is an interactive process through which there is an exchange of information that may occur verbally, non-verbally, in writing, or through information technology. Those who may be included in this process are the nurse, client, significant support person(s), other members of the health care team, and community agencies. Effective communication demonstrates caring, compassion, and cultural awareness, and is directed toward positive outcomes and establishing a trusting relationship.

Therapeutic communication is an interactive verbal and nonverbal process between the nurse and client that assists the client to cope with change, develop more satisfying interpersonal relationships, and integrate new knowledge and skills.

Sample Clinical Behaviors

COMMUNICATION COMPETENCIES:

Uses clear, open expression in dialogue; is engaged with clients, health care professionals, faculty and others.
Applies therapeutic communication skills appropriately, while caring for clients and families.
Elicits preferences and values from clients, clarifying understanding.
Listens attentively and respectfully without interruption.
Reports and documents accurate, relevant and complete information in a clear, concise and timely manner.
Produces clear, accurate, concise, and complete writing.
Uses appropriate channels of communication, including information technology to support and communicate delivery of patient care.
Maintains self-control and dignity; responds to situations professionally, without blame or aggressive behavior.

attributes and expected behaviors for graduates of the program and, with the help of a consultant, leveled those across the curriculum. Expected behaviors for the concepts are the same for all clinical courses and are broad enough to be used in all clinical settings with all patient populations. Performance levels increase with each subsequent clinical course, and graduates must receive a passing grade to progress to the next course. Critical behaviors are identified for each concept that must be met for each course. Examples of such critical behaviors include providing safe care, using appropriate infection control practices, and operating within ethical and professional boundaries. Exhibit 8.4 provides an example of clinical competencies that are derived from the concepts.

Program of Study

There are many practical matters of consideration in developing and revising nursing programs of study. Course sequencing, program length, prerequisite and corequisite courses, and admission criteria should be based on national and regional standards as well as any respective state board of nursing regulations. NLNAC (2008) standards state that the nursing program length must be congruent with the attainment of identified program outcomes and consistent with the policies of the governing organization, state and national standards, and best practices. As a degree-granting institution, the parent college or university establishes requirements for corequisite courses that must be included within the program of study.

ADN programs were designed at inception to require only 2 years of instruction, but currently they take a minimum of 3 years to complete (Orsolini-Hain & Waters, 2009). Although most programs require 4 semesters of instruction in nursing, prerequisite courses such as anatomy and physiology, microbiology, English, math, and nutrition generally take the student at least 1 year prior to admission to complete. Each program determines what students need to be successful in their program's nursing courses.

At TMCC's nursing program, the faculty created an integrated curriculum in which the traditional separations of medical–surgical, psychiatric, pediatrics, and maternity were woven into a comprehensive program of sequenced instruction. Large-credit courses were created, for example, Nursing Care 1, 2, 3, and 4—one for each of the 4 semesters of instruction within the program. Each of the courses has a theory and a clinical component, and the clinical course is graded on a pass/fail basis. Three courses were added that did not include a clinical component: Cultural Diversity in Nursing, Professional Behaviors, and Pathophysiology. Coupled with the credits required for prerequisite and corequisite courses, the associate degree program requires 75 credits to complete. Nursing courses comprise 68% of the total credits.

LEARNER OUTCOMES AND ASSESSMENT

NLNAC (2008) criteria require that nursing programs have student learning outcomes that are used to organize the curriculum, guide the delivery of instruction, direct learning activities, and evaluate student progress. Methods of evaluation must be established to measure the achievement of student learning and program outcomes (NLNAC).

EXHIBIT 8.5 Sample Course and Program Objective

Content Objective
Perform an accurate patient assessment and reassessment that addresses the psychosocial, developmental, physiological, nutritional needs of the individual.

Course Objective
The student will be able to document assessments, interventions, and client progress toward outcomes.

Related Program Outcome
Utilize comprehensive and accurate assessment, employing knowledge and concepts of evidence-based practice and critical thinking to provide effective care in meeting client needs and outcomes.

For each educational program within TMCC, The Northwest Accreditation Commission of Colleges and Universities (2003) requires establishing learner outcomes and assessing whether students achieve those outcomes. Regionally accredited colleges and universities must identify and publish the expected learning outcomes for each of their degree and certificate programs (NWCCU, 2009). Through regular and systematic assessment, each of the programs must demonstrate that students who complete their programs, no matter where or how they are offered, have achieved these outcomes. The institution must provide evidence that its assessment activities lead to the improvement of teaching and learning (NWCCU).

For nursing programs, this means that each course within a nursing curriculum has student learning objectives that guide student learning and instructional content as well as student learning outcomes that reflect the important and measureable behaviors or competencies for students. Level objectives for each semester or year are developed to assess the expected performance at that point. All objectives and program learning outcomes are measureable so that they can be assessed at each step within the program. If results are less than expected, program and instructional changes should be made that are based on evidence-based research. NLNAC (2008) standards and criteria can be used to establish a method of curriculum review that offers evaluation of both student learning and the curriculum itself. Exhibit 8.5 offers sample course objectives that relate to student outcomes.

SUMMARY

This chapter applied the components of the curriculum outlined in Chapter 7 to an ADN program. Details specific to ADN regulations and accreditation standards as well as community college education were provided. Examples were given using an existing curriculum in use at a public, state-supported community college. Curriculum development and evaluation, no matter what the setting, are a responsibility of the faculty. They are responsible for the development, implementation, and ongoing evaluation process. The examples provided here and the assessment process described in Chapter 7 can provide guidance for use by ADN programs and faculty.

DISCUSSION QUESTIONS

1. Define the term "concept" and discuss various concepts that might be used to develop an organizing framework for an ADN program.

2. Explore the NLNAC standards for ADN programs, Standard 4, which can be found at: http://www.nlnac.org/manuals/SC2008_ASSOCIATE.htm. Discuss whether the standards can be used to evaluate curriculum.

LEARNING ACTIVITIES

Student Learning Activities

1. Discuss entry-level programs into nursing and the differences among them. Debate the pros and cons for each type of program and ways in which graduates of each type of program function in the practice setting. Discuss career-ladder and continuing-education opportunities for each entry-level program.

2. Compare a curriculum chosen from an associate degree curriculum with the standards presented by the NCSBN's (2009) Model Nursing Practice Act and Model Nursing Administrative Rules. Determine whether the curriculum meets the standards and make recommendations for change if needed.

Faculty Learning Activities:

1. Compare the components of the curriculum to your nursing curriculum. Analyze and identify any gaps you find or components you need to revise to update the curriculum.

2. If you are an educator in an ADN program, compare your nursing curriculum with the NLN standards for accreditation.

REFERENCES

Abel, W. M., & Freeze, M. (2006). Evaluation of concept mapping in an associate degree nursing program. *Journal of Nursing Education, 45*(9), 356–364.

American Association of Colleges of Nursing. (2008). *2007–2008 Enrollment and graduations in baccalaureate and graduate programs in nursing.* Washington, DC: Author.

American Nurses Association. (1965). *A position paper.* New York: Author.

American Nurses Association. (2004). *Nursing: Scope and standards of practice.* New York: Author.

Carrieri-Kohlman, V., Lindsey, A. M., & West, C. (2003). *Pathophysiological phenomena in nursing: Human response to illness.* St. Louis, MO: Saunders.

Coxwell, G., & Gillerman, H. (Eds). (2000). *Educational competencies for graduates of associate degree nursing programs.* Sudbury, MA: Jones and Bartlett.

Giddens, J. F. (2007). The neighborhood: A web-based platform to support conceptual teaching and learning. *Nursing Education Perspectives, 28*(5), 251–256.

Giddens, J. F., & Brady, D. P. (2007). Rescuing nursing education from content saturation: The case for a concept-based curriculum. *Journal of Nursing Education, 46*(2), 65–69.

Giddens, J., Brady, D., Brown, P., Wright, M., Smith, D., & Harris, J. (2008). A new curriculum for a new era of nursing education. *Nursing Education Perspectives, 29*(4), 200–204.

Haase, P. T. (1990). *The origins and rise of associate degree nursing education.* Durham, NC: Duke University Press.

Institute of Medicine of the National Academies. (2003). *Who will keep the public healthy? Educating public health professionals for the 21st century (free executive summary).* Retrieved December 29, 2009 from http://www.nap.edu/catalog/10542.html

Ironside, P. M. (2004). "Covering content" and teaching thinking: Deconstructing the additive curriculum. *Journal of Nursing Education, 43*(1), 5–12.

Manthey, M. (2005). Associate degree nurses and the future of the profession. *Creative Nursing. 11*(1), 4.

National Council of State Boards of Nursing. (2009). *NCSBN model nursing practice act and model nursing administrative rules.* Retrieved December 29, 2009 from https://www.ncsbn.org/Model_Nursing_Practice_Act_December09_final.pdf

National League for Nursing. (2003). *Position statement: Innovation in nursing education: A call for reform.* Retrieved October 31, 2009 from http://www.nln.org/aboutnln/PositionStatements/innovation082203.pdf

National League for Nursing. (2005). *Position Statement: Transforming nursing education.* Retrieved September 30, 2009 from http://www.nln.org/aboutnln/PositionStatements/transforming052005.pdf

National League for Nursing. (2006). *NLN data reveal slowdown in nursing school admissions growth.* Retrieved December 28, 2009 from http://www.nln.org/newsreleases/databook_08_06.pdf

National League for Nursing Accrediting Commission. (2008). *NLNAC 2008 standards and criteria, associate degree programs in nursing.* Retrieved January 31, 2010 from: http://www.nlnac.org/manuals/SC2008_ASSOCIATE.htm

Northwest Accreditation Commission of Colleges and Universities. (2003). *Accreditation handbook.* Retrieved December 29, 2009 from http://www.nwccu.org/Pubs%20Forms%20and%20Updates/Publications/Accreditation%20Handbook.pdf

Oregon Consortium for Nursing Education. (2007). *OCNE at a glance.* Retrieved December 29, 2009 from http://ocne.org/at-a-glance.html

Orsolini-Hain, L., & Waters, V. (2009). Education evolution: A historical perspective of associate degree nursing. *Journal of Nursing Education, 48*(5), 266–271.

Tanner, C.A. (2007). The curriculum revolution revisited. *Journal of Nursing Education, 46*(2), 51–52.

Truckee Meadows Community College. (2009a). *TMCC mission, vision, and values.* Retrieved December 29, 2009 from http://www.tmcc.edu/about/mission.

Truckee Meadows Community College. (2009b). *Truckee Meadows Community College, nursing program handbook.* Retrieved December 29, 2009 from http://www.tmcc.edu/nursing/downloads/documents/NURSHandbook.pdf

U.S. Department of Health and Human Services, Health Resources and Services Administration. (2008). *Meeting the challenges. Challenges facing the nurse workforce in a changing health care environment of the new millennium.* Retrieved December 27, 2009 from http://bhpr.hrsa.gov/nursing/NACNEP/reports/sixth/default.htm

Vacek, J. E. (2009). Using a conceptual approach with a concept map of psychosis as an exemplar to promote critical thinking. *Journal of Nursing Education, 48*(1), 49–53.

Curriculum Planning for Baccalaureate Nursing Programs

Peggy Wros
Pamela Wheeler
Melissa Jones

OBJECTIVES

Upon completion of Chapter 9, the reader will be able to:

1. Summarize current trends in prelicensure baccalaureate nursing education.
2. Describe the integration of the American Association of Colleges of Nursing (AACN) Essentials as a foundation for developing a Bachelor of Science in Nursing (BSN) curriculum.
3. Describe the process of developing or revising an existing BSN curriculum.
4. Discuss innovation in nursing education, including models of clinical instruction.
5. Develop a plan for collaboration with a community/service organization to create a partnership model for clinical education.
6. Describe the relationship between generic Accelerated Bachelor of Science in Nursing (ABSN), and Registered Nurse to Bachelor of Science in Nursing (RN–BSN) programs.
7. Identify the challenges of new graduate residency programs that facilitate transition into practice.
8. Develop a curriculum plan and program of study for your institution.

OVERVIEW

Chapter 9 provides an overview of the process of curriculum development for BSN programs. It reviews the utilization of the AACN Essentials of Baccalaureate Education (2008) in curriculum development and discusses fast-track programs and RN to BSN programs. This chapter summarizes the advantages and challenges related to residency/externship programs for the new graduate. The following outlines the content of the chapter:

- When Is It Time for Curriculum Change?
  - Updated baccalaureate essentials
  - Recommendations for curriculum reform
  - Advances in educational technology

- Distance education
- High-fidelity simulation
- The learning-centered paradigm
- Curriculum Development
  - Conceptual framework
  - Curriculum outcomes
  - Identifying courses
- BSN Curriculum Design: Special Considerations
  - Content overload in nursing curricula
  - Integration of the curriculum
  - The inclusive curriculum: Paying attention to diversity
  - Transformative approaches to clinical education
  - Clinical Models
- Completing the Curriculum Development Process
- Transition to Practice
- Alternative BSN Pathways
  - Accelerated baccalaureate programs
  - Description of the ABSN program
  - ABSN students as experienced learners
  - Sample ABSN program
- RN–BSN Programs
  - Credit prior learning
  - Curriculum strategies
  - Clinical experiences
  - Inexperienced RN–BSN students
- Summary

WHEN IS IT TIME FOR CURRICULUM CHANGE?

Has there ever been a time in nursing education when so much is changing so quickly? Nursing is at the crossroads of major societal changes in health care reform, technology, and educational accountability to name only a few. The population is becoming more diverse, and baby boomers are aging. The country is at war and recovering from a recession. All of these factors affect the kind of programs that offered at schools of nursing, the content of the curricula, and the way that faculty teach in nursing education.

To prepare graduates of prelicensure nursing education programs for practice in an ever-changing health care environment, BSN curricula must be revised or updated on a regular basis. Nursing schools rely on a robust evaluation plan to provide information that guides curriculum revision. In addition, there are several compelling factors external to individual nursing programs that are currently influencing the need for curricular change within BSN nursing programs across the country. These include a recent revision of the *Essentials of Baccalaureate Education for Professional Nursing Practice* (AACN, 2008c), expressed concern with the quality of prelicensure nursing education by national health care organizations, advances in education technology, and educational research that has identified more effective teaching–learning strategies.

Updated Baccalaureate Essentials

The Essentials of Baccalaureate Education for Professional Nursing Practice (AACN, 2008c) have been updated to reflect changes in (a) health care, including expanded emphasis on quality and safety, patient technology, patient-centered care, population health, health care regulation, and globalization; (b) nursing education, with a focus on the liberal arts and information management; and (c) professional nursing practice, which is grounded in evidence-based practice, interprofessional communication and collaboration, and enduring social values. See Table 9.1 for a list of the revised *Essentials*.

These changes are supported by landmark documents such as the Institute of Medicine (IOM) reports (2001, 2003) and related Quality and Safety Education for Nurses (QSEN) competencies that include indicators for patient-centered care, teamwork and collaboration, evidence-based practice, quality improvement, safety, and informatics (Cronenwett et al., 2007). Other compelling and influential documents include *Healthy*

TABLE 9.1 The Essentials of Baccalaureate Education for Professional Nursing Practice

Essential I: Liberal Education for Baccalaureate Generalist Nursing Practice

- *A solid base in liberal education provides the cornerstone for the practice and education of nurses.*

Essential II: Basic Organizational and Systems Leadership for Quality Care and Patient Safety

- *Knowledge and skills in leadership, quality improvement, and patient safety are necessary to provide high quality health care.*

Essential III: Scholarship for Evidence Based Practice

- *Professional nursing practice is grounded in the translation of current evidence into one's practice.*

Essential IV: Information Management and Application of Patient Care Technology

- *Knowledge and skills in information management and patient care technology are critical in the delivery of quality patient care.*

Essential V: Health Care Policy, Finance, and Regulatory Environments

- *Health care policies, including financial and regulatory, directly and indirectly influence the nature and functioning of the healthcare system and thereby are important considerations in professional nursing practice.*

Essential VI: Interprofessional Communication and Collaboration for Improving Patient Health Outcomes

- *Communication and collaboration among healthcare professionals are critical to delivering high quality and safe patient care.*

Essential VII: Clinical Prevention and Population Health

- *Health promotion and disease prevention at the individual and population level are necessary to improve population health and are important components of baccalaureate generalist nursing practice.*

Essential VIII: Professionalism and Professional Values

- *Professionalism and the inherent values of altruism, autonomy, human dignity, integrity and social justice are fundamental to the discipline of nursing.*

Essential IX: Baccalaureate Generalist Nursing Practice

- *The baccalaureate graduate nurse is prepared to practice with patients, including individuals, families, groups, communities, and populations across the life span and across the continuum of healthcare environments.*

- *The baccalaureate graduate understands and respects the variations of care, the increased complexity, and the increased use of healthcare resources inherent in caring for patients.*

From AACN (2008c).

People 2010 (U.S. Department of Health and Human Services, 2000), the professional nursing study supported by the Carnegie Foundation for the Advancement of Teaching (Benner, Sutphen, Leonard, & Day, 2010), and numerous research and position papers authored by various key health care and educational organizations. The *Essentials* are the foundation for BSN curriculum development and will be referenced frequently throughout the discussion in this chapter.

Recommendations for Curriculum Reform

There has been significant concern with the preparedness of entry-level nurses to provide quality care within the complex and changing health care environments in which they practice. In addition, the shortage of nursing faculty and reduced capacity of clinical sites compel nurse educators to reconsider traditional models of prelicensure clinical education. A national survey conducted by the National League for Nursing (NLN) indicated that barriers to clinical education include lack of integration between theory and clinical components of the curriculum, inadequate preparation of clinical preceptors, and outdated clinical practice skills of supervising faculty (Jacobson & Grindel, 2006). The IOM (2001) clearly recommended a mandate for change in health care education, including nursing education, to improve quality and safety in the health care system. Benner et al. (2010) describe a practice–education gap that must be addressed by improving the quality of nursing education. The American Organization of Nurse Executives (AONE, 2004) takes the position that the nurse of the future will need different skills; BSN preparation will be necessary to meet the demands of practice, and BSN education must be "reframed" for graduates to be prepared. Additional reports from practice settings indicate that new graduates of prelicensure programs are not adequately prepared for nursing practice and therefore require additional development of clinical skills and professional competencies postgraduation (Forbes & Hickey, 2009; Hickey, 2009; Hofler, 2008).

Advances in Educational Technology

Advances in educational technology and Web-based learning have radically altered the process of prelicensure nursing education and affect the structure of the curriculum. As digital natives, students are often more technologically competent than faculty and expect current learning technology to be incorporated into the curriculum for interactive learning (Bleich, 2009; Skiba, 2007). Computer-based simulations such as the virtual neighborhood or community (Curran, Elfrink, & Mays, 2009; Giddens, 2007) are examples of innovations that are woven throughout the structure of the curriculum. Distance education and high-fidelity simulation learning strategies have been expanded and integrated into BSN programs.

Distance Education

Online learning is increasingly integrated into nursing education, although application of Web-based approaches varies widely among nursing programs. Faculty development and instructional design support are recommended to ensure the effective delivery of online course work (Anderson & Tredway, 2009; Little, 2009). The Web-enhanced classroom can be used to supplement learning through online activities such as discussion boards, resource-sharing, exams, videos, or other virtual programming (Creedy et al., 2007). Although specific nonclinical courses may be taught online or offered as an alternative method of delivery in prelicensure programs, they may be the primary pedagogy for BSN completion programs serving RN students (Anderson & Tredway). Distance applications include electronic classrooms and videoconferencing that facilitate inclusion of rural students and teaching across college campuses or to facilitate supervision for students involved in off-site practicum experiences. New applications are proliferating and significantly expand the resources available for educators. However, the use of Web-based resources in the curriculum has major implications for the development of student competency related to information literacy as part of the nursing program of study (Creedy et al.). The availability of distance education technologies and the related philosophy of an academic institution toward their use as a teaching–learning methodology have significant implications for the development of the program of study.

High-Fidelity Simulation

Although nursing educators have long employed low-fidelity and midfidelity simulation in nursing skills laboratories, high-fidelity simulation is quickly becoming the "gold standard" as schools of nursing incorporate this learning strategy into their curricula either to supplement or, in some cases, to replace clinical hours. Using this technology, faculty can create standardized and realistic clinical learning activities that ensure that all students get experience in critical patient-care situations in a low-risk and supportive environment (Nehring, 2008). The growing body of literature shows that high-fidelity simulation has the potential to improve student knowledge, skill performance, critical thinking, and self-confidence (Harder, 2009; Ironside, Jeffries, & Martin, 2009; Jeffries, 2005; Sinclair & Ferguson, 2009). Simulated learning experiences can be developed to support the progressive achievement of curriculum outcomes by intentionally spiraling core concepts and skills throughout the curriculum in increasingly more complex scenarios (Dubose, Sellinger-Karmel, & Scoloveno, 2010). Interdisciplinary simulations can provide an opportunity for students to learn about teamwork and collaboration and the roles of other health care professions (McGuire-Sessions & Gubrud, 2010). It must be noted, however, that there is little evidence regarding how high-fidelity simulation compares to traditional clinical approaches and that it is fairly costly and time intensive for faculty (National Council of State Boards of Nursing [NCSBN], 2009). In planning for use of simulation in a curriculum, schools are advised to check with their state board of nursing regarding regulations for percentage or replacement of clinical hours with high-fidelity simulation (Nehring, 2008). To make the best use of this technology, simulation must be approached with vision and intention in the curriculum development process (Harder, 2009).

The Learning-Centered Paradigm

There have been significant advancements in educational research that have improved understanding how students learn. For over a generation, college educators have been developing innovative approaches to interactive learning in higher education and there is a significant body of knowledge that provides evidence for the effectiveness of these practices (American Association of Colleges and Universities [AAC&U], 2007). Weimer

(2002) describes a paradigm shift in learning-centered education in which the power in the classroom is shared between teacher and students, content becomes less important than the reflective construction of knowledge, teachers become coaches, students assume responsibility for their learning, and authentic learning assessment is incorporated into the curriculum.

Nurse educators have made a case for moving away from the traditional content-laden behaviorist paradigm to a learning-centered model in which students are active participants. The traditional lecture and testing approach to instruction has been expanded to include narrative pedagogies, such as storytelling, reflective journaling, and literature (Brown, Kirkpatrick, Mangum, & Avery, 2008; Diekelmann, 2005; Ironside, 2006), and problem-based learning (Williams, 2001; Yuan, Williams, & Fan, 2008). The Carnegie Foundation's nursing education study supports significant innovation in prelicensure nursing education and recommends expansion of pedagogies that focus on patient experiences, such as clinical simulation scenarios, unfolding case studies, and clinical conferences focused on reflection about student experiences (Benner et al., 2010). These recommendations call for significant changes not only in the structure and organization of the program of study but also in the way the curriculum is delivered.

This is an exciting time in which nursing educators can seize the opportunity and challenge of developing new programs of study for prelicensure students for the 21st century and beyond. The creative wisdom of nursing faculty, grounded in educational expertise and experience and in collaboration with practice partners, has the potential to shape a more effective, more relevant, more responsive system of nursing education. Waiting for all the answers to come is pointless; innovation must start now.

CURRICULUM DEVELOPMENT

The curriculum reflects the heart and soul of a nursing faculty. For each school, at least some of the current faculty were most likely involved in developing the existing curriculum and are invested in its success. The curriculum expresses the faculty's values and beliefs about nursing and education, and reflects their professional identity. Faculty members have educated and mentored many students through the program and their courses have been the core of their daily work—in some cases, for many years. The curriculum is familiar and comforting. These factors mean that curriculum change is one of the most challenging undertakings for any faculty. It may prove difficult to build consensus about a new program based on different values and priorities among a diverse group of faculty members. Some faculty members have kept up with best practices and innovation in nursing education, whereas others are content with the status quo. Ideally curriculum revision is driven by the faculty and begins with an agreement by the faculty as a whole to enter into the process, but in reality, not all will be equally committed or involved in the effort.

Once a decision has been made to revise an existing curriculum or develop a new curriculum, next steps include selecting a work group or committee, developing a plan, and exploring best practices in nursing education. The composition of the group that will be leading the work of developing the curriculum is of primary importance to the success of the endeavor, and the members should be selected with intention. A strong team includes a diverse group of tenured and untenured faculty with various areas of expertise and backgrounds that are committed to the goal, are motivated to do the difficult work of curriculum development, and are able to work collaboratively through the process of change (Mawn & Reece, 2000). In addition to faculty with passion for curriculum, a balanced group includes both faculty members with current practice experience and those with expertise by virtue of their long teaching careers. Nursing students bring a unique and practical perspective to the work, and their participation enriches the curriculum development process. As the group organizes, a discussion about roles within the committee and ground rules facilitate the process. One strategy recommended by Hull, St. Romain, Alexander, Schaff, and Jones (2001) is for one member of the committee to assume the role of facilitator to make sure that the ground rules are followed and to mediate the inevitable conflicts. An early discussion of bias, territoriality concerns, and "sacred cows" contribute to the process. Other suggestions include a tentative plan and timeline to help the group to stay on schedule, and a plan for communicating the progress of the curriculum revision and points for feedback from the faculty as a whole.

The initial preparatory work of the curriculum development work group is to review program evaluation data and to plan various strategies to identify best practices in nursing education. The extent of this effort will depend on the time elapsed since the last curriculum revision and the extent of the planned revision. The following information and documents will inform the committee and provide data for difficult discussions and decision making:

- The *Essentials* (AACN, 2008c) document is foundational and should be made available to all members from the beginning. The document includes rationale, performance indicators, and sample content for each essential that are helpful in understanding the scope of each statement for application to a particular program of study.
- A comprehensive search of the literature identifies best practices and innovation in nursing education, and synthesizing the information for the faculty as a whole, facilitates shared understanding (Forbes & Hickey, 2009; Hull et al., 2001).
- A review of professional standards such as the American Nurses Association Code of Ethics (2005) and various published competencies for BSN graduates is important. Based on current issues and priorities in nursing practice, specific BSN level competencies have been developed for quality and safety (Cronenwett et al., 2007), cultural competency (AACN, 2008c), genetics and genomics (AACN, 2006), and geriatric nursing care (AACN & Hartford Foundation, 2000).
- A survey of other regional and national programs provides examples of model programs of study. Programs that have been recently updated and incorporate innovation, have similar missions, and have been recently accredited, may be of most value.
- Focus groups or surveys of stakeholders including students, faculty, and clinical or community partners, provide invaluable information regarding expectations and priorities and create an inclusive process. These surveys can provide meaningful local information about what was working and not working in the old curriculum, suggested changes or direction, new information and trends to be aware of, and priority knowledge and skills to include in the new curriculum.

Information in this chapter is relevant to the development or revision of curricula for several types of BSN programs that will be addressed in this chapter, including 4-year traditional nursing programs, transfer programs in which students complete prerequisites and general education courses before entering the nursing program, accelerated (or fast-track) BSN programs, and RN–BSN completion programs. If a school has more than one type of program, there must be consistency and congruency among programs. The suggested approach is to start with development of the generic prelicensure BSN program and then to develop modifications based on the core curriculum model. Examples of documents that describe the curriculum revision at Linfield-Good Samaritan School of Nursing (LGSSON) at Linfield College will be given throughout the chapter and supplemented by descriptions of innovations from other BSN programs.

The process of curriculum development is an iterative process of discovery, and the components of the curriculum package generally remain flexible until all parts are completed to allow for new insights and learning of the curriculum development team and the faculty. The curriculum development process begins with values clarification and development of a mission, vision, philosophy, and a specific goal or purpose of the program (as described in Chapter 7). These statements must be consistent with that of the parent institution and underlie all nursing programs at the school.

Conceptual Framework

The conceptual framework (or theoretical or organizational model) guides the development of the program of study and makes it unique; it unifies the curriculum and creates a coherent approach across courses and levels (Ervin, Bickes, & Schim, 2006). Although there are some curricular elements that are common among schools based on the *Essentials*, others define the particular identity of the program based on the characteristics of the parent institution and the philosophy of the particular nursing program. According to McEwen and Brown (2002), the use of a single theorist is an outdated approach and most nursing programs have an eclectic model that reflects their values and priorities. The metaparadigm for nursing that includes the key concepts of person, environment, health, and nursing is no longer an adequate foundation for an educational program (Webber, 2002). Theoretical models for BSN programs have shifted away from nursing process to critical thinking (McEwen & Brown, 2002) and reflect alternatives for the biomedical model that more closely reflect nursing concepts and values. If the theoretical model is basic and broad, it is possible for it to encompass and support various views of practice and education that may be held by faculty (Ervin et al., 2006) and allow for new developments in nursing and health care (Newman, 2008).

Webber (2002) designed a curriculum framework based on conceptual cornerstones in nursing: nursing knowledge, nursing skills, nursing values, nursing meanings, and nursing experience (KSVME). This model was used to organize outcomes for Associate Degree in Nursing (ADN), BSN, and Master of Science (MS) level programs and is flexible enough to accommodate the needs of various schools of nursing and ongoing changes in nursing. Some nursing programs have developed visual representations of their curriculum models that clarify the relationships between key concepts; examples include a theoretical framework integrating a multiple determinants of health paradigm and systems framework at Wayne State (Ervin et al., 2006), and a primary health care model at Mt. St. Joseph (Perkins, Vale, & Graham, 2001). See Figure 9.1 for a visual model of the LGSSON theoretical framework, which reflects the school's community-based philosophy.

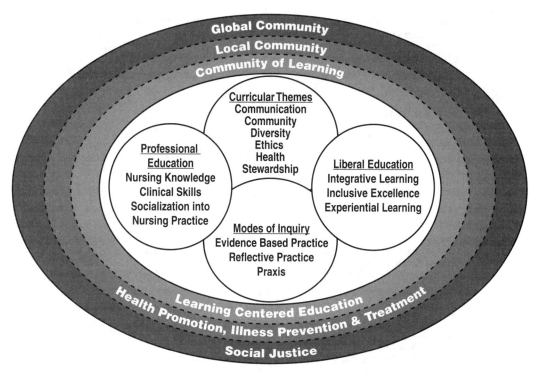

FIGURE 9.1 Linfield-Good Samaritan School of Nursing Theoretical Model for Community-Based Nursing Education. Reproduced with permission.

Curriculum Outcomes

The next step in the BSN curriculum development process is to identify level and terminal or end-of-program outcomes/student learning outcomes (or objectives or competencies), which must be directly related to the *Essentials* in the context of the school's philosophy. Whether a school uses outcomes, objectives, or competencies to create the curricular structure, the term must be defined, used consistently, and leveled across the program. The outcomes form the backbone of the curriculum and will be the foundation for program evaluation. Student Learning Outcomes (end-of-program outcomes) can be developed by reviewing each essential and writing outcome statements that address the key concepts. This task can either be completed by the curriculum development group or be more inclusive and involve the BSN faculty as a whole by assigning a small group of individuals to write outcomes for specific essentials. When all the outcome statements are reviewed and analyzed as a package, there will most likely be overlap and areas that need to be strengthened in preparing the final document. As the outcomes statements are combined and synthesized, some may address more than one essential, but all essentials must be addressed. Once the terminal outcomes are identified, the level outcomes are developed and spiraled to show students' progression throughout the program. Table 9.2 gives an example of curriculum outcomes as they relate to the *Essentials*.

TABLE 9.2 Linfield-Good Samaritan School of Nursing Mapping of Curriculum Outcomes and *Essentials (2008)*

Curriculum Outcomes	Essentials
1. Engages in ethical reasoning and actions that demonstrate caring and commitment to social justice in the delivery of healthcare to individuals and populations.	I: Liberal Education for Baccalaureate Generalist Nursing Practice V: Healthcare Policy, Finance, and Regulatory Environments VII: Clinical Prevention and Population Health VIII: Professionalism and Professional Values
2. Uses a range of information and clinical technologies to achieve healthcare outcomes for clients.	II: Basic Organizational and Systems Leadership for Quality Care and Patient Safety III: Scholarship for Evidence Based Practice IV: Information Management and Patient Care Technology IX: Baccalaureate Generalist Nursing Practice
3. Communicates effectively and collaboratively to provide client-centered nursing care in various healthcare communities.	I: Liberal Education for Baccalaureate Generalist Nursing Practice VI: Interprofessional Communication and Collaboration for Improving Health Outcomes VIII: Professionalism and Professional Values IX: Baccalaureate Generalist Nursing Practice
4. Applies principles of stewardship and leadership skills to support quality and safety within complex organizational systems.	II: Basic Organizational and Systems Leadership for Quality Care and Patient Safety
5. Provide effective nursing care that incorporates diverse values, cultures, perspectives and health practices	I: Liberal Education for Baccalaureate Generalist Nursing Practice VII: Clinical Prevention and Population Health VIII: Professionalism and Professional Values IX: Baccalaureate Generalist Nursing Practice
6. Incorporates a liberal-arts-based understanding of global healthcare issues to promote health, prevent disease and facilitate healing of clients across the lifespan.	I: Liberal Education for Baccalaureate Generalist Nursing Practice VII: Clinical Prevention and Population Health IX: Baccalaureate Generalist Nursing Practice
7. Apply sound clinical judgment and evidence-based practice in the provision of holistic nursing care	I: Liberal Education for Baccalaureate Generalist Nursing Practice III: Scholarship for Evidence Based Practice IV: Information Management and Patient Care Technology IX: Baccalaureate Generalist Nursing Practice
8. Integrate knowledge of healthcare policy, populations, finance, and regulatory environments that influence system level change within professional nursing practice	II: Basic Organizational and Systems Leadership for Quality Care and Patient Safety V: Healthcare Policy, Finance, and Regulatory Environments

Reproduced with permission.

There has been a recent resurgence in the use of competencies to structure curricula. Goudreau et al. (2009) identify the second-generation competency-based approach as grounded in a constructivist model that supports learning-centered approaches. Competencies are not constrained by the language of Bloom's taxonomy but are statements of "complex know-hows" specific to the discipline that "allows one to deal with different situations by drawing on concepts, knowledge, information, procedures, and methods" (Goudreau et al., 2009, p. 3). For example, the 10 competencies developed by the Oregon Consortium for Nursing Education (OCNE) are not grounded in the behaviorist tradition but reflect the complexity and integration of empirical knowledge and practical knowing. (Gubrud-Howe et al., 2003). The OCNE competency statements can be viewed at http://www.ocne.org/Curriculum%20Competency%20May%202009.pdf.

Identifying Courses

In the next step, essential knowledge, skills, and attitudes that students will need to accomplish related to each outcome are identified. This is the content that is then organized into coherent and logical groupings, which become courses. There are many possible ways to cluster the information, and the faculty should be guided by their previous research and philosophical work. The identification of new courses can be an exciting and creative activity but has the potential to be a phase of the curriculum development process that creates conflict. Issues of territoriality and "sacred cows" may assert themselves; it is sometimes difficult to think creatively and safer to regress to what is known (the old model). At this juncture, decisions must be made about which concepts to integrate and which to organize into a separate course. In the creation of a working course template, a program of study by semester begins to emerge. Table 9.3 shows the courses in the plan of study for the generic BSN curriculum at LGSSON.

TABLE 9.3 Linfield-Good Samaritan School of Nursing Generic BSN Program of Study*

Semester 1: Foundations for Community Based Nursing Practice	Credits	Semester 2: Chronic Health	Credits
Foundations of Community-based Nursing Practice	4	Nursing Care of Children, Adults, and Older Adults with Chronic Conditions	3
Professional Communication in Diverse Communities	2	Clinical Pathophysiology and Pharmacology for Nursing Practice I	2
Scholarship of Nursing	3	Mental Health and Illness Across the Lifespan	2
Integrated Experiential Learning I	6	Integrated Experiential Learning II	6
		Elective or General Education	3
	15		13–16

Semester 3: Acute Health	Credits	Semester 4: Stewardship for Health	Credits
Nursing Care of Children, Adults, and Older Adults with Acute Conditions	3	Leading and Managing in Nursing	3
Transitions and Decisions: Pregnancy, Birth and End of Life Care	2	Population-based Nursing in a Multicultural and Global Society	2
Clinical Pathophysiology and Pharmacology for Nursing Practice II	2	Integrated Experiential Learning IV	8
Integrated Experiential Learning III	6	Elective NCLEX-RN preparation course	1
Elective or General Education	3		
	13–16		13–14

Reproduced with permission.
*Approved by the school of nursing; in final approval process.

A program that relies on the biomedical model will tend toward a traditional course structure that adheres more closely to medical specialties, for example, pediatric nursing, psychiatric nursing, and medical–surgical nursing. A program that is organized according to a nursing framework may have more integrated courses, for example, a course focusing on chronicity in which students explore health issues and concerns of clients with chronic illness, including physical and mental health problems across the life span and including the entire health trajectory from prevention to end-of-life. The theoretical model should provide a framework for making decisions about the program of study. Once the program of study is drafted, faculty teams may begin work on course development (as described in Chapter 7).

BSN CURRICULUM DESIGN: SPECIAL CONSIDERATIONS

The nursing education literature identifies curriculum design issues that must be considered as faculty moves forward with development of the prelicensure program of study. These include the historical overloading of content in nursing curricula, integration of curriculum concepts, and consideration of the needs of diverse student body.

Content Overload in Nursing Curricula

Advances and trends in nursing science compel additions to the nursing curriculum in the areas of quality and safety, informatics, diversity, and cultural competence, genetics and genomics, and evidence-based practice. While these subjects are important for preparing BSN nurses of the future, how can faculty possibly add this content to an already packed curriculum? Nursing education has historically been plagued with "content overload." As health care and nursing practice change, nurse educators typically keep adding information to courses without taking anything out (Ironside, 2004; Tanner, 2007) As a result, both students and faculty are chronically overloaded and overworked with little time for reflection and real learning.

To facilitate meaningful learning, nursing faculty must reorient the curriculum, from what the students need to know to how they think in their developing nursing practice (Ironside, 2004; Tanner, 2006). Learning-centered approaches such as problem-based strategies, case studies, and narrative pedagogies (Benner et al., 2010; Diekelmann, 2005; Ironside, 2004) address issues of overload at the course level, but there are also curricular approaches to safeguard against it. Candela, Dalley, and Benzel-Lindley (2006) described learning-centered education as an approach to control content and suggested a systematic process for categorizing the importance of curricular content and eliminating all but the most essential. Giddens (2007) studied skills utilized by practicing nurses and determined that only a core set of skills taught in physical assessment classes were used in practice. Subsequently, Giddens and Eddy (2009) evaluated the content taught in physical assessment courses in ADN and BSN programs. Based on an apparent disconnect between skills taught in nursing education and those used in practice, they recommended that faculty teach fewer skills and only those most frequently used in practice. In similar fashion, nursing courses commonly teach management of clients with an exhaustive list of clinical disorders, many of them rare. In sorting essential content, only the most commonly encountered disorders should be used as exemplars within a nursing framework.

Tanner (2007) suggests that faculty cover few topics deeper to facilitate understanding of concepts most important for nursing practice.

The concept-based model for curriculum development is another way to reduce content saturation. In this approach, nursing faculty identifies, classifies, and defines concepts that subsequently provide the organizational framework for the curriculum and are threaded through courses (Giddens & Brady, 2007). For example, at LGSSON, the faculty identified six major themes that reflected the mission, vision, and philosophy of the school and were incorporated into the theoretical framework: communication, community, diversity, ethics, health, and stewardship. Essential concepts were identified for each of the themes and the concepts within each theme were spiraled from simple to complex and then leveled across 4 semesters. Although the emphasis on the themes varied from semester to semester, and new information for each theme was introduced each semester; the expectation was that knowledge and skills were cumulative throughout the program. Examples of the leveling of the concepts within three of these themes are provided in Table 9.4.

Within each semester, concepts from all themes were then organized into courses; as an example, the conceptual organization of the theory courses from the final 2 semesters of the program are shown in Table 9.5. By identifying more abstract concepts instead of content for each course, the faculty member is free to update and prioritize course content as it changes over time. For example, the concept of "environmental health," which is introduced in semester 4, does not specify specific content and allows the teacher to vary explanatory models and exemplars according to current research and community priorities.

Integration of the Curriculum

There are multiple meanings for the term "integrated learning," which has become part of the language of education; all are possible to incorporate within the BSN curriculum and influence the design of the program of study. In the broadest sense, the AAC&U (2004) describes the importance of integrated learning in undergraduate education, in which students connect their learning "across courses, over time, and between campus and community life." This includes applying knowledge and methods across fields, and from foundational humanities, social sciences, and science courses into the professional curriculum. This perspective is supported by the *Essentials* (AACN, 2008c), which clearly sets the standard for a liberal arts foundation in nursing programs. For example, the scientific method learned in prerequisite laboratory courses and the skill of building an argument in philosophy are fundamental to development of clinical thinking skills for nursing practice.

Integrated learning can refer to the seamless connection of nursing theory and practice. According to Benner et al. (2010), students learn better when they are in a classroom that integrates theory and clinical. Based on the results of the professional nursing education study, Benner et al. recommend that BSN curricula integrate three apprenticeships into the program of study: nursing knowledge, learned skills and clinical reasoning, and ethical comportment and formation. In this model, apprenticeships refer to situated learning and meaningful integration of theory and practice in which students learn through experiences within a "community of practice" (Benner et al., 2010, p. 25). Noone (2009)

TABLE 9.4 Linfield-Good Samaritan School of Nursing Community-based Curriculum Framework: Conceptual Organization Exemplars of Concepts Identified within Curriculum Themes: Communication, Diversity, Stewardship (3 of 6 themes)

	Semester 1: Foundations for Community-based Nursing Practice	Semester 2: Chronic Health	Semester 3: Acute Health	Semester 4: Stewardship for Health
	Curriculum Themes			
Communication Continuum: *student, client, family/group, team*	**Communication:** Therapeutic use of self-emotional intelligence Documentation Scholarly writing Interpersonal communication Interviewing Therapeutic communication	**Communication:** Interdisciplinary communication Collaboration Advocacy Family dynamics Group dynamics	**Communication:** Making a case	**Communication:** Conflict management Delegation, Teambuilding
Diversity Continuum: *cultural self, intercultural, multicultural, international*	**Diversity:** Cultural identity Cultural diversity Difference Cultural competence Racism Privilege Intercultural communication Spirituality Holism	**Diversity:** Culturally adaptive care Cultural health beliefs Integrative healthcare Cultural humility	**Diversity:** Cultural advocacy Cultural relativism	**Diversity:** Intercultural bridging Immigration Global health disparities Organizational cultural competence Universal cultural values
Stewardship Continuum: *professional nurse, organizational systems, professional leadership*	**Stewardship** Evolution of nursing Professionalism Self-care Lifelong learning Practice regulation	**Stewardship:** Care delivery Client outcomes	**Stewardship:** Organizational systems Cost consciousness QI/Patient safety	**Stewardship:** Leadership Management organizational culture Change Mentorship Continuous quality improvement Risk management Health care regulation Health care economics

Reproduced with permission.

suggests that educators develop curricula in which all three apprenticeships are integrated within each course.

Integration refers to the incorporation of concepts related to major curricular themes such as ethics, nursing research, or mental health nursing that have traditionally been stand-alone courses into broader, more comprehensive courses. Jayasekara,

TABLE 9.5 Linfield-Good Samaritan School of Nursing Organization of Curriculum Concepts into Theory Courses for the Final Two Semesters

Semester 3 (Fall): Acute Health	Semester 4 (Spring): Stewardship of Health
Nursing Care of Children, Adults, and Older Adults with Acute Conditions: acuity, crisis, trauma, clotting, perfusion, hemostasis, homeostasis, fluid & electrolytes, immunity, inflammation, infection, oxygenation, cell growth & regulation, hormonal regulation, generalizing experiences, adapting practice, cultural advocacy, organizational systems, QI/patient safety, cost consciousness, making a case, resource connecting, evidence-based client care: acute	**Leading and Managing in Nursing:** leadership, management, teambuilding, conflict management, organizational culture, organizational systems, healthcare economics, mentorship, quality improvement, risk management, healthcare regulation, organizational ethics, organizational cultural competence, collective action, health policy, responsible action, change, evidence-based organizational change, delegation.
Transitions and Decisions: Pregnancy, Birth, and End-of-Life	**Population-based Nursing in a Multicultural and Global Society:** healthy communities, epidemiology, immigration, community education, community outreach, environmental health, sustainability, emergency preparedness, universal cultural values, global health, global consciousness, global nursing ethics, global health disparities, complex health situations, evidence-based aggregate care.
Care: family coping, pregnancy, childbirth, midwifery, death & dying, loss & grief, good nurse, quality of life, self-determination, comfort care, moral distress, healthcare ethics, case analysis, healthcare ethics, genetics/genomics, cultural relativism.	**Integrated Experiential Learning IV (7–8 credits)**
Clinical Pathophysiology and Pharmacology II: inflammation/immunity/infection; alterations in cell growth; alterations in fluid, electrolyte, and acid-base balance; alterations in ventilation and diffusion; alterations in perfusion.	
Integrated Experiential Learning III (6 credits)	

Reproduced with permission.

Schultz, and McCutcheon (2006) used the term to describe the integration of subjects or concepts into courses across semesters or across the program in nontraditional ways. In a synthesis of evidence related to undergraduate nursing curriculum models, the only meaningful finding was that a combination of integrated and subject-centered models may be most effective; concepts and program components that were more effectively taught in an integrated manner included those related to aging and liberal education, and technical concepts like assessment were better presented in a separate course.

The Inclusive Curriculum: Paying Attention to Diversity

There is a national call to increase the enrollment of students from underrepresented populations in schools of nursing, and recent reports show that some progress is being made (U.S. Department of Health and Human Services, Health Resources and Services Administration, 2010). Learning-centered education generally addresses diverse learning styles, and there is a growing body of literature regarding effective teaching and assessment strategies for nursing students from underrepresented populations (Bosher & Pharris, 2009). However, schools of nursing typically have not considered the needs of students who are minorities, low income students, first-in-family to attend college, or multilingual, nonnative English speakers in developing the plan of study or the curriculum structure. Ideally, the curriculum should be creative and flexible, and it should reflect the multicultural perspectives of our pluralistic society (Warda, 2008). If diversity and cultural competence is part of the mission or philosophy of the school, related concepts should be included in the theoretical framework, explicit in program and level outcomes, and reflected in concepts/content threaded throughout the curriculum (Crow, 1997). For example, at tribal colleges, curriculum is structured to focus on important elements of the Native American culture.

The AAC&U promotes *inclusive excellence,* an approach, which is based on the understanding that becoming an educated person in a pluralistic society includes developing the ability to communicate and interact with individuals and populations that are different from themselves (Williams, Berger, & McClendon, 2005). This philosophy compels faculty members to facilitate the success of all students, including those with diverse backgrounds and learning styles. Swaner and Brownell (2008) recommend high impact strategies for the success of underrepresented minority students, including learning communities, service learning, undergraduate research, first year seminars, and capstone projects that could readily be incorporated into the structure of nursing programs. Faculty may not be aware of how programmatic organization affects students differentially. For example, the practice of "front-loading" theory in a curriculum or a particular course prior to engagement in clinical practice disadvantages tactile and kinesthetic learners, and this is the preferred learning style for many ESL students (Reid, 1987). In a theory-first model, students who are having difficulty with theory miss the opportunity to reinforce classroom learning in the most effective way possible—through hands-on learning in the real world (Bosher, 2007). These learners would best achieve academically in a curriculum model that more closely integrate theory and clinical experience.

Other ways of demonstrating inclusiveness in curriculum planning include consideration of pre-entry nursing courses, parallel academic support courses, culture-focused or special interest general education courses or electives, and international experiences as part of the program of study from the beginning rather than as an afterthought. The cocurriculum can play an important role in supporting and validating underrepresented students on the campus. Other ideas include development of clinical models that facilitate multicultural clinical experiences and intentionally threading exemplars throughout the curriculum that address health care issues experienced by particular ethnic or cultural groups. Another strategy is to institute a curriculum requirement that assures that students have various experiences with populations or clients that are different from themselves. One best practice in nursing education identified in a study of California nursing programs included organizing and scheduling the program of study to accommodate working students, which could include options for evening and/or part-time course work (Buchbinder, 2007). And finally, admission and progression requirements for incoming students that disadvantage those who were educated in another country or are multilingual nonnative English speakers will shape the student body and affect the quality of learning for all the students.

Transformative Approaches to Clinical Education

One of the most challenging aspects of curriculum revision is designing an approach to students' clinical experiences that reflects the school's theoretical model and integrates new learning pedagogies in the context of local realities related to the availability of qualified clinical faculty and availability of clinical sites. Whereas clinical experience is essential in preparation for practice, what constitutes clinical experience? What kinds of clinical learning activities and how much time in what kind of health care settings is most effective for BSN students to meet generalist competencies and transition successfully into practice? The "NLN Think Tank on Transforming Clinical Nursing Education" (National League for Nursing, 2008) made recommendations for the ideal clinical education model that described integrative experiences, including cross-disciplinary experiences; new relationships within learning communities, including innovative relationships with clinical partners; and reconceptualized learning experiences in which all students do not have clinical experiences in traditional rotations. While there are scarce data about the effectiveness of either traditional or new clinical models, it is incumbent on nurse educators to develop and test models and approaches and contribute to the database. Each school of nursing needs to develop an approach that best utilizes its resources and fits its theoretical model.

Clinical Models

The traditional clinical education model in which a nursing faculty member provides direct supervision and oversight for a small group of students on a hospital unit is no longer practical or effective for several reasons:

- Shortened patient lengths of stay make it difficult for students to collect information from the medical record and prepare for patient care prior to the clinical experience, and often patients are discharged sooner than anticipated.
- Students miss experiences when they are dependent on clinical faculty and are obligated to wait for them before engaging in particular skills or situations.
- Students spend too much of their clinical time in repetitive tasks and not enough on higher level thinking activities (Ironside & McNelis, 2009).
- The total patient care model for a limited number of patients does not provide the breadth of experiences with authentic nursing activities required for preparation for generalist practice.
- The traditional role that faculty plays in sequentially supervising skills (like passing medications) is not responsive to the rapidly changing and competing demands of clinical practice and does not focus on development of students' clinical thinking skills.
- Given the reduced capacity of clinical sites, faculty logistically cannot attend to all students with placements at various community clinical sites or even on different units at a hospital.

In response to the changing reality, MacIntyre, Murray, Teel, and Karshmer (2009) made recommendations to strengthen academic-service relationships and create new models for clinical education that:

> 1. *reenvision nursing student-staff relationships; 2. reconceptualize the clinical faculty role; 3. enhance development for school-based faculty and staff nurses working with students; 4. reexamine the depth and breadth of the clinical component; and 5. strengthen the evidence for best practices in clinical nursing education* (p. 448).

The need for new clinical models was driven in large part by the lack of availability of clinical sites and increased enrollments in nursing programs in response to the projected nursing shortage. In addition, nursing faculty members are challenged to find meaningful and predictable clinical experiences for students in health care facilities where there is less staff caring for higher acuity patients. As previously discussed, many schools are using simulated learning activities in the classroom and the learning laboratories to prepare students for clinical experiences and, in some cases, to substitute for clinical hours (NCSBN, 2009). Some other innovative approaches are described as follows:

In lieu of the traditional model, OCNE developed a new approach to expand clinical capacity that proposed five elements of clinical learning that defined a set of activities that build on one another throughout the curriculum. The new model includes focused direct client care, concept-based experiences, case-based experiences, intervention skill–based experiences, and integrative experiences (Gubrud-Howe & Schoessler, 2008). In this approach, traditional comprehensive patient care is only one strategy among others that supports students to meet course outcomes. Research to evaluate the efficacy of these models is in progress.

At LGSSON, overcrowding and complex scheduling of limited laboratory space and decreasing (and sometimes competing) clinical opportunities resulted in the development of an integrated experiential learning (IEL) model, in which concepts introduced in multiple corequisite theory courses in a particular semester are applied and synthesized in a single course that includes field experiences, laboratory, simulation, and clinical experiences. Each clinical course includes some experience with clients in a primary, secondary, and tertiary site according to the theoretical model. The details of the IEL model are in development.

The University of Delaware developed a nurse residency model, which is a senior-year clinical immersion experience that meets 3 days per week during the last semester along with clinical integration seminars. What is unique about this model is that during the first 3 years of the program, students do not have traditional acute care clinical experiences. Students instead demonstrate readiness by successful completion of didactic courses and progressive development of knowledge and competence through laboratory and simulation, field experiences, teaching assistantships, and a work requirement. (Diefenbeck, Plowfield, & Herrman, 2006; Herrman & Diefenbeck, 2009). In this innovative approach, practice is decoupled from theory in course work, and the definition of clinical education is expanded to include the alternative experiences. In the context of the new definition, the total number of clinical hours increased in the residency model although less faculty resources were required (Diefenbeck et al., 2006).

Another approach to clinical education relies on community partnerships in which student cohorts stay primarily in one health care system so that they do not have to spend precious learning time repeatedly reorienting to different organizations (Joynt & Kimball, 2008). For example, the University of North Florida's BSN program utilizes a clinical model in which the school partners with communities to develop ongoing relationships in service to the community's specific issues and agendas. Students are assigned to a home base during their first year and participate in collaborative activities during their entire nursing program. While students have other clinical experiences, the long-term relationship with the community agency and gradual progression of clinical experiences resulted in positive learning experiences for students (Kruger, Roush, Olinzock, & Bloom, 2009).

The dedicated education unit (DEU) is another education–practice collaborative model that relies on ongoing partnerships with clinical agencies. In this model, nurses, faculty, and students working together create an optimal teaching environment, while continuing the commitment to quality patient care. Staff nurses on identified patient care units assume the direct teaching role with support from faculty who facilitate development of their expertise in teaching. Because the unit is utilized exclusively by students from the partner school, the nurses become adjunct faculty members and are oriented to the curriculum and specific learning outcomes (Moscato, Miller, Logsdon, Weinberg, & Chorpenning, 2007). The DEU model utilizes scarce faculty resources in an efficient manner that significantly increases the capacity for student placements (Moscato et al., 2007).

These innovative approaches to clinical education are grounded in new pedagogy and make creative use of scarce resources to help students achieve curriculum outcomes. They rely on more focused clinical experiences that maximize faculty resources, collaborative relationships with clinical agencies, and student learning potential. Evaluation of the effectiveness of models such as these, including cost/benefit, will inform and influence the quality of nursing education in the future.

COMPLETING THE CURRICULUM DEVELOPMENT PROCESS

Concurrent with the development of the program of study, additional work must be completed as part of the comprehensive curriculum package. A glossary defines terms that have special meaning within the mission, vision, and philosophy, theoretical model, and curriculum plan, including concepts that provide the organizational framework for the curriculum. Prerequisites, including humanities, science, and social science courses that serve as foundation for the nursing course work must be identified and negotiated with various other departments. These will include collegewide requirements such as general education. Progression issues must be considered, including minimum GPA for admission into the school of nursing, a description of how students will progress from semester to semester, and prerequisites and corequisites for each course. The curriculum development group will need to work with the administrative team to cost out the curriculum, including faculty and other resources that will be needed to manage the new curriculum. Often, old and new curricula will be offered simultaneously for a time until the students in the old program graduate, which may require additional resources. The curriculum package must be approved by the nursing faculty and be directed through academic channels for approval. The new curriculum must be submitted to the state board of nursing and the national accrediting body.

TRANSITION TO PRACTICE

Transition of new BSN graduates into clinical practice is recognized as an issue since *Reality Shock* was first published (Kramer, 1974). Capstone or integrative clinical experiences have been shown as one curriculum strategy that contributes to the socialization of graduate nurses into practice (Butler & Hardin-Pierce, 2005; Tanner, 2006). In addition, a synthesis of recommendations from national reports about transition from the academic environment to nursing practice environment showed significant support for the formation of academic and service partnerships to develop standardized internship and residency programs (Hofler, 2008). In support of programs that are offered through academic-service partnerships, the Commission on Collegiate Nursing Education (CCNE, 2008) recently implemented accreditation for postbaccalaureate nurse residency programs.

The goal of transition programs are primarily to mediate "reality shock" and assist the new graduate to develop clinical competency as well as improve recruitment and retention and reduce orientation costs for the employer. Programs may be situated prior to graduation or following, and include educational and psychosocial support strategies such as mentoring, preceptor training, clinical coaching, expanded orientation, clinical and professional skill development, classes, and other learning activities targeted at the needs of the developing professional (Bratt, 2009; Herdrich & Lindsay, 2006; Rosenfeld, Smith, Iervolino, & Bowar-Feres, 2004).

Although quantitative results were equivocal, qualitative evaluation of an externship program for BSN students between their 3rd and 4th years of study showed that participants felt more a part of their clinical units, were more familiar with the environment and available resources, and understood the role and responsibilities of the professional nurse. Overall, graduates benefitted from the program, which proved to be an effective recruitment and retention tool, but they were not spared the realities of transition into practice (Cantrell & Browne, 2005; Cantrell & Browne, 2006; Cantrell, Browne, & Lupinacci, 2005). Results of an evaluation of a for-credit summer internship program reported by Barger & Das (2004) demonstrated stronger student clinical skills during senior year, improved recruitment to the agency, less time in orientation, and less turnover.

Model postgraduation programs show similar results and are reported to be particularly successful in building capacity and community for rural hospitals (Bratt, 2009). Additional benefits include improved confidence and critical thinking ability, development of leadership skills, professional growth, improved job performance and satisfaction, and role socialization (Altier & Krsek, 2006; Butler & Pierce, 2005). Participants in residence programs scored higher on core competencies and were higher functioning team members (Blanzola, Lindeman, & King, 2004). In one study, less satisfaction was documented among nonwhite program participants (Altier & Krsek, 2006). One major challenge in residency program management is preparing and maintaining committed and effective mentor/preceptors (Eigsti, 2009; Fitzgerald, 2009; Rosenfeld et al., 2004). Achievement of quality indicators is important to justify program continuation in the context of the current economic downturn and climate of scarce resources; evaluation should include not only the cost–benefit analysis related to retention of new graduates but also factors such as quality indicators of professional achievement of nurse residents (Bratt).

ALTERNATIVE BSN PATHWAYS

Accelerated Baccalaureate Programs

The first accelerated baccalaureate program was initiated at St. Louis University in 1971 and by 1990 there were 31 such programs (Lindsey, 2009). Since then, the numbers have proliferated and by fall 2009, totaled 230 programs (AACN, 2009c) with others in various stages of development. The more recent, rapid development of programs has been a response to the projected shortage of nurses and is viewed as a viable option to help meet that need (Cangelosi, 2007; Penprase & Koczara, 2009). Graduates from ABSN programs are highly valued by employers because they tend to be more mature, learn quickly, have well-developed clinical skills, and stay longer at their first job than generic students (AACN, 2009b; Brewer et al., 2009; Raines & Sipes, 2007).

Description of the ASBN program

Accelerated BSN (ABSN) programs offer students who completed a bachelor's degree in another discipline the opportunity to obtain a degree in nursing in a shorter time frame than those in traditional baccalaureate nursing programs. Accelerated programs are generally offered as intensive full-time courses of study with no breaks between semesters or terms and most programs are 11 to 18 months in length, including prerequisites (AACN, 2009b).

It is difficult to identify a standardized design model for accelerated programs. Curriculum outcomes should be the same as those of the other prelicensure programs at a particular school, but course structure and pedagogical approaches may vary. ABSN programs require students to take prerequisites although the school's liberal arts and general education requirements are usually waived (DeBasio, 2005). Some schools maintain accelerated and traditional students as separate cohorts, whereas others integrate them at some point during their educational process. ABSN programs may conform to the standard undergraduate academic schedule or define their own without standard breaks. By building on prior learning, students in ABSN programs are able to complete the same curriculum outcomes in a program with less overall credits. Although the number of didactic or theory hours/courses may differ between the traditional BSN and the ABSN program at a school, the number of clinical hours generally remains the same. (AACN, 2009b).

ABSN Students as Experienced Learners

Students in accelerated programs have been characterized as adult learners (Raines, 2009) who return to school with high expectations of themselves (Raines & Sipes, 2007). Because many had a career following their first degree, they bring an increased depth of life experience and knowledge that broadens their perspectives and enriches their learning (Korvick, Wisener, Loftis, & Williamson, 2008). They are eager to learn (Hegge & Hallman, 2008) and expect to be actively engaged in their learning (Teeley, 2007). The critical thinking skills of ABSN students, when compared to those of traditional students, are higher (Cangelosi, 2007), which enables them to understand complex information faster and move through a nursing curriculum more quickly (Raines & Sipes). In a study conducted by Korvick et al., students in an accelerated program performed better academically than those in a traditional program. They also have a higher first-time NCLEX-RN pass rate than generic graduates (Brewer et al., 2009; Korvick et al., 2008; Raines & Sipes, 2007).

Having successfully completed a prior baccalaureate degree, students in accelerated programs are experienced learners who understand the challenges of college and have learned how to effectively navigate through the system. These skills, grounded in their previous college experiences, help them cope with the rigors of a professional program. Not only are they self-directed learners and highly motivated (Walker et al., 2007), they are also critical consumers of education and clear in what they want from their second degree: the knowledge and skill sets to become effective nurses in a program that is well-organized, relevant, and considerate of their learning styles. However, as mature and motivated as they might be, these students have also reported high levels of stress

(Penprase & Koczara, 2009) as they struggle to return to the role and expectations of being a student, while balancing the demands of family, work, and finances. An orientation to the challenges and demands of an accelerated program may be key to student success (Kohn & Truglio-Londrigan, 2007). Utley-Smith, Phillips, and Turner (2007) describe a model they developed and implemented to help those enrolled in an ABSN program to understand the culture of nursing and begin their socialization into the profession. The model describes various phases students might experience and find challenging, and identified strategies that will help them be successful in their educational process.

ABSN students have high expectations of themselves, their faculty, and the learning environment. They enjoy the opportunity to ask questions in the classroom (Lindsey, 2009) and benefit from learning strategies that employ interaction between themselves as well as faculty (Kohn & Truglio-Londrigan, 2007). They are more apt to question assignments that are perceived as busy work (Lindsey, 2009), which may lead faculty to feel as if they are being challenged. Clinical experiences are highly anticipated as a means to learn (AACN, 2009b), and students report that they learn from the stories faculty tell regarding their own clinical experiences (Walker et al., 2007). Although ABSN students look to their faculty to determine what they need to know (Teeley, 2007; Walker et al., 2007), they prefer a more collegial relationship with faculty, who serve as guides to and facilitators of learning. Kohn and Truglio-Londrigan (2007) note that it is important to match students in ABSN programs with faculty who have an affinity and an interest in teaching adult learners.

Students in accelerated programs do well in learning environments that are dynamic. Courses in which technology such as Web-based teaching modalities, simulation, and case studies are integrated as well as face-to-face classroom activities serve them well (Hegge & Hallman, 2008; Teeley, 2007; Walker et al., 2007). Hegge and Hallman discuss the need for an environment in which collaborative learning occurs, noting that it lends itself to fostering students' "self-esteem, academic excellence, and social support" (p. 554).

Sample ABSN Program

At LGSSON, the ABSN program was developed as part of a comprehensive curriculum revision. The mission, vision, and philosophy; theoretical model; and curriculum outcomes are the same as those for the BSN program, but the plan of study is different. At Linfield, the college calendar provides annually for two 14-week semesters, a January interim semester, and no summer courses. In contrast, the ABSN curriculum (Table 9.6) was designed in four 12-week terms throughout the year so that students could go to school without breaks and finish within a year.

As engaged and motivated adult learners, ABSN students and graduates can offer important insights as part of the planning group during curriculum redesign initiatives. For example, during the curricular redesign process at LGSSON, students in the ABSN program were surveyed to determine their perspectives and suggestions regarding the scheduling of the ABSN curriculum. When asked how important it was to maintain a continuous program of study without breaks, 97 of 107 students (91%) responded that it was either "important" or "very important." Many of the students took time off from previous careers to return to school and were anxious to complete the program to restore their income and spend more time with their families. Based in part on the survey results, the decision was made to implement the 4-term program of study.

TABLE 9.6. Linfield-Good Samaritan School of Nursing Accelerated BSN Program of Study*

January–March (12 weeks) **	April–June (12 weeks)	July–September (12 weeks)	October–December (12 weeks)
Foundations of Community-based Professional Nursing 4	Lifespan Chronic Illness Care 4	Lifespan Acute Illness Care 4	Population-based Nursing in a Multicultural and Global Society 2
Scholarship of Nursing 3	Pathophysiology and pharmacology for Nursing Practice 3	Integrated Experiential Learning III: Acute Care 6	Leading and Managing in Nursing 3
Integrated Experiential Learning I: Foundations 6	Integrated Experiential Learning II: Chronic Care 6	Elective	Integrated Experiential Learning IV 8
13 credits	13 credits	10–13 credits	13 credits

Reproduced with permission.
*Approved by the school of nursing; in final approval process.
**Course Sequencing: 1-year Equal Terms

Courses in the ABSN program can be different from those in the traditional program based on the characteristics of the ABSN students as highly motivated, self-directed, adult learners with previous degrees and life experiences. For example, in the LGSSON ABSN curriculum, some of the theory courses in the generic program were combined and content-integrated in the first 3 semesters of the program for less overall theory credit. The total number of clinical hours remained the same for both the traditional and ABSN programs. It is the outcome and concept-based curriculum that remain consistent throughout both programs of study.

There is a growing body of literature about ABSN programs and it is incumbent on nurse educators to continue to study this population to determine which educational approaches are most effective and facilitate the greatest learning with this population of students. Postgraduation evaluation of the professional experiences of ABSN graduates provides insight into the facility of their transitions into the workplace and subsequent effects on client care and nursing.

RN–BSN PROGRAMS

RN completion programs, also called RN-to-BSN programs, are designed for registered nurses (RNs) who are graduates of accredited associate degree or hospital-based diploma programs and who seek a BSN degree. Based on research demonstrating improved performance on quality and safety outcomes when nurses are educated at the baccalaureate level or higher, the AACN maintains that the BSN degree should be the minimum educational requirement for professional nursing practice (AACN, 2009a).

While graduates can begin practice as RNs with associate degrees or hospital-based diplomas, the BSN degree is essential for nurses seeking to perform at the case-manager or supervisory level or move across employment (AACN, 2004). Nurses generally enter RN–BSN programs to advance their careers (Megginson, 2008) and the BSN degree is the gateway to graduate education and subsequent roles in advanced practice, nursing education, and research. The BSN has become the preferred preparation for practice in all health care settings and many organizations, including Magnet

TABLE 9.7 Linfield-Good Samaritan School of Nursing RN to BSN Program of Study*

Semester 1: Foundations for Community Based Nursing Practice	Credits	Semester 2: Stewardship of Health	Credits
Transition to Professional Nursing Practice**	6	Scholarship of Nursing	3
Professional Communication in Diverse Communities	2	Leading and Managing in Nursing	3
		Population-based Nursing in a Multicultural and Global Society	2
	8		**8**

Semester 3: Stewardship of Health Experiential Learning	Credits
Integrated Experiential Learning IV	8
	8

Reproduced with permission.
*Approved by the school of nursing; in final approval process.
**Includes 30 credits for prior learning after completion of the first RN–BSN class

hospitals and academic health care organizations, require the baccalaureate for specific nursing roles (AACN, 2009a).

Although RN–BSN students are generally experienced in nursing practice, the purpose of the completion program is to assist students to develop higher level critical-thinking skills, broaden their scope of practice, and understand the social, cultural, economic, and geopolitical context of health care to assume expanded professional roles (AACN, 2009a). The mission, vision, and philosophy, theoretical model, and student learning outcomes for a RN–BSN program will be the same as those for the generic BSN program at a particular school, although the program of study may look very different. See Table 9.7 for an example of an RN–BSN program. Program credits and length are variable between schools, and the design of the curriculum often offers part-time and online options to meet the needs of working nurses.

Credit for Prior Learning

As the nursing workforce is challenged to meet the increasingly complex needs of the current and future health care system, nursing programs across the country are challenged to encourage RNs to return to school for BSN completion. Nursing programs responded to this challenge by acknowledging that the RN holds knowledge, skills, and abilities related to prior work experience that can be applied to the current degree they are seeking. It is typical for RN-to-BSN completion programs to require introductory courses that are designed to validate this prior knowledge and to "bridge" or "transition" the RN from diploma or associate degree preparation. In addition to providing an opportunity to validate prior knowledge and skills, these introductory courses offer learning experiences, such as professional portfolio activities, that assist with the role transition and socialization to the BSN level of preparation. The nurse is granted credit for selected prelicensure courses offered at the upper division level once the transition course is successfully completed.

For example, at the Linfield-Good Samaritan School of Nursing RN-to-BSN program, credit for prior learning equates knowledge demonstrated through experience with actual Linfield College courses and is awarded 36 semester credits of nursing course work that includes many of the clinical courses in the generic curriculum. See Table 9.7 for the program of study. Course outcomes and related learning assessments in the transition course focus on evaluation of the nursing knowledge, skills, and professionalism that the nurse brings to the program from prior work experience and demonstration of readiness for subsequent courses in the curriculum.

Curriculum Strategies

The RNs who enroll in completion programs are adult learners who bring to the academic arena a repertoire of clinical knowledge and skills, a structured background of educational preparation, and employment experiences (Cangelosi, 2006). In the typical RN-to-BSN curriculum, the nurse is prepared for an expanded professional role through course work focused on enhancing professional communication, theoretical perspectives, community and population-based nursing care, and leadership. The senior practicum hours are spent working with nurse-preceptors in acute care settings as well as in community-based settings where the nurses can build on previous knowledge and enhance their effectiveness across the continuum of care. Many programs incorporate professional projects designed to meet the needs of the clinical agency from an evidence-based perspective, whereas other activities include projects related to nursing leadership, health promotion, disease prevention, and the care of vulnerable populations. Overall, the BSN enhances nurses' concepts of the profession and provides a wider range of experiences, allowing them to better adapt to an ever-changing health care environment (Jacobs, Dimattio, Bishop, & Fields, 1998).

With a growing awareness about the positive outcomes associated with advancing to higher levels of education and increasing encouragement from employers who provide tuition support for RN-to-BSN programs, more and more nurses are returning to school to complete a baccalaureate degree (Raines & Taglaireni, 2008). From 2006 to 2007, enrollments in RN to baccalaureate programs increased by 11.5% or 5,188 students, which makes this the fifth consecutive year of enrollment increases in these degree completions programs (Raines & Taglaireni). To meet the demand for BSN completion, nursing programs responded by offering curricula delivered using online and distance learning, the traditional classroom setting, or by using combined methods (AACN, 2009a). Distance education provides RN students, who are usually employed and juggling multiple roles, with greater accessibility to attend class at times of the day that meet their needs.

Clinical Experiences

The increasing enrollment in RN–BSN programs creates additional strain on scarce clinical practicum sites and faculty. However, the fact that RN–BSN students are licensed, as compared to the BSN student, allows for placement of licensed nurses in various traditional and nontraditional clinical sites. This ability generates opportunities for students to provide nursing care in settings in which they can begin to view caring in new ways, awakening a sense of advocacy, civic responsibility, and concern for political action (Hunt, 2007). A sense of responsibility is gained from various types of experiential and service-learning experiences that extend beyond the singular nurse–client relationship to embrace the client's family, community, and society (Hunt). Clinical experiences designed for service in community-based settings assist the nurse in adopting a broader, global view of nursing practice.

RN-to-BSN students benefit from being able to explore areas of interest for their clinical experiences as well as collaborating with faculty to identify creative ways to meet their goals for learning. There is the potential for deep engagement and mutuality for preceptors and staff in clinical sites within the student's community. RN-to-BSN students often choose experiences in public and community health, school-based health settings, correctional nursing, mental and behavioral health centers, addiction treatment and homeless shelters, geriatric settings, and home health and hospice settings. In addition, RN-to-BSN students are uniquely suited for participation in global health care delivery when interested in opportunities related to international travel and meeting the needs of the vulnerable and underserved.

International clinical placements provide nursing students with valuable experiences and understanding of nursing in the global community (Grant & McKenna, 2003). In addition to the opportunity to explore different cultures, these experiences provide the student with the ability to explore how health care systems vary greatly among countries and how this influences the manner health care is delivered within any particular country (Grant & McKenna). RN-to-BSN students who complete international clinical experiences describe meaningful learning related to awareness of diversity and cultural competence in nursing, enhanced skills in intercultural communication, an increased awareness of social and political injustices, and a greater understanding of poverty.

Inexperienced RN–BSN Students

As the trend toward hiring "BSN preferred" nurses continues, it is anticipated that more nurses will enter RN-to-BSN completion programs immediately following graduation from associate degree and diploma programs. To meet admission requirements for RN-to-BSN completion programs, applicants must pass the NCLEX examination for licensure and obtain an RN license. Because the RN-to-BSN curriculum is developed to build upon the prior work experience of the RN, nurses just beginning nursing practice require special consideration related to their relative lack of clinical experience. In the current economic climate, some of the students may have not found jobs following completion of their initial degree, and they have no work experience, which challenges some of the assumptions of many RN–BSN programs. Depending on the structure of the curriculum, inexperienced completion students may have difficulty engaging in classroom activities designed for experienced nurses where nurses are consistently asked to apply new knowledge and insights to their current practice. In the clinical setting, the less experienced RN requires additional oversight and support by faculty and preceptors, beyond that usually provided for licensed students.

Research suggests that RN students, in their quest for higher education, seek to attain professional credibility, career mobility, personal achievement, and longevity in nursing (Megginson, 2008). The RN–BSN completion program provides a rich and supportive environment for nurses returning to school. Nurse faculty members have the opportunity to mentor and role-model professional behaviors that assist in building positive connections and influence the learning of their students.

SUMMARY

Robust baccalaureate nursing education programs are foundational to the health of the profession and the population. Curriculum development and revision is both a challenge and an opportunity to shape the future. Now is the time for schools of nursing to collaborate within faculties between schools and with health care service organizations to innovate and find local solutions in a new age of health care reform. It is incumbent upon nurse educators to try new curricular approaches, evaluate their efficacy, and to share the results with the professional community.

The authors would like to acknowledge the Curriculum Committee at LGSSON for their hard work and commitment in developing the new curriculum and their willingness to share their work with the nursing community.

DISCUSSION QUESTIONS

1. Identify your primary partners in service or education. What is the nature of those relationships and how could they be expanded to create innovative clinical experiences for nursing students?
2. What are the most common groups of underrepresented students in your region? How could your curriculum be changed to be more inclusive of these groups?
3. What are the barriers to prelicensure graduates' successful transition into practice? Describe strategies in your curriculum that help to mediate "reality shock." What are some new ideas that could be developed?
4. How will health care reform affect your prelicensure program?

LEARNING ACTIVITIES

Student Learning Activities

1. Interview the chair of the undergraduate curriculum committee at your school to determine if there is a plan for curriculum revision.
2. Using the Candela, Dalley, and Benzel-Lindley (2006) approach for categorizing content, review a course in the BSN curriculum and identify which content (knowledge, skills, and attitudes) is most essential.
3. Create an innovative clinical education model that meets the criteria outlined by MacIntyre et al. (2009).

Nurse Educator/Faculty Development Activities

1. Map your curriculum outcomes according to the new *Essentials*. What changes need to be made to update your program?
2. Create a visual representation of your school's theoretical model.

   Invite a colleague to coffee and discuss the "sacred cows" at your institution that could be barriers to innovative curriculum revision.

REFERENCES

Altier, M. E., & Krsek, C. A. (2006). Effects of a 1-year residency program on job satisfaction and retention of new graduate nurses. *Journal for Nurses in Staff Development, 22*(2), 70–77.

American Association of Colleges of Nursing. (2004). Your nursing career: A look at the facts. Retrieved from http://www.aacn.nche.edu/education/career.htm

American Association of Colleges of Nursing. (2006). *Essential nursing competencies and curricula guidelines for genetics and genomics.* Silver Spring, MD: American Nurses Association. Retrieved from http://www.aacn.nche.edu/Education/pdf/Genetics%20%20Genomics%20Nursing%20Competencies%2009-22-06.pdf

American Association of Colleges of Nursing. (2008a). Accelerated programs: The fast-track to careers in nursing. Retrieved from http://www.aacn.nche/edu/Publications/issues/Aug02.htm

American Association of Colleges of Nursing. (2008b). *Cultural competency in baccalaureate nursing education.* Retrieved from http://www.aacn.nche.edu/Education/pdf/competency.pdf

American Association of Colleges of Nursing. (2008c). *The essentials of baccalaureate education for professional nursing practice.* Retrieved from http://www.aacn.nche.edu/Education/pdf/BaccEssentials08.pdf

American Association of Colleges of Nursing. (2009a). *Degree completion programs for registered nurses: RN to master's degree and RN to baccalaureate programs.* Retrieved from http://www.aacn.nche.edu/media/factsheets/DegreeCompletionProg.htm

American Association of Colleges of Nursing. (2009b, February). *Fact sheet: Accelerated baccalaureate and master's degrees in nursing.* Retrieved from http://www.aacn.nche.edu/Media/FactSheets/AcceleratedProg.htm

American Association of Colleges of Nursing. (2009c). *Schools that offer accelerated programs for non-nursing college graduates.* Retrieved from http://www.aacn.nche.edu/Education/pdf/aplist.pdf

American Association of Colleges of Nursing and the John A. Hartford Foundation Institute for Geriatric Nursing (2000). *Older Adults: Recommended Baccalaureate Competencies and Curricular Guidelines for Geriatric Nursing Care.* Retrieved from http://www.aacn.nche.edu/Education/gercomp.htm

American Association of Colleges and Universities. (2004). A statement on integrative learning. Retrieved from http://www.aacu.org/integrative_learning/pdfs/ILP_Statement.pdf

American Association of Colleges and Universities. (2007). *College learning for the new global century. A report from the National Leadership Council for Liberal Education & America's Promise.* Retrieved from http://www.aacu.org/leap/documents/GlobalCentury_final.pdf

American Nurses Association. (2005). *Code of Ethics for nurses with interpretive statements.* Silver Spring, MD: Author.

American Organization of Nurse Executives. (2004).*Guiding principles for the role of the nurse in future health care delivery.* Retrieved from http://www.aone.org/aone/resource/practiceandeducation.html

Anderson, G. L., & Tredway, C. A. (2009). Transforming the nursing curriculum to promote critical thinking online. *Journal of Nursing Education, 48*(2), 111–115.

Barger, S. E., & Das, E. (2004). An academic-service partnership: Ideas that work. *Journal of Professional Nursing, 20*(2), 97–102.

Benner, P., Sutphen, M., Leonard, V., & Day, L. (2010). Educating nurses: A call for radical transformation. San Francisco, CA: Jossey-Bass.

Blanzola, C., Lindeman, R., & King, M. L. (2004). Nurse internship pathway to clinical comfort, confidence, and competency. *Journal for Nurses in Staff Development, 20*(1), 27–37.

Bleich, M. R. (2009). Technology: An imperative for teaching in the age of digital natives. [Editorial]. *Journal of Nursing Education, 48*(2), 63.

Bosher, S. (2007). *Recommendations for meeting the needs of ESL nursing students.* Unpublished report for Linfield-Good Samaritan School of Nursing, Linfield College, Portland Oregon.

Bosher, S. D., & Pharris, M. D. (2009). *Transforming nursing education: The culturally inclusive environment.* New York: Springer.

Bratt, M. M. (2009). Retaining the next generation of nurses: The Wisconsin nurse residency program provides a continuum of support. *The Journal of Continuing Education in Nursing, 40*(9), 416–425.

Brewer, C. S., Kovner, C. T., Poornima, S., Fairchild, S., Kim, H., & Djukic, M. (2009). A comparison of second-degree baccalaureate and traditional-baccalaureate new graduate RNs: Implications for the workforce. *Journal of Professional Nursing, 25*(1), 5–14.

Brown, S. T., Kirkpatrick, M. K., Mangum, D., & Avery, J. (2008). A review of narrative pedagogy strategies to transform traditional nursing education. *Journal of Nursing Education, 47*(6), 283–286.

Buchbinder, H. (2007). *Increasing Latino participation in the nursing profession: Best practices at California nursing programs.* Los Angeles, CA: Tomás Rivera Policy Institute.

Butler, K. M., & Hardin-Pierce, M. (2005). Leadership strategies to enhance the transition from nursing student role to professional nurse. *Nursing Leadership Forum, 9*(3), 110–117.

Candela, L., Dalley, K., & Benzel-Lindley, J. (2006). A case for learning-centered curricula. *Journal of Nursing Education, 45*(2), 59–66.

Cangelosi, P. (2006). RN-to-BSN Education: Creating a context that uncovers new possibilities. *Journal of Nursing Education, 45*(5), 177–181.

Cangelosi, P. R. (2007). Accelerated second-degree baccalaureate nursing programs: What is the significance of clinical instructors? *Journal of Nursing Education, 46*(9), 400–405.

Cantrell, M. A., & Browne, A. M. (2005). The impact of a nurse externship program on the transition process from graduate to registered nurse. Part II. Qualitative findings. *Journal for Nurses in Staff Development, 21*(6), 249–256.

Cantrell, M. A., & Browne, A. M. (2006). The impact of a nurse externship program on the transition process from graduate to registered nurse. Part III. Recruitment and retention effects. *Journal for Nurses in Staff Development, 22*(1), 11–14.

Cantrell, M. A., Browne, A. M., & Lupinacci, P. (2005). The impact of a nurse externship program on the transition process from graduate to registered nurse. Part I. Quantitative findings. *Journal for Nurses in Staff Development, 21*(5), 187–195.

Commission on Collegiate Nursing Education. (2008). *Standards for accreditation of post-baccalaureate nurse residency programs.* Retrieved from www.aacn.nche.edu/Accreditation/PubsRes.htm

Creedy, D. K., Mitchell, M., Seaton-Sykes, P., Cooke, M., Patterson, E., Purcell, C., et al., (2007). Evaluating a Web-enhanced bachelor of nursing curriculum: Perspectives of third-year students. *Journal of Nursing Education, 46*(10), 460–467.

Cronenwett, L., Sherwood, G., Barnsteiner, J., Disch, J., Johnson, J., Mitchell, P., et al., (2007). Quality and safety education for nurses. *Nursing Outlook, 55*(3), 122–131.

Crow, K. (1997). Interpreting transcultural knowledge into nursing curricula: An American Indian example. In A. I. Morey & M. K. Kitano (Eds.), *Multicultural course transformation in higher education* (pp. 211–228). Boston, MA: Allyn & Bacon.

Curran, C. R., Elfrink, V., & Mays, B. (2009). Building a virtual community for nursing education: The town of Mirror Lake. *Journal of Nursing Education, 48*(1), 30–35.

DeBasio, N. O. (2005). *Accelerated nursing programs.* Washington, DC: AACN. Retrieved from http://www.aacn.nche.edu/Education/nurse_ed/AccelArticle.htm

Diefenbeck, C. A., Plowfield, L. A., & Herrman, J. W. (2006). Clinical immersion: A residency model for nursing education. *Nursing Education Perspectives, 27*(2), 72–79.

Diekelmann, N. (2005). Engaging the students and the teacher: Co-creating substantive reform with narrative pedagogy. *Journal of Nursing Education, 44*(6), 249–252.

Dubose, D., Sellinger-Karmel, L. D., & Scoloveno, R. L. (2010). Baccalaureate nursing education. In W. M. Nehring & F. R. Lashley (Eds.) *High fidelity simulation in nursing education* (pp. 189–209). Sudbury, MA: Jones & Bartlett.

Eigsti, J. E. (2009). Graduate nurses' perceptions of a critical care nurse internship program. *Journal for Nurses in Staff Development, 25*(4), 191–198.

Ervin, N. E., Bickes, J. T., & Schim, S. M. (2006). Environments of care: A curriculum model for preparing a new generation of nurses, *Journal of Nursing Education, 45*(2), 75–80.

Fitzgerald, B. (2009). Educating novice perioperative nurses. *Perioperative Nursing Clinics, 4*(2), 141–155.

Forbes, M. O., & Hickey, M. T. (2009). Curriculum reform in baccalaureate nursing education: Review of the literature. *International Journal of Nursing Education Scholarship, 6*(1), 1–16.

Giddens, J. F. (2007). The neighborhood: A Web-based platform to support conceptual teaching and learning. *Nursing Education Perspectives, 28*(5), 251–256.

Giddens, J. F., & Brady, D. P. (2007). Rescuing nursing education from content saturation: The case for a concept-based curriculum. *Journal of Nursing Education, 46*(2), 65–69.

Giddens, J. F., & Eddy, L. (2009). A survey of physical examination skills taught in undergraduate nursing programs: Are we teaching too much? *Journal of Nursing Education, 48*(1), 24–29.

Goudreau, J., Pepin, J., Dubois, S., Boyer, L., Larue, C., & Legault, A. (2009). A second generation of the competency-based approach to nursing education. *International Journal of Nursing Education Scholarship, 6*(1), 1–15.

Grant, E., & McKenna, L. (2003). International clinical placements for undergraduate students. *Journal of Clinical Nursing, 12*(4), 529–535.

Gubrud-Howe, P., & Schoessler, M. (2008). From random access opportunity to a clinical education curriculum. [Editorial]. *Journal of Nursing Education, 47*(1), 3–4.

Gubrud-Howe, P., Shaver, K. S., Tanner, C. A., Bennett-Stillmaker, J., Davidson, S. B., Flaherty-Robb, M. et al. (2003). A challenge to meet the future: Nursing education in Oregon, 2010. *Journal of Nursing Education, 42*(4), 163–167.

Harder, B. N. (2009). Use of simulation in teaching and learning in health sciences: A systematic review. *Journal of Nursing Education, 7*, 1–6.

Hegge, M. J., & Hallman, P. A. (2008). Changing nursing culture to welcome second-degree students: Herding and corralling sacred cows. *Journal of Nursing Education, 47*(12), 552–556.

Herdrich, B., & Lindsay, A. (2006). Nurse residency programs: Redesigning the transition into practice. *Journal for Nurses in Staff Development, 22*(2), 55–62.

Herrman, J. W., & Diefenbeck, C.(2009). The nurse residency model: A clinical immersion model for curriculum change. *Dean's Notes, 30* (4), 1–2.

Hickey, M. T. (2009). Preceptor perceptions of new graduate nurse readiness for practice. *Journal for Nurses in Staff Development, 25*(1), 35–41.

Hofler, L. D. (2008). Nursing education and transition to the work environment: A synthesis of national reports. *Journal of Nursing Education, 47*(1), 5–12.

Hull, E., St. Romain, J. A., Alexander, P., Schaff, S., & Jones, W. (2001). Moving cemeteries: A framework for facilitating curriculum revision. *Nurse Educator, 26*(6), 280–282.

Hunt, R. (2007). Service-learning: an eye-opening experience that provokes emotion and challenges stereotypes. *Journal of Nursing Education, 46*(6), 277–281.

Institute of Medicine. (2001). *Crossing the quality chasm.* Washington, DC: National Academies Press.

Institute of Medicine. (2003). *Health professions education: A bridge to quality.* Washington, DC: National Academies Press.

Ironside, P. M. (2004). "Covering content" and teaching thinking: Deconstructing the additive curriculum. *Journal of Nursing Education, 43*(1), 5–12.

Ironside, P. M. (2006). Using narrative pedagogy: Learning and practicing interpretive thinking. *Journal of Advanced Nursing, 55*(4), 478–486.

Ironside, P., Jeffries, P., & Martin, A. (2009). Fostering patient safety competencies using multiple-patient simulation experiences. *Nursing Outlook, 57*(6), 332–337.

Ironside, P., & McNelis, A. (2009). NLN clinical education survey. In N. Ard & T. M. Valiga (Eds.), *Clinical nursing education: Current reflections* (pp. 25–38). New York: National League for Nursing.

Jacobs, L., DiMattio, M., Bishop, T., & Fields, D. (1998). The baccalaureate degree in nursing as an entry-level requirement for professional nursing practice. *Journal of Professional Nursing, 14*(4), 225–233.

Jacobson, L., & Grindel, C. (2006). What is happening in pre-licensure RN clinical nursing education? Findings from the faculty and administrator survey on clinical nursing education. *Nursing Education Perspectives, 27*(2), 108–109.

Jayasekara, R., Schultz, T., & McCutcheon, H. (2006). A comprehensive systematic review of evidence on the effectiveness and appropriateness of undergraduate nursing curricula. *International Journal of Evidence-Based Healthcare, 4*(3), 191–207. doi: 10.1111/j.1479-6988.2006.00044.x

Jeffries, P. R. (2005). A framework for designing, implementing, and evaluating simulations used as teaching strategies in nursing. *Nursing Education Perspectives, 26*(2), 96–103.

Joynt, J., & Kimball, B. (2008). Blowing open the bottleneck: Designing new approaches to increase nurse education capacity. Retrieved from http://championnursing.org/sites/default/files/1695_BlowingOpentheBottleneck.pdf

Kohn, P. S., & Truglio-Londrigan, M. (2007). Second-career baccalaureate nursing students: A lived experience. *Journal of Nursing Education, 46*(9), 391–399.

Korvick, L. M., Wisener, L. K., Loftis, L. A., & Williamson, M. L. (2008). Comparing the academic performance of students in traditional and second-degree baccalaureate programs. *Journal of Nursing Education, 47*(3), 139–141.

Kramer, M. (1974). Reality shock: Why nurses leave nursing. St. Louis, MO: Mosby.

Kruger, B. J., Roush, C., Olinzock, B. J., & Bloom, K. (2009). Engaging nursing students in a long-term relationship with a home-based community. *Journal of Nursing Education, 7:* 1–7.

Lindsey, P. (2009). Starting an accelerated baccalaureate nursing program: Challenges and opportunities for creative educational innovations. *Journal of Nursing Education, 48*(5), 279–281.

Little, B. B. (2009). The use of standards for peer review of online nursing courses: A pilot study. *Journal of Nursing Education, 48*(7), 411–415.

MacIntyre, R. C., Murray, T. A., Teel, C. S., & Karshmer, J. F. (2009). Five recommendations for prelicensure clinical nursing education. *Journal of Nursing Education, 48*(8), 447–453.

Mawn, B., & Reece, S. M. (2000). Reconfiguring a curriculum for the new millennium: The process of change. *Journal of Nursing Education, 39*(3), 101–108.

McEwen, M., & Brown, S. C. (2002). Conceptual frameworks in undergraduate nursing curricula: Report of a national survey. *Journal of Nursing Education, 41*(1), 5–14.

McGuire-Sessions, M., & Gubrud, P. (2010). Interdisciplinary simulation center. In W. M. Nehring & Lashley, F. R. (Eds.), *High-Fidelity Patient Simulation in Nursing Education* (pp. 303–322). Sudbury, MA: Jones & Bartlett.

Megginson, L. A. (2008). RN-BSN education: 21st century barriers and incentives. *Journal of Nursing Management, 16*(1), 47–55.

Moscato, S. R., Miller, J., Logsdon, K., Weinberg, S., & Chorpenning, L. (2007). Dedicated education unit: An innovative clinical partner education model. *Nursing Outlook, 55*(1), 31–37.

National Council of State Boards of Nursing. (2009). Report of findings from the effect of high-fidelity simulation on nursing students' knowledge and performance: A pilot study. *NCSBN Research Brief, 40.* Chicago: Author.

National League for Nursing. (2008). Final report of the 2008 NLN think tank on transforming clinical nursing education. Retrieved from: http://www.nln.org/facultydevelopment/pdf/think_tank.pdf

Nehring, W. M. (2008). U.S. boards of nursing and the use of high-fidelity patient simulators in nursing education. *Journal of Professional Nursing, 24*(2), 109–117.

Newman, D. (2008). Conceptual models of nursing and baccalaureate nursing education. [Editorial]. *Journal of Nursing Education, 47*(5), 199–200.

Noone, J. (2009). Teaching to the three apprenticeships: Designing learning activities for professional practice in an undergraduate curriculum. *Journal of Nursing Education, 48*(8), 468–471.

Penprase, B., & Koczara, S. (2009). Understanding the experiences of accelerated second-degree nursing students and graduates: A review of the literature. *The Journal of Continuing Education in Nursing, 40*(2), 74–78.

Perkins, I., Vale, D. J., & Graham, M. S. (2001). Partnerships in primary health care: A process for re-visioning nursing education. *Nursing and Health Care Perspectives, 22*(1), 20–25.

Raines, C., & Taglaireni, M. (2008). Career pathways in nursing: Entry points and academic progression. *The Online Journal of Issues in Nursing: A Scholarly Journal of the American Nurses Association, 13*(3). Retrieved from www.nursingworld.org

Raines, D. A. (2009). Competence of accelerated second degree students after studying in a collaborative model of nursing practice education. *International Journal of Nursing Education Scholarship, 6*(1), 1–12. doi: 10.2202/1548-923X.1659.

Raines, D. A., & Sipes, A. (2007). One year later: Reflections and work activities of accelerated second-degree bachelor of science in nursing graduates. *Journal of Professional Nursing, 23*(6), 329–334. doi:10.1016/j.profnurs.2007.10.011

Raines, C., & Taglaireni, M. (2008). Career pathways in nursing: Entry points and academic progression. *The Online Journal of Issues in Nursing: A Scholarly Journal of the American Nurses Association, 13*(3). Retrieved from www.nursingworld.org

Reid, J. M. (1987). The learning style preferences of ESL students. *TESOL Quarterly, 21*(1), 87–111.

Rosenfeld, P., Smith, M. O., Iervolino, L., & Bowar-Feres, S. (2004). Nurse residency program: A 5-year evaluation from the participants' perspective. *Journal of Nursing Administration, 34*(4), 188–194.

Sinclair, B., & Ferguson, K. (2009). Integrating simulated teaching/learning strategies in undergraduate nursing education. *International Journal of Nursing Education Scholarship, 6*(1), 1–11.

Skiba, D. J. (2007). Emerging technologies center. Faculty 2.0: Flipping the novice to expert continuum. *Nursing Education Perspectives, 28*(6): 342–344.

Swaner, L. E., & Brownell, J. E. (2008). Outcomes of high impact practices for underserved students: A review of the literature. Retrieved from http://www.aacu.org/inclusive_excellence/documents/DRAFTProjectUSALiteratureReview.pdf

Tanner, C. A. (2006). Thinking like a nurse: A research-based model of clinical judgment in nursing. *Journal of Nursing Education, 45*(6), 204–211.

Tanner, C. A. (2007).The curriculum revolution revisited. *Journal of Nursing Education, 46*(2), 51–52.

Teeley, K. H. (2007). Designing hybrid Web-based courses for accelerated nursing students. *Journal of Nursing Education, 46*(9), 417–422.

U.S. Department of Health and Human Services. (2000). *Healthy People 2010* (2nd ed.). Vols 1–2. Washington, DC: U.S. Government Printing Office.

U.S. Department of Health and Human Services, Health Resources and Services Administration. (2010). *The Registered Nurse Population: Initial Findings from the 2008 National Sample Survey of Registered Nurses.* Retrieved from http://bhpr.hrsa.gov/healthworkforce/rnsurvey/initialfindings2008.pdf

Utley-Smith, Q., Phillips, B., & Turner, K. (2007). Avoiding socialization pitfalls in accelerated second-degree nursing education: The returning-to-school syndrome model. *Journal of Nursing Education, 46*(9), 423–426.

Walker, J. T., Martin, T. M., Haynie, L., Norwood, A., White, J., & Grant, L. (2007). Preferences for teaching methods in a baccalaureate nursing program: How second-degree and traditional students differ. *Nursing Education Perspectives, 28*(5), 246–250.

Warda, M. R. (2008). Curriculum revolution: Implications for Hispanic nursing students. *Hispanic Health Care International, 6*(4), 192–199. doi: 10.1891/1540.6.4.192

Webber, P. B. (2002). A curriculum framework for nursing. *Journal of Nursing Education, 41*(1), 15–24.

Weimer, M. (2002). *Learner-centered teaching.* San Francisco, CA: Jossey-Bass.

Williams, B. (2001). Developing critical reflection for professional practice through problem-based learning. *Journal of Advanced Nursing, 34*(1), 27–34.

Williams, D. A., Berger, J. B., & McClendon, S. A. (2005). Toward a model of inclusive excellence and change in postsecondary education. Washington, DC: AAC&U. Retrieved from http://www.aacu.org/inclusive_excellence/documents/Williams_et_al.pdf

Yuan, H., Williams, B. A., & Fan, L., (2008). A systematic review of selected evidence on developing nursing students' critical thinking through problem-based learning. *Nurse Education Today, 28*(6): 657–663.

10 Curriculum Planning for Master's Nursing Programs

Sarah B. Keating

OBJECTIVES

Upon completion of Chapter 10, the reader will be able to:

1. Discuss the process of curriculum development for master's programs in nursing including the:
   a. Generalist master's degree
   b. Entry-level Masters of Science in Nursing (MSN)
   c. Clinical nurse leader (CNL)
   d. Advanced practice programs
   e. Functional roles (e.g., case management, community health nursing, nursing administration or leadership, and nurse educator)
2. Review recommendations from accrediting, professional specialty and educational organizations, and certification agencies for curriculum development.
3. Analyze issues surrounding graduate-level nursing at the master's level including:
   a. Entry into practice
   b. Terminal degrees and advanced practice
   c. Post-master's certificates
   d. Certification, licensure, and regulation

OVERVIEW

As nursing education matured in the academic world and the profession grappled with the issue of defining itself as a discipline, graduate education in nursing evolved. Nursing leaders recognized the need for additional education to be prepared for faculty and administrator roles. Because there was a dearth of graduate nursing programs, nurses often sought degrees in other disciplines such as education, business, and health care administration. Nurses in practice were focusing their services on clinical specialties such as pediatrics, obstetrics, medical/surgical nursing, and intensive care; and they, too, felt the need for additional specialty training; many seeking nondegree certification. In community settings, it was recognized that public health nurses needed knowledge in epidemiology and the public health sciences, and the specialty roles of nurse midwives and nurse anesthetists, required advanced educational preparation. Many of these programs were first offered in baccalaureate programs or as certificate programs to expand on knowledge and skills from basic nursing programs; however, all eventually moved into the graduate level.

In the 1970s, schools of nursing in higher degree institutions were developing master's degree programs that focused on the preparation of nursing faculty, administrators and some of the classic specialties such as pediatrics, maternity, community health, and mental health/psychiatric nursing. These latter specialties became clinical specialties and as they were developing, the advent of the nursing role in primary care began with the introduction of nurse practitioners. With acute care rising in complexity, it became apparent that nurses with blended specialty role preparation were indicated such as the acute care nurse practitioner.

See Chapter 1 for a history of graduate nursing education to gain an appreciation for how nursing evolved in its role in health care to match the needs of the health care system with its growing demands for well-educated providers of care. Out of all of these changes and demands came master's degrees that focus on the specialties, primary care, management/administration, and education.

Chapter 10 breaks the various master's level programs in nursing into groups from the entry-level master's to that of the advanced generalist and specialty roles that are available in today's graduate programs. Each group is reviewed and its role in graduate nursing and the profession are discussed. Some of the major issues related to master's level nursing education are discussed.

THE GENERALIST MASTER'S DEGREE

There are many master's programs that offer generalist degrees without specializations. However, these programs, to receive national accreditation, usually include at least nursing theory, research, and health care policy courses. The purpose for the generalist degree is to provide advanced nursing knowledge that can serve as a baseline for nursing roles in leadership positions. Students are usually free to choose electives that meet their special interests such as courses in business, education, counseling, and so forth. The degree neither prepares them for advanced practice nor qualifies them for specialty certification, administrative, or education roles. However, many graduates complete post-master's certification programs to qualify them for these roles.

ENTRY-LEVEL (GENERIC) MASTER'S DEGREE PROGRAMS IN NURSING

Raines and Taglaireni (2008) list various ways that people can apply to nursing and among them are **entry-level master's in nursing** programs for college graduates. They cite the increasing interest in nursing on the part of the public owing to the shortages in nursing and its attractiveness as a viable career that offers a stable income. They state that the numbers of entry-level programs are increasing across the country and in 2007; the American Association of Colleges of Nursing (AACN, 2008) reported 56 entry-level master's programs across the country and more in the process of development. The first program for college graduates was founded by Yale University in 1974 (AACN, 2010a). California alone has 19 entry-level programs that began with the first in 1988 at San Francisco State University (California Board of Registered Nursing, 2010).

Entry-level master's programs have two major programs of study to reach licensure (registered nurse [RN]) requirements and a graduate degree in nursing. The first program provides basic nursing knowledge and skills courses specifically designed for college graduates and taught at the post-baccalaureate level. Included in the program or required as prerequisites are the usual sciences, social sciences, and liberal arts courses. Examples of classic prerequisites for any entry-level nursing program (associate's, baccalaureate, and master's degree) are Anatomy, Chemistry, English, Genetics, Human Development, Mathematics/Statistics, Microbiology, Nutrition, Physiology, Psychology, Sociology, and Speech/Communications. Students complete nursing theory and clinical courses and a capstone experience that can be a thesis, project, and/or comprehensive examination. Schools of nursing differ in their preparation of these graduates by offering either a generic or generalist master's degree for entry into practice or a specialist track to prepare graduates for advanced levels of nursing practice.

The other entry-level curriculum is for students to complete courses equivalent to or the same as existing courses in baccalaureate-level nursing programs. They are not necessarily specifically revised for college graduates. As with the first program, students either must have the prerequisite sciences and liberal arts courses or complete them in the program. After completion of the baccalaureate-level courses, students enter into the master's program to complete either an advanced generalist role such as the Clinical Nurse Leader (CNL) track, or a specialty track such as case management, clinical specialist, nurse anesthetist, nurse midwife, and nurse practitioner.

The track record for the graduates of entry-level master's programs is excellent. Students in the programs bring their life experiences, previously earned higher degrees, and most programs require at least a 3.0 GPA in the undergraduate program for admission. National Council Licensure Exam (NCLEX) pass rates exceed 90% (author) for entry-level MSN graduates.

The Clinical Nurse Leader

The CNL program was developed by the AACN (2010b) in response to the need for health care providers to manage clients or groups of clients at the point of care. It applies to all settings of health care. The program is at the master's level and lends itself very well to entry-level master's programs as well as post-baccalaureate in nursing programs. AACN (2007) provides the following description of the role of the CNL:

> The CNL is a leader in the health care delivery system; not just the acute care setting but in all settings in which health care is delivered. The implementation of the CNL role, however, will vary across settings. The CNL role is not one of administration or management. The CNL assumes accountability for client care outcomes through the assimilation and application of research-based information to design, implement, and evaluate client plans of care. The CNL is a provider and manager of care at the point of care to individuals and cohorts of clients within a unit or health care setting. The CNL designs, implements, and evaluates client care by coordinating, delegating and supervising the care provided by the health care team, including licensed nurses, technicians, and other health professionals. (p. 10)

The Veterans Administration (VA) system was one of the first to use CNL services in the interest of cost-effectiveness and coordination of safe and quality care for clients. An article by Ott et al. (2009) reported on a study of CNLs in the VA system and their impact on quality of care and cost-effectiveness. Although the authors found that a specific instrument for collecting data on the CNL role is needed, owing to the newness of the role, their findings about the effect of CNLs at the point of care were significant. Among other findings, rates of patient falls, hours of sitters necessary to stay with confused patients, pressure ulcers, pneumonia, and discharge follow-up all improved. According to the authors, it is the intention of the VA system to integrate the role and services of the CNL into the system to transform nursing practice. Other health care systems could benefit from the VA experience.

There are close to 80 accredited nursing programs that provide the CNL major at the master's level at the time of this writing (AACN, 2010b). AACN has a certification program for CNLs who apply after graduation (AACN, 2010c). Based on the support the VA system has for the role of the CNL and the effect it has on improving care, it is anticipated that more nurses will be prepared for this advanced generalist role in the near future.

ADVANCED PRACTICE MASTER'S DEGREE PROGRAMS IN NURSING

The classic advanced practice roles encompass the clinical specialist, nurse anesthetist, nurse midwife, and nurse practitioner. As discussed in Chapter 1 on the history of master's education, the advanced practice roles emerged in the 1960s and 1970s. Nurse anesthetists (certified registered nurse anesthetists [CRNAs]) and nurse midwives predated these programs by many years (centuries for midwives and 150+ years for CRNAs), however their move into higher education/graduate education occurred about the same period as did the clinical specialist and nurse practitioner roles. A few advanced practice nurses still have a certificate to practice depending on state licensure laws; although, most states now require the master's degree for entry into advanced practice. With the advent of the Doctor of Nursing Practice (DNP) degree, many of these nurses will continue their education to earn a DNP (see Chapter 11 for discussion of the DNP). The AACN (2010e) issued a statement that the DNP will be the entry level for advanced practice in nursing by 2015, which has implications for the future when many master's programs for advanced practice will be phased out and moved into the DNP.

All master's degree programs that prepare advanced practice nurses require a baccalaureate in nursing or in rare cases, its equivalent, and some have additional prerequisites for example, the CRNA programs often require more than one or two Chemistry courses. Both the clinical specialist and nurse practitioner programs have sub-specialties. For example, adult, cardiovascular, family, geriatric, pediatrics, psychiatric/mental health, women's health, and so forth. In addition, there are blended roles such as the adult nurse practitioner. Fulton (2005) writes in her editorial that the blended roles require many more hours of course work and practice that surpasses the usual 401 requirements for an advanced practice master's in nursing. In addition, there is some confusion about the definition of these roles and no specific competencies or standards as yet that are specific to the blended role. Rather, graduates are eligible for national certification for both roles.

The 2008 consensus model for APRN regulation (AACN, 2010d) limits the blended role of primary and acute care foci to adult–geriatric and pediatric roles only and specifies that graduates must be nationally certified for both the primary (practitioner) and acute care (clinical specialist) roles. The consensus model was a product of meetings with the leading professional nursing organizations, specialty organizations, accrediting bodies, nursing education organizations, certification agencies, and the national council of state boards. It was the intention of the group to clarify advanced practice roles for the profession and the public and to begin an initiative for consistent licensing, certification, and regulation across the various states in the nation.

Advanced practice nurses have a key role in the delivery of quality care. To provide some evidence of the impact they have on the health care delivery system, the following reports from the literature verify this statement. Bourbonniere et al. (2009) conducted a review of the literature on the outcomes of patient care and costs in nursing homes that used services of advanced practice nurses (clinical specialist and nurse practitioners). Their findings affirmed that patient outcomes were improved such as reductions in falls, pressure ulcers, incontinence and improved patient, and family satisfaction. In addition, the consultation and education that these nurses offered for staff led to less absenteeism and increased job satisfaction. Cost-effectiveness studies demonstrated that advanced practice nurses save the system money in unnecessary hospitalizations for the residents of nursing homes. Although reimbursement for advanced practice nurses is based on medical services, indirect costs such as referrals and staff and patient education are not billable. The panel that studied the effects of advanced practice nurses in nursing homes concluded that there is need for increased services of this kind in these facilities, that new financial systems need to be set for their services, and that it is essential that geriatric content be included in nursing curricula and that geriatric specialties in the advanced roles would be beneficial.

McCorkle (2006) reported on the use of advanced practice nurses to support cancer patient and their caregivers in home care agencies. After refining several instruments to measure symptom distress and enforced social dependency, McCorkle and others conducted several studies to observe the effects of advanced practice nursing interventions on dying patients and their caregivers, many of whom were spouses. The researchers compared patients and their caregivers who received the services of advanced practice nurses to those who received the usual types of care. They found that providing support throughout the dying process for both the patient and the caregiver resulted in lessening of symptoms for the patients and less psychological stress for the caregivers during and after the patient's death. An interesting finding was that caregivers with pre-existing medical conditions when the patient was diagnosed had more psychological difficulties than those who were relatively healthy. It was McCorkel's conclusion that using advanced practice nurses to assess and provide interventions during these episodes of illness and dying result in better outcomes for the patients and their caregivers.

Delgado-Passler and McCaffrey (2006) reviewed the literature for studies to compare the use of RNs to advanced practice nurses for follow-up of heart failure patients. Although the number of studies was limited, they found that advanced practice nurses were more effective in managing posthospitalized heart failure patients owing to their advanced knowledge in care management and with the physician could individualize discharge and follow-up at home, which resulted in fewer readmissions to the hospital. This in turn resulted in cost savings.

Parrish and Peden (2009) reviewed the literature for studies that reported on depressed clients' outcomes when cared for by advanced practice psychiatric nurses (APPN). They found 10 studies that met their criteria for the review. The studies compared the outcomes of APPNs care to other psychiatric/mental health professionals care for depressed patients. Overall, the studies found that the most effective treatment for depressed clients is a combination of psychotherapy and medications, which APPNs can provide. In addition, they found that patients were satisfied with the care they received from APPNs. It was concluded by the authors that APPNs are effective providers of care for patients owing to their expertise, availability of time to spend with the patients, and they can be cost-effective, if it is only necessary for one professional to provide care.

In summary, the traditional role for advanced practice continues to play an important role in the delivery of high quality, safe, and cost-effective care. Nursing continues to find it necessary to illustrate this to not only the health care industry but the public as well. Kleinpell (2007) labels advanced practice nurses in the hospital setting as "invisible" and makes the case for nurse managers and administrators to demonstrate their contributions to the health care system. She offers several recommendations and outlines for gathering the information to promote the role of advanced practice nurses.

MASTER'S DEGREES IN NURSING FOR FUNCTIONAL ROLES

There are other roles and specialties for nurses with master's degrees not included in the advanced practice and advanced generalist roles. They include case management, community/public health nursing, nursing administration, nurse educator, staff development/patient education, and other leadership roles. Nurses prepared for these roles usually have nursing theory, health care policy, and research as core courses along with the courses that focus them into a specific function within the health care system. The following discussion presents a few examples of the programs that prepare nurses for specific roles.

Case Management

The educational preparation for roles in case management in nursing usually requires at least a baccalaureate in nursing with a master's preferred. Case managers provide coordination of services for aggregates in many health care settings. They work closely with other health care professionals. The role began in the 1970s with its purpose to work with patients to individualize care, avoid duplication of services, enhance the quality of care, and promote cost-effectiveness (White & Hall, 2006). White and Hall reviewed the literature to identify journals in the literature that pertain to case management and found three source journals for the specialty; although, the topic is mentioned in many other health-related journals. There are approximately 20 schools of nursing that offer case management master's degrees. The American Nurses Credentialing Center (ANCC, 2010) offers certification, which requires 2000 hours of clinical practice in case management, RN licensure, practice as an RN for 2 years, and 30 hours of continuing education in case management in the last 3 years.

Community/Public Health Nursing

Community/public health nursing master's programs prepare nurses for advanced roles in community settings. There are some schools of nursing that offer a joint degree awarding both the Master of Science in Nursing and the Master of Public Health (MPH). Others have community health nursing as a clinical specialty. The ANCC (2010) offers a public health nurse-advanced certification for graduates of masters in nursing with a specialty in community health nursing or nurses (BSNs) who hold an MPH. Other graduate degrees might be eligible but they must have a baccalaureate degree in nursing.

Swider et al. (2006) reviewed the core competencies recommended by the Quad Council (2004) that include Analytic Assessment Skills, Basic Public Health Sciences Skills, Cultural Competency Skills, Communication Skills, Community Dimensions of Practice Skills, Financial Planning and Management Skills, Leadership and Systems Thinking Skills, and Policy Development/Program Planning Skills. The authors compared the competencies to Rush University's curriculum and found that the competencies provide a framework for the community/public health nursing practice at an advanced level and recommended that other schools may wish to consider this model as well as when planning their programs. Swider et al. (2009) discuss DNP as an educational option for master's degree–prepared nurses with community/public health nursing backgrounds. They surveyed leaders in community health nursing practice and although community health nursing is considered as clinical specialty, it is not always recognized when listing advanced practice nurses. The respondents to the survey raised issues such as their belief that the DNP would not result in salary differentials and they felt that the Doctorate in Public Health is the more accepted degree in their field. They also raised some concerns about nurses in the community and their roles in school health, home care, and hospice. These issues need to be addressed in the near future as the DNP gains recognition in the profession and the health care system.

Nursing Administration

The most common master's degrees in nursing to prepare nurse leaders are the master's in nursing administration or leadership. Some programs offer joint master's degrees with nursing such as Master Business Administration (MBA) or health care administration. The graduates of these programs are not prepared for advanced practice roles such as clinical specialists and nurse practitioners, but rather, have education in the management of health care systems including staffing, human resources, finances, budgeting and administration. There are several ways for nurse administrators to receive national certification through the American Organization of Nurse Executives (AONE) (2010) for executive nursing or as nurse manager and leader. The latter requires only a baccalaureate in nursing, whereas the executive certification requires a master's. ANCC (2010) also has a national certification exam for nurse executives. In addition to these roles in management and administration, there are other leadership certifications for quality control, legal nurse consultants, risk managers, and infection-control nurses. These certifications occur through specialty organizations and for the most part, require or prefer that nurses have a master's degree as well as continuing education for the specific role.

Nurse Educator

The role of the nurse educator in health care agencies includes staff development and patient education. There are programs in schools of nursing that specifically prepare nurses for this role at the master's level. With the recent growth of nursing education programs to help relieve the shortage of nursing faculty, many of the programs offer a track for nurse educators in health care settings and some offer post-master's certificates in nursing education. The National Nursing Staff Development Organization (NNSDO; 2010) recommends that staff developers become credentialed by ANCC for the nursing clinical specialty for which they are prepared.

The shortage in nursing faculty continues. According to the AACN (2010f) report on enrollments, 49,948 qualified applicants to nursing schools were turned away in 2008–2009 and two thirds of the schools reported that faculty shortages contributed to the turndowns. Owing to the shortage, there has been a surge of master's programs that prepare nurses for faculty roles. In addition, there are many post-master's certificate programs in education.

It is recommended that faculty should have at least the same degree level for the type of program in which they teach and it is highly recommended that they have one degree higher. Therefore, faculty teaching in associate's degree programs should have a master's degree, whereas those teaching in baccalaureate and higher degree programs should have a doctorate. However, with the shortage in nursing, it is not uncommon for master's degree–prepared nurses to teach clinical courses in specialties that match their expertise and in some state, Boards of Nursing allow nurses with baccalaureate degrees in nursing to teach under the supervision of an experienced educator.

Beres (2006) discusses her transition from a staff development role in the practice setting to that of faculty. She points out that her experiences and knowledge gained in andragogy and curriculum/program development contributed to her transition into the academic role and suggests that nurse educators in agencies are a good source for helping to ease the shortage.

There is a continuing debate about whether nursing faculty need to have special courses in education since they are specialists in their fields. There is no question that there is a separate body of knowledge related to curriculum development, instructional design and strategies, instructional technology, and program and student evaluation (Beres, 2006). Without this knowledge, many instructors in nursing neither have the background in learning theories that support best practices in education for meeting the needs of learners, nor do they have the curriculum planning and evaluation background to connect the program to the actual implementation (teaching) of the program. Such knowledge ensures the quality of the program so that learning experiences are linked to the mission and goals of the program. The same is true for evaluation of program review to measure outcomes and student evaluation to measure student's progress in the program. At the same time, it is equally important that nursing faculty have the content knowledge and theory on the materials they are teaching. To further support these statements, the National League for Nursing (NLN, 2010) offers national certification for nurse educators. Eligibility qualifications require a master's or doctorate degree in nursing and courses in curriculum development and evaluation, instructional design, principles of adult learning, assessment/measurement and evaluation, principles of teaching and learning, and instructional technology.

SUMMARY

Chapter 10 reviewed common master's degree programs in nursing and the differences among the majors available in nursing at the master's degree level. Roles for master's degree–prepared nurses were discussed and postgraduate certification possibilities were reviewed. Some issues were raised such as the advent of the DNP and its impact on advanced practice master's programs, entry into practice at the master's level, expectations of educational preparation for nursing faculty, and the place for the advanced generalist master's degree in the health care system.

DISCUSSION QUESTIONS

1. Debate the pros and cons of entry into practice at the master's level versus second baccalaureate for college graduates.
2. How should nursing differentiate between advanced practice roles and advanced knowledge roles such as nurse administrators, case managers, risk managers, and so forth?
3. Why or why not is it important for nurse educators in the practice setting and in schools of nursing to have graduate degrees and what levels of advanced education are necessary? Explain your answer.

LEARNING ACTIVITIES

Student Learning Activities

1. Review the literature and Web sites for nursing education to identify how many possible majors there are for master's degrees in nursing. Compare these majors to the job market for these specialties in your region. Discuss the pros and cons for the continuation or discontinuation of some of the programs.
2. Go to the Web sites of various credentialing and certification organizations for nursing and identify how many require at least a master's degree in nursing. Discuss why or why not certification for advanced roles should continue.

Nurse Educator/Faculty Development Activities

1. Review the latest follow-up survey of the graduates of your master's program for data on the employment of the graduates in settings where they use the focus of their graduate degree. Determine if your program prepares the graduates for the needs of the health care system and why or why not. Consider the

effect of your findings on curriculum revision or, possibly, development of new programs.
2. Discuss among yourselves your beliefs about master's education for advanced practice or roles in leadership and if the master's degree serves your graduates as a terminal degree and/or pathway to doctoral studies.

REFERENCES

American Association of Colleges of Nursing. (2007). *White paper on the education and role of the clinical nurse leader.* Washington, DC

American Association of Colleges of Nursing. (2008). *2007–2008 Enrollment and Graduations in Baccalaureate and Graduate Programs in Nursing.* Washington, DC: Author.

American Association of Colleges of Nursing. (2010a). *Accelerated BSN and MSN programs. The fast track to careers in nursing.* Retrieved from http://www.aacn.nche.edu/Publications/issues/Aug02.htm

American Association of Colleges of Nursing. (2010b). *Clinical Nurse Leader Master's Degree Programs.* Retrieved from http://www.aacn.nche.edu/CNL/CNLWebLinks.htm

American Association of Colleges of Nursing. (2010c). *CNL certification.* Retrieved from: http://www.aacn.nche.edu/CNC/index.htm

American Association of Colleges of Nursing. (2010d). *Consensus model for APRN Regulation: licensure, accreditation, certification, & education.* Retrieved July 7, 2008, from http://www.aacn.nche.edu/education/pdf/APRNReport.pdf

American Association of Colleges of Nursing. (2010e). *Position statement on the practice doctorate in nursing. October 2004.* Retrieved October 2004, from http://www.aacn.nche.edu/DNP/DNPPosition-Statement.htm

American Association of Colleges of Nursing. (2010f). *Nursing faculty shortage fact sheet.* Retrieved from http://www.aacn.nche.edu/Media/factsheets/FacultyShortage.htm

American Nurses Credentialing Center. (2010). *Board certification of nurses makes a difference.* Retrieved from http://www.nursecredentialing.org/default.aspx

American Organization of Nurse Executives. (2010). *Credentialing Center.* Retrieved from http://www.aone.org

Beres, J. (2006). Staff development to university faculty: Reflections of a nurse educator. *Nursing Forum, 41*(3), 141–145.

Bourbonniere, M., Mezey, M., Mitty, E. L., Burger, S., Bonner, A., Bowers, B., et al. (2009). Expanding the knowledge base of resident and facility outcomes of care delivered by advanced practice nurses in long-term care: Expert panel recommendations. *Policy, Politics, & Nursing Practice, 10*(1), 64–70.

California Board of Registered Nursing. (2010). *Entry-level master's degree programs.* Retrieved from http://www.rn.ca.gov/schools/rnprograms.shtml#msn

Delgado-Passler, P., & McCaffrey, R. (2006). The influences of postdischarge management by nurse practitioners on hospital readmission for heart failure. *Journal of the American Academy of Nurse Practitioners, 18*(4), 154–160.

Fulton, J. S. (2005). Calling blended role programs to account. *Clinical Nurse Specialist: The Journal for Advanced Nursing Practice, 15*(5), 221–222.

Kleinpell, R. (2007). APNs: Invisible champions? *Nursing Management, 38*(5), 18–22.

McCorkle, R. (2006). Leadership and professional development. A program of research on patient and family caregiver outcomes: Three phases of evolution. *Oncology Nursing Forum, 33*(1), 25–31.

National League for Nursing. (2010). *Certification for nurse educators.* Retrieved from http://www.nln.org/facultycertification/index.htm

National Nursing Staff Development Organization. (2010). *Become a Staff Educator.* Retrieved from https://www.nnsdo.org

Ott, K. M., Haddock, K. S., Fox, S. E., Shinn, J. K., Walters, S. E., Hardin, J. W., et al. (2009). The clinical nurse leader (SM): Impact on practice outcomes in the veterans health administration. *Nursing Economics, 27*(6), 363–370.

Parrish, E., & Peden, A. (2009).Clinical outcomes of depressed clients: A review of current literature. *Issues in Mental Health Nursing, 30*(1), 51–60.

Quad Council of Public Health Nursing Organizations. (2004). Public health nursing competencies. *Public Health Nursing, 21*(5), 443–452.

Raines, C., & Taglaireni, M. (2008). Career pathways in nursing: Entry points and academic progression. *Online Journal of Issues in Nursing, 13*(3).

Swider, S., Levin, P., Ailey, S., Breakwell, S., Cowell, J., McNaughton, D., et al. (2006). Matching a graduate curriculum in public/community health nursing to practice competencies: The Rush University experience. *Public Health Nursing, 23*(2), 190–195.

Swider, S., Levin, P., Cowell, J., Breakwell, S., Holland, P., & Wallinder, J. (2009). Community/public health nursing practice leaders' views of the doctorate of nursing practice. *Public Health Nursing, 26*(5), 405–411.

White, P., & Hall, M. E. (2006). Mapping the literature of case management nursing. *Journal of the Medical Library Association, 94*(2 Suppl.), E99–E106.

The Doctor of Nursing Practice

Sarah B. Keating

OBJECTIVES

Upon completion of Chapter 11, the reader will be able to:

1. Describe the role(s) of the Doctor of Nursing Practice (DNP) in practice and in the health care system.
2. Analyze the recommended components of the DNP educational program according to American Association of Colleges of Nursing (AACN).
3. Differentiate between applied practice/professional doctorates and research-focused degrees.
4. Explain the potential impact of the DNP on the nursing profession, education, and the health care system.

OVERVIEW

The movement toward a doctorate in nursing for advanced practice and leadership roles has grown tremendously over the past decade. According to the AACN, the DNP is the highest level of advanced nursing practice (AACN, 2010a). In 2010, AACN reported 120 existing DNP programs with another 161 planning to open. There were 35 states in the nation with DNP programs. The expansion of programs was no doubt in response to AACN's goal of the doctorate as preparation for advanced practice nursing by 2015. Chapter 11 reviews the DNP, its role in health care, the essentials for the degree as recommended by AACN, its differences from research-intensive degrees, and the potential impact of DNPs on the profession, education, and the health care system.

THE ROLE OF THE DOCTOR OF NURSING PRACTICE IN PRACTICE

When the notion of a professional/applied practice doctoral degree in nursing was first introduced in the late 1990s and early 2000s, there was much controversy about it from the profession and outside of the profession. Among the issues raised by nursing when the program was fairly new were the many different nursing doctoral degree programs and titles that confuse the public and nursing such as ND, DNSc, DNS, DSN, PhD, and so forth.. Objections to the use of the title *doctor* were raised for fear the public would assume that the provider was a medical doctor. Chism (2009) provides definitions of the term doctor and points out that nurses who earn the degree are entitled to use it;

however, she reports that some professional organizations suggest using a title such as "Dr. Jane Doe, Nurse–Midwife" to indicate that it is a nursing degree. The Unified Statements (2008) by organizations representing nurse practitioners and faculty for nurse practitioner programs clearly state that nurses who earn the DNP have a right to title themselves as doctor as no one profession has the right to this title (Nurse Practitioner Roundtable, 2008).

McCabe (2006) summarized some of the controversy about the DNP and its place in nursing. She stated that there is a need for nurses prepared at advanced levels for the increasing complexity of health care, informatics, technology, patient safety, and quality assurance. She raised the issue about the advanced role and if it is necessary to keep some of nursing's traditional functions in curricula because there is an ever-expanding knowledge base to include. She advocated for innovative approaches to curriculum development that makes room for and incorporates new knowledge. Although there has been controversy over the DNP role, the fact that nearly 300 programs are established or in the process of development across the nation speaks to its acceptance in the nursing profession (AACN, 2010c).

There are several major roles for DNP-prepared nurses in the health care system. One role is in advanced practice including clinical specialists, nurse anesthetists, nurse midwives, and nurse practitioners; however, this is not limited only to these roles and could include others, for example, advanced practice community health nurses. The DNP is considered the terminal degree for advanced practice. Another essential role for DNPs is to apply research to bring about change in evidence-based nursing and health care. A major role is for systems leadership in public policy to improve health care. Although the focus of the DNP is not to prepare nurse educators, graduates of DNP programs will be involved in the clinical education of nurses and AACN recommends that DNP graduates who wish to have faculty roles should complete education courses to prepare for the teaching role (AACN, 2010b; Chism, 2009).

EDUCATIONAL PREPARATION FOR THE DOCTOR OF NURSING PRACTICE

DNP educational programs follow the recommendations of AACN's (2010b) document, *The Essentials of Doctoral Education for Advanced Nursing Practice*. The following are the eight essentials defined in this document:

1. Scientific underpinnings for practice
2. Organizational and systems leadership for quality improvement and systems thinking
3. Clinical scholarship and analytical methods for evidence-based practice
4. Information systems/technology and patient care technology for the improvement and transformation of health care
5. Health care policy for advocacy in health care
6. Interprofessional collaboration for improving patient and population health outcomes
7. Clinical prevention and population health for improving the nation's health
8. Advanced nursing practice

Each of these essentials is described in detail by AACN and specific learning objectives are listed under each essential. AACN discusses the incorporation of specialty competencies for programs that prepare DNPs for advanced practice roles such as clinical specialists, nurse practitioners, nurse midwives, nurse anesthetists, and others. Program developers are directed to specialty organizations for the lists of competencies expected for national certification in advanced nursing roles.

Fain, Asselin, and McCurry (2008) discuss not only the advanced practice role of the DNP-prepared nurses, but also the leadership they provide to promote change in the health care system. DNPs have the knowledge and experience to work with interprofessional teams, translate research, develop new evidence-based practice interventions, act as change agents to bring about improvements in the health care system and health policy, and provide visionary leadership.

Currently, there are two major types of DNP programs. The first is the post-master's DNP program that admits nurses with master's degrees who are nationally certified for advanced practice including nurse anesthetists, midwives, practitioners, and clinical specialists. Additionally, nursing administrators, managers, and other nurse leaders with or without national certification enroll in DNP programs to gain additional education and experiences for leadership in the health care system. Many of these programs were first initiated to meet the needs of master's degree–prepared nurses wishing to earn a doctorate to advance their practice, act as change agents in the health care system, increase interprofessional collaboration, and gain professional credibility in a system with most of the major disciplines prepared at the doctoral level, for example, medical doctor (MD), doctor of pharmacy (PharmD), doctor of physical therapy (DPT), doctor of psychology (PsyD), and so forth. Although it is expected that advanced practice nurses currently in practice who do not have the DNP will be "grandparented in" for licensure to practice in the states in which they are licensed and recognized, it is anticipated that many will wish to have the DNP credential. This is validated by the high enrollment in post-master's DNP programs (AACN, 2010c).

The other route to the DNP is to move the baccalaureate (Bachelor of Science in Nursing [BSN])-prepared nursing generalist into the DNP program. These programs prepare BSNs for advanced-practice roles similar to the programs for advanced practice nurses at the master's level, for example, advanced community health nurses, certified registered nurse anesthetists, clinical specialists, nurse midwives, and nurse practitioners. Additional course work related to health care systems management and leadership is included. In addition to the traditional advanced practice roles, DNP programs offer other options such as informatics and technology, health care management, and/ or administration roles. Supervised clinical experiences are included and must account for more than 1,000 hours of practice to meet professional accreditation and/or certification standards. As well as completion of the specialty role, students have courses that include the content of the eight essentials recommended by AACN (2010b). Graduates are eligible for national certification depending on the program of study's specialization and meeting of eligibility requirements.

DIFFERENCES BETWEEN PROFESSIONAL AND RESEARCH-BASED DOCTORATES

Although nursing has a history for developing various titles for its doctoral programs, academe recognizes two types of degrees. The first is the research-focused *PhD* program or in the case of nursing, the PhD, DNS, or DNSc. These degrees emphasize nursing theory and research, educate nurses prepared to conduct research, and foster the development of new knowledge in health care and nursing. Nurse educators in higher education prefer the PhD for faculty who wish to teach in tenure-track positions. The rationale for this is that research-extensive and -intensive institutions prefer a faculty prepared to develop new knowledge and theories in the respective disciplines. Academe in these institutions and other colleges or universities with productive research records award tenure to faculty who demonstrate research productivity through publications and other scholarly works that advance knowledge in their disciplines. This results in keeping the curriculum up-to-date and prepares graduates who are abreast of changes in their disciplines.

The second is the *professional doctorate degree*, including the DNP, which prepares graduates for application of research to practice or another way to say it is to translate research into practice. The role of graduates of the DNP has been mentioned previously. Nursing education programs are sometimes reluctant to hire DNPs into tenure-track positions owing to its focus on applied research as compared to active research for discovering new knowledge. However, the profession and educators are beginning to recognize the role of DNP graduates in providing clinical instruction and teaching in DNP programs owing to their expertise in evidence-based clinical practice and in translational research. Many DNP graduates can demonstrate extensive research in practice that makes them eligible for tenure-track positions. DNP graduates who expect to teach in schools of nursing should compare tenure-track policies in potential employing institutions to other tracks that are not research-focused but still offer academic ranks from instructor to professor and the potential for job stability over time. For both the research-focused degree (PhD, DNSc, DNS) and the DNP, AACN (2010b) strongly recommends taking courses in education if graduates intend to teach.

Loomis, Willard, and Cohen (2006) reviewed the literature on DNP programs to ascertain the profession and students' perspectives on the DNP, its role in health care and nursing education, and its difference from research-related degrees (PhD and DNSc). They found that early in its development, nursing education leaders feared that the DNP would decrease the applicant pool for research-oriented programs and thereby, decrease the numbers of faculty prepared for tenure-track positions in schools of nursing. One nurse educator leader responded to these concerns by stating that schools will eventually have two tenure-track pathways to include those educators focused on nursing research, whereas others would focus on the application of clinical research. The authors found that students in DNP programs preferred the DNP to the PhD program for its emphasis on practice that matched their career goals to provide the best care for their patient populations. A majority included teaching as a goal and considered the DNP as preparation for a blending of the role of clinician and educator. With the aging of the nursing faculty workforce, the authors recommended follow-up studies to determine the average age of students in DNP programs and the observation that BSN to DNP programs may result in a lowering of the average age of graduates and therefore, potential faculty.

PROGRAM EVALUATION AND ACCREDITATION

Program evaluation and accreditation are essential to the quality of DNP programs. Each school of nursing that has a DNP program usually has a master plan of evaluation for all programs and the DNP is included. DNP programs, in addition to the usual layers of approval within the home institution, are subject to the institution's govern-ing board's approval and if they are preparing entry-level advanced practice nurses, they must undergo program approval by their state board of nursing. Because the DNP is a relatively new degree, most programs must also have regional accreditation as a new degree is considered a substantive change. See Chapters 14 and 15 for more details on program evaluation and accreditation.

Specific to the DNP is the role of the Commission on Collegiate Nursing Education (CCNE; 2010) in accrediting DNP programs. The Commission determined that it would only accredit doctoral degrees that reflected the terminal practice degree in the profes-sion. This is in line with other professional or applied practice doctoral degrees in other disciplines. To be eligible for accreditation, DNP programs must have students enrolled for at least 1 year before hosting an on-site evaluation by CCNE with a self-study sub-mitted to CCNE prior to the visit. Action on accreditation takes place after the visit and during the next scheduled CCNE Board of Commissioners' meeting. This usually means that students enrolled in the program will graduate from an accredited program.

Kaplan and Brown (2009) present an overview of the evaluation plan used by the University of Washington to assess its DNP program. They provide the measures used to evaluate program outcomes including benchmarks such as student GPA, retention and graduation, completion of the capstone project, and a synthesis practicum. Other evaluation measures included student, faculty, and employer satisfaction with the pro-gram, and comparisons of the implementation of courses to the AACN's (2010) *Essentials*. The evaluation plan described by Brown and Kaplan should be very helpful for the assessment of DNP programs.

Program evaluation provides the data for assessing the effectiveness and quality of the program. Developing evaluation plans that incorporate all of the parameters of the program for assessment are important but it is also essential that plans are in place to implement the assessment. The methods for collecting and analyzing the data, the persons responsible, and when and how the findings from the analysis are used for program improvements are key factors to include.

IMPACT OF THE DOCTOR OF NURSING PRACTICE

Education

AACN's (2010b) *Essentials of Doctoral Education for Advanced Practice Nursing* provides the guidelines for schools of nursing that develop DNP programs. The essentials are the prod-uct of collaboration between nursing leaders and educators and is a consensus document. Although the DNP is an applied/professional or terminal degree for advanced practice, it does not emphasize research that leads to the development of new knowledge for the dis-cipline. Yet the issue arises as to who will conduct research for practice? Who will teach in DNP programs? Who are the experts for transmitting clinical knowledge and skills for nurses in practice and for students of nursing? Some of these issues have been raised in the literature and will continue into the future. However, with the growth of so many DNP programs, these issues should be resolved within the next decade or sooner.

Webber (2008) addresses the issue of the preparation of DNPs for research. She describes the DNP graduate's preparation for applying research to evidence-based practice rather than using research processes to investigate clinical practice and develop new knowledge and modalities. Her impression from the literature related to the DNP is that research in nursing is left to an elite few nurses prepared at the PhD, DNSc, or DNS levels and that this poses possible gaps in the discipline's need for research. To address this issue, she promotes the integration of research into baccalaureate, master's, and research-focused and applied-practice doctoral degree programs alike, to create collaborative research across the various levels. She urges further discussion by key professional and educational organizations on the role of research in DNP programs for the sake of nursing and its need for continued research in the discipline.

A coalition of nurse practitioner organizations omitted research skills in its description of DNP education, certification, and titling (Nurse Practitioner Roundtable, 2008). AACN's (2010b) *Essentials* refers to translational research applied to evidence-based practice. In its statement as follows:

> Research- and practice-focused doctoral programs in nursing share rigorous and demanding expectations: a scholarly approach to the discipline, and a commitment to the advancement of the profession. Both are terminal degrees in the discipline, one in practice and one in research. However, there are distinct differences between the two degree programs. For example, practice-focused programs understandably place greater emphasis on practice, and less emphasis on theory, meta-theory, research methodology, and statistics than is apparent in research-focused programs. Whereas all research- focused programs require an extensive research study that is reported in a dissertation or through the development of linked research papers, practice-focused doctoral programs generally include integrative practice experiences and an intense practice immersion experience. Rather than a knowledge-generating research effort, the student in a practice-focused program generally carries out a practice application-oriented "final DNP project," which is an integral part of the integrative practice experience. (p. 3)

This statement and the one from the Nurse Practitioner Roundtable reiterate Webber's point that DNPs are not expected to conduct research, but rather to apply it for evidence-based practice and clinical applications.

The Profession and Effects on Practice

The explosive growth of DNP programs over the past 10 years had significant effects on nursing education, the profession, and the health care system. One of the arguments cited frequently for the development of the DNP is for nursing to achieve parity with other professions who require the doctorate as entry-level into the profession. Upvall and Ptachcinski (2007) compare the development of the DNP to that of pharmacy's PharmD. They report that it took quite some time for the pharmacy profession to approve the PharmD as the entry-level into practice; finally achieving the requirement by the 1990s. Upvall and Ptachcinski argue that rather than seeking parity with other health professions for entry into practice, the purposes for the PharmD were to recognize the expanding roles of pharmacologists in the health care system and the growing numbers and complexities of pharmaceuticals. They also point out that many pharmacy schools have faculty and administrators prepared at the PharmD level and they are recognized as academicians contrary to some of the issues raised by nursing about the role of DNPs in academia. The authors discuss the differences between the PharmD and the DNP and that nursing needs to look at reasons other than parity with other health professionals such as the effect of advanced practice nurses on the health care system. (There is documentation of improved patient outcomes related to the services of advanced practice nurses.) Another point is that the DNP and the PharmD are not alike. The PharmD is an entry-level professional degree and the DNP is not.

Brown-Benedict (2008) analyzed several other health professions for their development of the doctorate level for practice. Included in the analysis were audiology, chiropractic, law, nutrition, physical therapy, and nutrition. Most of these programs have the doctorate as entry into advanced clinical practice somewhat similar to nursing's DNP but not other roles in nursing such as the generalist BSN and the advanced generalist CNL. Some of the doctorates require a residency, which is another issue that nursing may wish to consider. Brown-Benedict urges nursing to continue with its vision for the DNP and work on solving the titling, credentialing, and licensure issues revolving around it. She reinforces nursing's role in the delivery of compassionate holistic care, patient advocacy, evidence-based practice, leadership in health care policy, and the need to retain and strengthen these as nursing's niche in the health care system.

Johnson (2008) reviews the American Medical Association's (AMA) objections to the DNP. In 2008, the AMA presented two major resolutions at their meeting against the DNP urging passage for the use of the title *doctor*; confining it only to MDs. The other resolution was for DNPs to be under the supervision of physicians. Her editorial exhorts readers to promote the focus of the DNP on evidence-based practice and the effects it can have on best practices and improved patient outcomes. She urges nurses to remain vigilant and to support professional nursing organizations as the DNP develops and its effects are felt within the health care system and the health policy arena.

SUMMARY

Chapter 11 reviewed the growth of DNP programs in the nation and the role of DNPs in the health care system including evidence-based advanced practice and leadership in the health care system and health policy. Many of the issues pertaining to the preparation of DNPs, research versus translational research, the question of what level of academic degree is necessary for advanced practice, and the controversies among health care professional on the professional or applied doctorate degree were discussed. References for guidelines on the development of DNP curriculums and suggestions for evaluating the programs were listed.

DISCUSSION QUESTIONS

1. To what extent do you believe the DNP as the terminal degree for advanced practice has on reaching consensus on the doctorate as entry into practice?
2. Debate research-focused degrees as contrasted to professional degrees and how research activities differ or are the same. What effect do you believe this debate has on the profession of nursing as a discipline?

LEARNING ACTIVITIES

Student Learning Activities

Review the latest research and literature (the past 2 years) to identify the state of debate on the DNP and its role in research and academe.

Nurse Educator/Faculty Development Activities

If your school of nursing has a DNP program, analyze its curriculum for its congruence with the AACN's *Essentials* document. If your school does not have a DNP program, find a school that does and review its program of study to compare to the *Essentials*.

REFERENCES

American Association of Colleges of Nursing. (2010a). *AACN position statement on the practice doctorate in nursing.* Retrieved, from http://www.aacn.nche.edu/DNP/DNPPositionStatement.htm

American Association of Colleges of Nursing. (2010b). *The essentials of doctoral education for advanced nursing practice.* Retrieved, from http://www.aacn.nche.edu/DNP/pdf/Essentials.pdf

American Association of Colleges of Nursing. (2010c). *Press release.* Retrieved, from http://www.aacn.nche.edu/Media/NewsReleases/2010/enrollchanges.html

Brown-Benedict, D. J. (2008). The doctor of nursing practice degree: Lessons from the history of the professional doctorate in other health disciplines. *Journal of Nursing Education, 47*(10), 448–57.

Chism, L. A. (2009). Toward clarification of the doctor of nursing practice. *Advanced Emergency Nursing, 31*(4), 287–297.

Commission on Collegiate Nursing Education. (2010). *DNP: Program accreditation information.* Retrieved, from http://www.aacn.nche.edu/Accreditation/DNPaccred.htm

Fain, J. A., Asselin, M., & McCurry, M. (2008). The DNP: Why now? Several broadscale health care factors influenced nursing policy makers to roll out the doctorate of nursing practice degree in the midst of a national shortage. *Nursing Management, 39*(7), 34–37.

Johnson, P. J. (2008). The DNP storm. *Neonatal Network, 27*(5), 297–298.

Kaplan, L., & Brown, M. (2009). Doctor of nursing practice program evaluation and beyond: Capturing the profession's transition to the DNP. *Nursing Education Perspectives, 30*(6), 362–366.

Loomis, J. A., Willard, B., & Cohen, J. (2006). Difficult professional choices: Deciding between the PhD and the DNP in nursing. *Online Journal of Issues in Nursing, 12*(1), 6.

McCabe, S. (2006). What does it take to make a nurse? Considerations of the CNL and DNP role development. *Perspectives in Psychiatric Care, 42*(4), 252–255.

Nurse Practitioner Roundtable. (June, 2008). *Nurse practitioner DNP education, certification and titling: A unified statement,* Washington, DC: Author. Retrieved, from http://www.nonpf.com/associations/10789/files/DNPUnifiedStatement0608.pdf

Upvall, M. J., & Ptachcinski, J. (2007). The journey to the DNP program and beyond: What can we learn from pharmacy? *Journal of Professional Nursing, 23*(5), 316–321.

Webber, P. B. (2008). The Doctor of Nursing Practice degree and research: Are we making an epistemological mistake? *Journal of Nursing Education, 47*(10): 466–472.

Curriculum Planning for Doctor of Philosophy and Other Research-Focused Doctoral Nursing Programs

Nancy A. Stotts

OBJECTIVES

Upon completion of Chapter 12, the reader will be able to:

1. Describe the research-focused doctorate in nursing.
2. Compare the curriculum of an existing research-focused doctoral program with the recommended American Association of Colleges of Nursing (AACN) components of a research-focused doctoral degree.
3. Describe strategies used to evaluate the quality of research-focused doctoral programs.
4. Identify common issues faced by research-focused doctoral programs.

OVERVIEW

Nurse scientists are the major product of research-focused doctoral programs, including the Doctor of Philosophy (PhD) and Doctor of Nursing Science (abbreviated both as DNS and DNSc) programs. The goal of these programs is to enhance the health of the population by preparing graduates to conduct, disseminate, and translate research. This chapter addresses the role of the research-focused doctoral program in nursing, the curriculum, and evaluation of program quality. Issues common to research-focused programs also will be discussed.

THE ROLE OF THE RESEARCH-FOCUSED DOCTORAL PROGRAM IN NURSING

Research-focused doctoral programs, including both PhD and DNS programs, are designed to prepare students to pursue intellectual inquiry and conduct independent research that results in extension of knowledge (AACN, 2001). From a theoretical perspective, PhD programs are theory based and focus on testing theory, whereas the DNS programs are oriented more toward clinical practice research (Keithley et al., 2003; Robb, 2005). However, it is often difficult to tell the difference in the programs based on their curricula. Clearly, the commonality between the two program designations is the focus on original research that has potential to contribute to the body of knowledge in the field. Graduates are scholars (Walker, Golde, Jones, Bueschel, & Hutchings, 2008), although the nature of the knowledge and how it contributes to the field is unique to each candidate and possibly to each school.

In reality, the designation as a PhD or DNS program is often determined by the school's specific mission and philosophy as well as by institutional criteria for PhD/DNS program approval. Although holding the highest academic degree in the field, nurses from research-focused institutions are prepared and expected to be leaders in nursing as demonstrated by their role in knowledge generation and dissemination, professional organizations, and policy. In fact, graduates of PhD/DNS program have been called the *stewards of the discipline*, those entrusted with the preserving the past as the basis for the future of the discipline (Walker et al., 2008, pp. 13–14).

Enrolled are 4,177 students; 567 graduated in 2009. The number has increased only 5.1% ($n = 201$) in the past year; a small increase in comparison with the DNP that increased by 51.2% ($n = 1,750$) over the same period (AACN, 2009a). The student body in these schools is somewhat homogeneous. It is mostly White and female. Ethnic minorities are increasing and have reached 23% whereas male students comprise 7.3% of the research-focused doctoral program student body (AACN, 2009a). The average student is middle-aged (mean 42.7 years for full time and 44 years for part-time; AACN, 2009b).

There remains a shortage of faculty, illustrated by the fact that qualified students at all levels of nursing education (entry into practice as well as graduate school) are not being accepted into programs and the 61.7% of schools indicate the reason they are not accepting qualified applicants is lack of faculty (AACN, 2009a). In addition, the faculty in nursing education is aging. Across the various levels of nursing programs, the mean age of professors is 59.1 years, associate professors is 56.1 years, and assistant professors is 51.7 years (AACN, 2009c). Clearly, a cadre of new faculty is needed to replace the aging and soon-to-be-retiring faculty (Meleis, 2005; Meleis & Dracup, 2005).

Most graduates from research-focused programs work in academia where scholarly activity/research, service to the university and profession, professional competence, and teaching are core criteria for tenure and promotion (Faculty Handbook, 2009). There are two types of academic programs where PhD/DNS graduates work: research-intensive universities and teaching-intensive universities. In the research- intensive university, the most highly rewarded activity is research and scholarship. The expectation is that new PhD/DNS faculty members will develop a program of research that is externally funded, publish in peer-reviewed journals, develop a national and eventually international reputation as a scholar, provide scientific critique and review for journal articles and grants, and influence policy (AACN, 2001). The expectation is that they will mentor and teach PhD/DNS students that subsequently will go on to become faculty that will be research scientists. They will provide leadership to the profession, have a national reputation, and provide service to their institution (e.g., serve on committees).

In teaching-intensive programs, PhD/DNS faculty members teach and mentor prelicensure students as well as graduate students. Scholarly activity is required but may be more broadly defined than in the research-intensive university and in addition to externally funded research, may include writing textbooks, conducting education-focused studies, and publishing clinically focused papers. Committee service in the university and leadership in professional organizations are also usual expectations in these schools.

Some graduates will work in industry, government, and policy. Their roles vary but they are hired for their expertise and leadership capacity, much of which is the product of their doctoral education. In industry, they may work in clinical research and direct or monitor research studies. In government, they may assume a role in the National Institute of Nursing Research as well as various other agencies (e.g., Veterans Administration). Doctorally prepared nurses may work in policy to affect public, industry, or government opinion on health-related issues (e.g., smoking).

Postdoctoral work often follows graduation from a research-focused doctoral program (Nolan et al., 2008). The postdoctoral program is focused on learning a new method, extending expertise in substantive content, publication of papers from the dissertation, and writing of research grants to set the direction for future research. Those who have completed a postdoctoral program are better prepared to enter academia and successfully complete the research-related milestones of obtaining external funding and publishing in peer-reviewed journals than PhD-/DNS-prepared nurses who have not gone on for further preparation (National Research Council, 2005).

THE CURRICULUM

The core content of the PhD/DNS program is course work in philosophy of science, history of nursing science, research methods, processes of theory development, substantive nursing knowledge, and role related content (e. g., academic, research, practice, policy; AACN, 2001). Cognates from supporting disciplines, such as sociology or physiology, are often required. From a process perspective, most programs require a formal evaluation of substantive knowledge prior to the student undertaking their original research project. All programs have a process by which the research topic is approved by the faculty and the quality of the dissertation project is evaluated.

Table 12.1 is the modal curriculum at the University of California San Francisco (*Faculty Handbook*, 2009). The fit of this program with AACN criteria is shown by the superscripts after course titles indicating whether they focus on history and philosophy of science (*A*), research (*B*), theory (*C*), substantive nursing (*D*), or are role related (*E*). Review of the modal program reveals a preponderance of research-focused course work.

PROGRAM EVALUATION

The quality of research-focused doctoral nursing programs is established and maintained by the individual programs. There is not an external accreditation that is used for research-focused doctoral programs.

There are quality indicators provided by AACN (2001) available to evaluate research-focused doctoral programs. Criteria for evaluation are divided into categories of faculty, program of study, resources, students, and evaluation. Table 12.2 provides examples of indicators cited in the AACN (2001) document. Programs often supplement these measures with their own indicators. For example, for a state-supported program, one rubric might be the proportion of state residents in the student body.

At times, the larger institution in which the program or school is located has internal processes for ensuring quality of their programs. For example, within the University of California 10-campus system, an external review is conducted every 5 years for PhD programs to ensure program quality. Reviewers from similar doctoral programs within the discipline use a set of established criteria to evaluate the program. The review

TABLE 12.1 Modal Curriculum of the University of California, San Francisco

YEAR 01: FALL

N209A Comparative Qualitative Research Design[B]

N209B Comparative. Quantitative Research Design[B]

N269A Human Health and Nursing Systems[D]

N2XX Theory Course[C] (choice of N221.01 Theories Related to Nursing Care; N253 Theories of the Policy Process; N290 Family Theory/Research in Health)

YEAR 01: WINTER

N229 Philosophy of Nursing. Science[A]

B187 Introduction to Statistics[B]

XXX (3) Cognate

YEAR 01: SPRING

N212A Data Collection & Ethics[B]

N212B Quantitative Measurement & Theory[B]

B192 Introduction to Linear Models[B]

YEAR 02: FALL

N285A Advanced Qualitative Methods I[B] OR N289A Advanced Quantitative Methods I[B]

XXX Cognate

NXXX Advanced Nursing Seminar in _____ (e.g., N232ABC Symptom Management, N240.01/.02/.03 Biomarkers, N240.05 Vulnerable Women, N240.12 Research in Aging)[B, C, D]

YEAR 02: WINTER

N285B Advanced Qualitative Methods II[B] OR N289B Advanced Quantitative Methods II[B]

N276 Research Rotation[B]

NXXX Advanced Nursing Seminar (as above)[B, C, D]

YEAR 02: SPRING

N276 Research Rotation[B]

NXXX Advanced Nursing Seminar (as above)[B, C, .D]

N291 Applied Statistical Methods[B]

YEAR: 03

Additional cognates, advanced nursing seminars, and specialized methods courses as needed; teaching residency.

Qualifying examination and advancement to candidacy.

Proposal approval.

YEAR: 04

Dissertation research (data collection, analysis).

Dissertation defense.

Note: Data in this table are from *A Faculty Handbook for Success: Advancement and Promotion at UCSF*, 1999, San Francisco: Regents of the University of California. Copyright 1999 by Regents of the University of California. Reprinted with permission.

[A], history and philosophy of science
[B], research
[C], theory
[D], substantive nursing
[E], role related

TABLE 12.2 Examples of Quality Indicators in Research-Focused Doctoral Programs in Nursing

Faculty

- Extramural research grants
- Peer-reviewed publications
- Presentations of research or theory at national meetings

Program of Study

- Dissertation is an original contribution.
- Employers report satisfaction with leadership and scholarship.
- Graduates' scholarship and leadership are recognized in awards, honors, and external funding within 3–5 years.

Resources

- Office of research exists.
- Internal research funds are awarded.

Students

- Selected from a pool of highly qualified applicants that represent diverse populations
- Student goals and objectives are congruent with faculty research.

Evaluation

- Evaluation is systematic and ongoing.
- Process and outcome data are obtained related to indicators of quality.

involves a self-study as well as in-person meetings with the program and school's administration, faculty, students (i.e., predoctorals, graduates, postdoctorals). This culminates in a report to the campuswide committee responsible for graduate education. Program directors then are charged to address the items identified in the review. Overall, it is a positive process and helps maintain parity both of the nursing program nationally and the doctoral programs within the larger University of California system.

COMMON ISSUES FACED BY RESEARCH-FOCUSED DOCTORAL PROGRAMS

Internal and external forces create issues for research-intensive programs. The shrinking availability of funding for higher education is one of the external issues that caused ripples in academia. As state dollars are stretched and colleges and universities receive less state funding and fewer funds are available to both public and private schools because of the national/international monetary downturn, there is a change in many schools about how faculty members are funded. Increasingly, the expectation is that faculty will bring in their own salary from grants, as well as fund the salary and tuition of their PhD/DNS students. Although requiring grants to provide doctoral/postdoctoral student salary is a long-standing norm in the basic sciences, only recently has it become explicit in nursing. To make matters more challenging, there is an increasing competition for National Institutes of Health funds, as well as private foundation grants, as the number of research-focused graduates increases. Schools have entire departments that focus on fund-raising and this seems partially effective. Increasingly, nursing programs have looked to collaboration with industry as another source of revenue for their studies; this has raised questions of conflict of interest. New faculty members are advised to be cautious when obtaining funding from commercial vendors to avoid even the perception of bias or tainted scientific objectivity (Nolan et al., 2008). A new business model for research-focused doctoral programs is emerging and how the model is shaped will have profound effect on the number and nature of future research-focused nursing doctoral programs.

Clear differentiation of the product of research and practice-focused doctoral programs is needed as the Doctor of Nursing Practice (DNP) becomes more widely accepted as the nursing parallel of the Doctor of Medicine (MD) or Doctor of Dental Science (DDSc). It will be important for the discipline and the profession that nursing speak as a single voice as to the nature of education to avoid divisiveness, such as that which existed with the issue of entry into practice (Meleis & Dracup, 2005). This is a perfect time to rethink, clarify, change, and reaffirm the pivotal tasks of the various levels of nursing education. Following a national study of nursing education funded by the Carnegie Foundation, there is a call for "radical transformation" in nursing education (Benner, Sutphen, Leonard, & Day, 2009). It is time to step up to the plate and take on the challenge, especially in research-focused doctoral programs.

Several issues could be rolled into such a reevaluation, change, and reaffirmation package. The issue of pedagogy (i.e., how to teach, the role of active learning, distance approaches to learning) needs increased attention. The nature of the students also needs to be addressed. At the moment, the normative expectation is that the doctoral preparation is built on the foundation of expertise attained in a master's program. Only 60% ($n = 72$) of programs admit students who have only baccalaureate preparation (AACN, 2009b) and even fewer admit nonnurses. The nature of those admitted for PhD/DNS education needs further attention if nursing is to move into parity with doctoral programs in other fields. One dimension of this issue is how to recruit racial/ethnic minority nurses into research-focused doctoral programs (Nnedu, 2009). To date, fewer than one in four enrolled students are minority students (AACN, 2009a); more are needed if nurse scientists are going to reflect the characteristics of the population they serve.

Finally, there needs to be clearer delineation of how interdisciplinary education can be mounted in research-focused programs. Discussion needs to center on various issues beyond the practical issues of cross-discipline teaching and scheduling. Topics that might be addressed include the ethics that underlie work produced by multiple persons and how interdisciplinary work informs the science differently than a single discipline perspective. Much progress has been made in enhancing interdisciplinary learning, but most has been on an individual basis. Nursing has much to give and gain from inter-disciplinary research. It would behoove us to better define our expectations in research- focused doctoral programs.

SUMMARY

Research-based doctoral programs produce scientists. Most work in academia after graduation and balance research/scholarship/creative activity, teaching, and service to the university and profession. Research-focused doctoral programs emphasize developing skills as a researcher/scholar and include course work in history and philosophy of science, research methods, theory development, substantive nursing knowledge, and role-related content. A sample curriculum illustrates one approach to operationalizing these areas of course work. Although robust in the number of programs and students enrolled, these doctoral programs face ongoing issues having to do with funding, clear differentiation of research and practice-focused doctoral programs, the nature of applicants to be admitted for future PhD/DNS programs, and the role of interdisciplinary education in research-focused programs.

DISCUSSION QUESTIONS

1. Propose how interdisciplinary research might be supported and developed as part of a PhD/DNS program.
2. What are the strengths and limitations of having students admitted to a PhD/DNS with only a baccalaureate?

LEARNING ACTIVITIES

Student Learning Activities

Compare a selected PhD/DNS program with the recommended curriculum components from AACN (2001).

Nurse Educator/Faculty Development Activities

Review the literature to identify the most efficient and effective strategies to teach students in PhD/DNS programs. Compare the findings with how you are teaching students in your program. Consider how you would make change, if that is appropriate.

REFERENCES

American Association of Colleges of Nursing. (2001). *Indicators of quality in research-focused doctoral programs in nursing.* Washington, DC: Author.
American Association of Colleges of Nursing. (2009a). *Amid calls for more highly educated nurses, new AACN data show impressive growth in doctoral nursing programs.* Washington, DC: Author.
American Association of Colleges of Nursing. (2009b). *Annual report: Advancing higher education in nursing.* Washington, DC: Author.
American Association of Colleges of Nursing. (2009c). *Nursing faculty shortage. Fact sheet.* Washington, DC: Author.
Benner, P., Sutphen, M., Leonard, V., & Day, L. (2009). *Educating nurses: A call for radical transformation.* San Francisco: Jossey-Bass.
"A Faculty Handbook for Success: Advancement and Promotion at UCSF." (2009). San Francisco: Regents of the University of California.
"Faculty Handbook: 2009." (2009). San Francisco: UCSF School of Nursing.
Keithley, J. K., Gross, D., Johnson, M. E., McCann, J., Faux, S., Shekleton, M., et al., (2003). Why Rush will keep the DNSc. *Journal of Professional Nursing, 19*(4), 223–229.

Meleis, A. I. (2005). Shortage of nurses means shortage of nurse scientists. *Journal of Advanced Nursing*, *49*(2), 111.

Meleis, A. I., & Dracup, K. (2005). The case against the DNP: History, timing, substance, and marginalization. *Online Journal of Issues in Nursing*, *10*(3), 3.

National Research Council. (2005). *Advancing the nation's health needs*. Washington, DC: National Academics Press.

Nnedu, C. C. (2009). Recruiting and retaining minorities in nursing education. *ABNF Journal*, *20*(4), 93–96.

Nolan, M. T., Wenzel, J., Han, H. R., Allen, J. K., Paez, K. A., & Mock, V. (2008). Advancing a program of research within a nursing faculty role. *Journal Professional Nursing*, *24*(6), 364–370.

Robb, W. J. (2005). PhD, DNSc, ND: The ABCs of nursing doctoral degrees. *Dimensions of Critical Care Nursing*, *24*(2), 89–96.

Walker, G. E., Golde, C. M., Jones, L., Bueschel, A. C., & Hutchings, P. (2008). *The formation of scholars: Rethinking doctoral education for the twenty-first century*. San Francisco, CA: Jossey-Bass.

13 Curriculum Development and Evaluation in Staff Development

Jennifer Richards

OBJECTIVES

Upon completion of Chapter 13, the reader will be able to:

1. Analyze the role of the staff development educator in the practice setting.
2. Apply learning theories and research to the development of staff development programs.
3. Conduct a needs assessment of internal and external frame factors as it relates to staff development programs.
4. Apply the components of curriculum development to staff development and programs.
5. Realize the importance of budget planning as it applies to staff development.
6. Apply program evaluation concepts to staff development.
7. Consider the issues and trends in staff development programs.

INTRODUCTION

This chapter applies the previous information on curriculum development and evaluation in academic settings to staff development programs in health care organizations. The staff development function involves the postlicensure education of nurses in health care organizations to ensure that members of the nursing staff have the most current, evidence-based knowledge and skills for nursing practice. In large health maintenance organizations (HMOs), university medical centers, major county hospitals, and other health care agencies, the staff development function is often centralized with responsibilities for the training and professional development of all personnel from custodial staff and unlicensed health care workers to nurses, physicians, managers, and administrators. For the purposes of this chapter, the term *staff development educator* will be used. Some other terms to describe educators with a staff development role include clinical nurse educator, hospital-based educator, education specialist, and education coordinator.

Activities of staff development educators often include new graduate programs, orientation, competency assessment, cross training, new product and technology training, specialty practice education, research utilization education, leadership development, and continuing education to encourage lifelong learning. Additionally, staff development educators are often involved in providing ongoing education to ensure that health care providers have up-to-date information on standards and guidelines set by government and regulatory agencies such as state health departments and the Joint Commission, also known as the Joint Commission on Accreditation of Health-care Organizations (JCAHO). In accordance with the mission of a health care organization, additional areas of education may include quality improvement processes, interpersonal relationships, customer service, information technology, and health care economics. Through the provision of initial and ongoing support and education, staff development educators play a key role in the retention of nurses and other health care providers within an organization.

Most health care facilities have a major educational plan for staff development services. Curriculum development in staff development often involves revisions to the plan based on changes in health care delivery, population demographics, emerging health risks and health problems, advances in practice and technology, and program feedback from the recipients of educational programs. The intended impact of staff development is quality patient care by a well-prepared staff with an ultimate outcome of improved health and quality of life in the patient population served by the agency. Information in this chapter includes roles and responsibilities of nurse educators in the practice setting, adult learning theories appropriate for staff development programs, the emphasis on quality assurance and patient safety as it applies to staff education, a needs assessment of external and internal frame factors relevant to developing or revising staff development programs, adaptation of curriculum components to the practice setting, evaluation strategies, preparing and managing budgets, and issues in nursing education in the practice setting.

QUALIFICATIONS, RESPONSIBILITIES, AND FUNCTIONS OF NURSE EDUCATORS IN STAFF DEVELOPMENT PROGRAMS IN HEALTH CARE AGENCIES

In addition to nursing and health care knowledge, the staff development educator needs knowledge and skills in program and curriculum development, learning theories, instructional design, teaching strategies, program evaluation, and budget management. Excellence in communication is critical to building support for the program, interacting with the public and vendors, and fostering relationships with administrators, advisory boards, staff, academic faculty and students, other agency personnel, patients, families, and the community. Although many of these qualifications come with experience, additional education is recommended, preferably at the master's or doctorate level. According to the *Scope and Standards of Practice for Nursing Professional Development* (American Nurses Association [ANA], 2000), staff development educators should have graduate education in nursing or a related specialty. If the graduate degree is in a related specialty, the baccalaureate degree must be in nursing. Ideally, administrators of staff development programs have a doctoral degree in nursing or a related field, such as education. Additionally, it is preferable for nurses working in staff development roles to be certified in their specialties and/or in continuing nursing education or nursing professional development (NPD). Information on specialty certification can be found at http://www .nursecredentialing.org (American Nurses Credentialing Center, 2010).

The current standards for NPD were published by the ANA in 2000. It is important to note that at the time of this writing, the 2010 version of the *Scope and Standards of*

Practice for Nursing Professional Development are not yet published. According to an update published on *Health Leaders Media* in December 2009, a task force commenced in March of 2008 to review and revise the scope and standards document. Proposed changes to the document were then posted for public comment from members of various professional organizations including the ANA and the National Nursing Staff Development Organization (NNSDO) (Health Leaders Media, 2009). In the 2000 version, the scope of practice for NPD was expanded to include the roles of educator, facilitator, change agent, consultant, researcher, and leader. Areas addressed in the standards of practice for NPD include assessment, diagnosis (or analysis to determine target audience and learner needs), identification of educational outcomes, planning, implementation, and evaluation. Areas addressed in the standards of professional performance for NPD are performance appraisal, education, collegiality, ethics, collaboration, research, management and resource utilization, and leadership (ANA, 2000).

Just as nurses have a responsibility to lifelong learning to maintain and increase competence in their practice, so do staff development educators (ANA, 2000). In terms of ongoing professional development for staff development educators, the education standard in the *Scope and Standards of Practice for Nursing Professional Development* requires that in order to maintain current knowledge and competency, the educator must do the following:

1. Participate in ongoing educational activities related to practice knowledge and professional issues.
2. Acquire knowledge and skills appropriate to the specialty area, practice setting, and cultural competence.
3. Seek experiences that reflect current theories and methods of teaching, learning, and delivery.
4. Maintain a professional portfolio that documents ongoing continuing professional nursing competence.
5. Seek certification when eligible. (ANA, 2000, p. 17)

The role of the staff development educator is multifaceted and can vary on a daily, sometimes even on an hourly basis. Activities of staff development educators often include preparation and support of new graduate programs, orientation, competency assessment, cross training, new product and technology training, specialty practice education, research utilization education, leadership development, and continuing education to encourage lifelong learning. In an ever-changing health care environment with a renewed focus on patient safety and quality outcomes, staff development educators play a key role in ensuring that nurses and other health care professionals have the knowledge and resources to provide evidence-based care. Through the provision of initial and ongoing support and education, staff development educators play a key role in the retention of nurses and other health care providers within an organization.

With the renewed focus on patient safety and quality outcomes in health care organizations, the nursing profession is held accountable for nursing-sensitive quality indicators such as skin integrity and patient falls. The application of research utilization and evidence-based practice in nursing highlights one of the many roles of nurse educators in the practice setting and their potential to impact patient safety and outcomes. Acting as change agents, nurse educators in staff development roles are key to creating a culture of inquiry, promoting research utilization, and preparing nurses and other health care providers to seek out and evaluate the evidence, and ultimately improve the quality of care within their organizations (Krugman, 2003; Strickland & O'Leary-Kelley, 2009). In addition, with regard to patient safety and quality outcomes, nurse educators are responsible for educating nurses about the "measurement, improvement, and benchmarking of clinical costs, quality, and outcomes specific to nursing" (Gallagher, 2005, p. 39). To this end, nurse educators must be engaged in data gathering and evaluation activities and more importantly, in communicating findings and benchmarking information to nursing staff. It is difficult, if not impossible, to change practice and improve outcomes if knowledge about current performance and progress is not shared with the nurses who are actually providing interventions and evaluating patient care at the bedside. Nurse educators are challenged to implement teaching methodologies that prepare bedside nurses to continually question the effectiveness of their interventions, determine if the evidence supports their practice, and use their clinical judgment to impact the outcomes of the care they are providing (Durham & Sherwood, 2008).

The responsibilities and functions of the staff development educator include program planning, implementation, and evaluation. If the educator is the sole person responsible for the educational program, other nursing staff members and/or health care providers are consulted for their content expertise in developing educational sessions and the management staff for infrastructure support. In contrast, a large health care system will have an administrator or director of the staff development program, administrative staff, and educators to implement the program. In either case, all of the components of educational program development, implementation, management, and evaluation apply.

LEARNING THEORIES

Chapter 3 describes in detail the classic and postmodernistic learning theories applied to nursing education. For the health agency setting, adult learning theories usually prevail in educational programs, especially for staff development. The terms *pedagogy* and *andragogy* are especially relevant to these practice-setting situations. Pedagogy is defined as the art, science, or profession of teaching (Merriam-Webster, 2010). Although the root of pedagogy (ped-) implies education of children, its use in the United States became more generic and applied to all ages of learners. However, as continuing education needs became apparent and especially after World War II with the return of America's war veterans, the term andragogy became popular to differentiate the learning needs of students of different ages and to develop strategies that were consistent with adult learning theories. Malcolm Knowles, an influential leader in the field of adult education, popularized the concept of andragogy in the United States. From his perspective, the premise of andragogy was based on differences in characteristics between child and adult learners (Knowles, Holton, & Swanson, 1998). The five assumptions described by Knowles are outlined as follows:

1. Self-concept—with maturity, self-concept moves from dependent to self-directed.
2. Experience—with maturity, a person's life experiences become a resource for learning.
3. Readiness to learn—with maturity, readiness to learn becomes linked to the "developmental tasks of social roles."

4. Orientation to learning—with maturity, perspective changes from "postponed application of knowledge to immediacy of application" and learning shifts from subject-centered to problem-centered.

5. Motivation to learn—with maturity, motivation to learn becomes internal.
(Smith, 2002, p. 7)

NEEDS ASSESSMENT

Curriculum development for staff development programs begins with a needs assessment that examines the frame factors that are both external and internal to the organization and that have an impact on the curriculum (Johnson, 1977). Chapters 5 and 6 provide a comprehensive discussion of the adaptation of the Johnson model to current curriculum development activities. The discussion to follow applies these same frame factors to a needs assessment for developing and revising curricula for staff development educators.

External Frame Factors

External frame factors to consider are the community, including changes in population demographics; health needs of the population served by the health care agency; the physical, social, and economic environment; the health care system; the nursing workforce; regulations and accreditation requirements for staff development programs; resources for staff education programs; and the need for program development or revision. See Table 13.1 for a summary of the external frame factors to consider.

Description of the Community

An assessment of the community or geographical area served by the health care agency yields a great deal of information useful for developing and/or revising staff development programs. Exhibit 13.1 identifies elements of data collection for conducting a community needs assessment.

Urban and suburban areas may have several community characteristics and resources that enrich staff. A well-developed public transportation system provides convenient access to the health care organization. On the other hand, the lack of a well-developed public transportation system means that staff development educators need to address this barrier for those without any means of transportation. Technology support systems such as the Internet, e-mail, and videoconferencing offer access to health education materials for people who might otherwise not have access; however, lack of access to these technological resources or an inability to use them is a potential barrier. Other existing health resources, such as hospitals, clinics, public health services, voluntary health organizations, public libraries, and other social service organizations in the community may be tapped for support and collaborative partnerships in providing staff education.

Compared to urban and suburban communities, rural areas may not have the infrastructure for easy access to health care, such as public transportation, and may lack other social service and auxiliary health care resources beyond a local hospital. Additionally, continuing education and ongoing professional development may be challenging in rural areas. Staff educators in rural areas need to develop creative

TABLE 13.1 Guidelines for Assessing External Frame Factors

Frame Factor	Questions for Data Collection	Desired Outcomes
Description of the Community	Is the community served by the health care facility urban, suburban, or rural? What community services are available to patients seeking health care and health information, such as transportation, libraries, childcare and other health care and social service organizations?	Hospital staff, patients, and families have access to the health care facility by public transportation; other resources in the community can be tapped to support patients and families seeking health care and health education.
Demographics of the Population	What are the characteristics of the population served by the health care facility, such as gender, race, ethnicity, and age distribution across the life span; family and household characteristics; employment data and income level; education, languages spoken, and literacy level?	Staff development programs are developed or revised to address the current shift in population demographics.
Health Needs of the Populace	What are the measures of health and wellness in the population served by the health care facility? What are the risk factors and measures of morbidity and mortality in this population? What health problems are emerging in the population? What percentage of the population live at or below poverty level? What percentage has health insurance?	Staff development programs are developed or revised to address current and emerging major health risks, health problems, diseases, and injuries in the community; health education programs provide outreach to unserved and underserved populations in the community.
The Health Care System	What are the major health insurance programs and entitlement programs within the population served by the health care facility, such as HMOs, Medicare, Medicaid, Supplemental Security Income, General Assistance, and Veterans Administration benefits? What are other health care and social service resources in the community such as hospitals, clinics, home care and long-term care agencies, public health services, voluntary health organizations?	Patients and families have health insurance coverage to provide access to health care, including patient and family teaching; community outreach health education and entitlement programs support the basic prerequisites for health, such as income, housing, food, childcare and transportation.
The Nursing Workforce	What are the numbers of nurses in the region served by the health care facility? Is there a shortage of nurses, and if so, what are the specific areas of severe nursing shortages, such as emergency room, critical care, gerontology, and long-term care? Among the nursing staff at the health care facility, what is the level of education? How many are prepared for and certified in advanced practice roles, such as nurse practitioner, clinical nurse specialist, nurse-midwife, and nurse anesthetist?	Staff development programs are tailored to the educational level, job responsibilities and learning needs of the nursing workforce. Creative staff development approaches address the shortage of nurses.

(Continued)

TABLE 13.1 Guidelines for Assessing External Frame Factors *Continued*

Frame Factor	Questions for Data Collection	Desired Outcomes
Regulations and Accreditation	What are the state regulations governing approval of continuing education curricula and course offerings for nurses? What are the ANA standards for professional development of staff?	Staff development and continuing education programs offered in the health care facility meet state requirements for approval of continuing education offerings and the ANA Standards for Nursing Professional Development programs.
Need for Development or Revision of the Program	Has there been a major shift in population demographics? Are there major changes in health risks, morbidity, and mortality in the population served by the health care facility? Do the external and/or internal program evaluation findings reveal areas for improvement? Are staff education programs culturally, linguistically, and educationally appropriate for the intended recipients? Are staff education programs and teaching methods based on the latest research evidence? Are there newer technologies for delivery of effective staff education?	Staff development and patient education programs address changing demographics and emerging health risks, morbidity and mortality Program revisions address areas identified for improvement by program from internal and external evaluations. Program revisions are based on current research findings on teaching methods and learning strategies, including effective use of advances in technology in delivering educational programs.

approaches for overcoming barriers to learning, such as making low-cost staff development videos available for rent or purchase, developing Web-access and e-mail or list-serve services, and forming partnerships with other communities in the area to purchase distance-learning technology and share access to resources.

Community assessment involves an examination of environmental factors that promote or impede good health, and therefore have an impact on health care services. The physical environment may have health hazards, such as poor air quality, water, soil, and food source contamination, lead poisoning in older homes, poor street lighting, and unsafe playgrounds and street crossings. A social environment in an inner city marked

EXHIBIT 13.1 Data Collection for the Community Needs Assessment

1. A description of the community, including size, community services such as transportation systems and communication mechanisms, major industries, educational and religious institutions, political parties, and local government

2. Population demographics—gender, race/ethnicity and age distribution across the life span

3. Employment information, income levels, and percentage of health insurance coverage

4. Education and literacy levels and languages spoken

5. Family and household characteristics

6. Health and wellness measures in the client population served by the clinical agency, including risk factors, health problems, and morbidity and mortality data

7. Health care and social service agencies, such as hospitals, clinics, home care agencies, long-term care agencies, public health services, voluntary health organizations, and other community-based organizations

by inadequate housing, lack of job training, high unemployment, poverty, and weak social ties among residents must have the basic needs for food, shelter, income, and social support met before attempting to address health issues. On the other hand, clean air and water, safe food sources, good nutrition, and community resources such as subsidized housing, good schools, job training, and availability of childcare, transportation, and health care services contribute significantly to the health of the community.

Demographics of the Population

Census data allow health care organizations to anticipate and plan for meeting the health needs associated with gender, age, and socioeconomic status, and to forecast the number of persons at risk for poor health outcomes. Family and household characteristics reveal the number of homeless persons and/or number of single-parent families who are more vulnerable to poor health outcomes. Information on employment and income indicates the percentage of persons living at or below poverty level, the single most important variable associated with poor health outcomes. The percentage of the population without health insurance provides approximate information on the size of the underserved and unserved populations. Information on race and ethnicity, level of education and literacy, and language skills identify important elements to consider in planning programs that prepare health care providers to provide educationally and culturally appropriate care to the intended target population. Census data, including trends and projections for the future, are often available online from city, county, state, and the federal government (U.S. Census Bureau, 2010). The Web site for the latter is http://www.census.gov.

Health Needs of the Populace

Health status reports provide data on current or emerging health risks and health problems as well as existing morbidity and mortality data in a given region or specific patient population. Health status reports relevant to the population served by health care organizations are usually available in print form from local libraries or online from city, county, and state departments of health, or the federal government. The U.S. Department of Health and Human Services publication *Healthy People* (2010) is an excellent resource for targeting major health problems in the populace and strategies for promoting health and preventing disease (http://www.healthypeople.gov). More than likely, the health care agency itself has demographic and health status data available on the client population served in recent years, such as the most common diagnoses, diagnoses-related groups (DRGs), injuries, and surgeries, thus providing a basis for determining current needs and projecting trends in the future.

The Health Care System and Nursing Workforce

An assessment of major health care providers in the area, such as managed care systems, health insurance programs, public health services, hospitals, clinics, voluntary health care organizations, other health care facilities, and social services in the area reveal community resources that may be tapped for staff development support as well as potential partners for collaboration. This assessment should include the nursing workforce in the area served by the health care organization, number of nurses employed by the health care organizations, level of education from the licensed practical/vocational nurse to nurses prepared at the doctorate level, numbers of advanced practice nurses by type (nurse practitioner, clinical nurse specialist, nurse-midwife, nurse anesthetist), and critical areas of nursing shortage in the health care organization.

Regulations and Accreditation Requirements

As an integral part of program development or revision, the most current regulations, standards of practice, and accreditation criteria governing staff development are reviewed to ensure that new and revised programs are in compliance. Staff development educators in states with mandatory continuing education for nurses need to review their state regulations for receiving approval for continuing education offerings. The current standards for NPD include continuing education, staff development, and academic education as areas in which nurses may take advantage of professional development opportunities.

Need for Program Development or Revision

Because most staff development departments have a major education plan in place, it is rare that a staff development educator actually develops a new staff education program from the ground up. The need for program revision often arises from the changing demographics and health status in the population served by the health care organization and in response to emerging threats to the health of the community. In addition, feedbacks from staff, patients, families, health facility managers, and administrators indicate areas of program weakness needing change and improvement. Prior evaluations of staff education programs provide information on the satisfaction of program recipients and the extent to which the program goals of each were achieved.

Internal Frame Factors

Internal frame factors to consider in developing staff education curricula are the mission, philosophy, and goals of the institution; characteristics of the health care setting such as organizational structure, including the decision-making structure, particularly as it applies to staff development; institutional economics, including resources for staff development; the characteristics and learning needs of staff; and potential educators for staff development programs. See Table 13.2 for a summary of the internal frame factors to consider.

Mission, Philosophy, and Goals of the Health Care Setting

The health care facility's mission, philosophy, and goals provide the overall framework and direction for the organization. Therefore, the mission, philosophy, and goals of the staff education programs should be closely aligned with those of the parent organization. Staff educators should have a solid understanding of the organizational structure and decision-making processes as they relate to staff education programs.

TABLE 13.2 Guidelines for Assessing Internal Frame Factors

Frame Factor	Questions for Data Collection	Desired Outcomes
Mission, Philosophy, and Goals of the Health Care Organization	Do the mission, philosophy, and goals of the institution speak to staff development and curricula? Are the mission, philosophy, and goals of the staff development program congruent with the institutions?	The mission, philosophy, and goals of the institution address the professional development of staff. The mission, philosophy, and goals of the staff development programs are congruent with those of the health care organization.
Characteristics and Educational Needs of Staff	What are the educational needs of staff? What are important characteristics of staff to consider in developing appropriate and effective educational programs?	Educational needs of staff are assessed using multiple sources of information. Characteristics of staff affecting access to education and having impact on learning are taken into consideration in developing educational programs.
Institutional Economics and Resources for Staff Development	What is the present financial health of the institution? What are the existing and potential resources staff education programs? What are creative strategies for increasing resources for educational programs?	Creative strategies, such as collaborating with other experts from nearby health and social service organizations in the community and recruiting course faculty from among the in-house professional staff are implemented. Resources are sufficient for developing and implementing needed staff education programs.

Final decisions regarding program course offerings for staff education programs, including the commitment of resources to them, are made with consideration for the extent to which the offerings will support the goals of the overall organization. Successful staff education programs are those that prepare health care providers to meet the needs of the community and population served, and the goals and priorities of the health care organization.

Educational Needs Assessment Specific to Staff Development

The characteristics and needs of the learners need to be considered in developing and revising staff development curricula. The characteristics of staff members are their level of education and scope of practice, work experience, present level of knowledge and skills, particularly in relationship to new or changing job responsibilities, and clinical practice expectations. It is not unusual for staff development educators to have the responsibility for the staff development of nonnursing/ancillary staff, nursing assistants, and various levels of licensed and certified personnel. Therefore, part of the educational needs assessment must include the identification of knowledge and skills that are common to the various types of staff and their differences in learning needs.

The educator then develops strategies to enhance the best learning environment for each type of staff member through group work, small classes, individual learning modules, and/or online learning modalities.

Staff members may have additional needs and skills arising from other demands and situations in their lives. For example, they may have family responsibilities that at times, take priority over the employment setting. Some may have multilingual skills and represent various cultural and ethnic groups, and thus have additional knowledge to contribute to the care of clients. The availability of staff to attend professional development programs outside of scheduled work shifts may be limited among those with family responsibilities or those who live a long distance from the health care organization. Using advanced technology, such as distance education technology and other online learning modalities, can ameliorate some of the problems associated with staff access to professional development programs.

There are several methods for assessing the educational needs of staff. Educational needs are defined as "any gap between needed and actual knowledge, skills, and behaviors, which can be remedied by an educational intervention" (Burk, 2008, p. 227). Sources of data include chart audits and quality improvement/benchmarking reports, occurrence reports, performance evaluations of staff, and input from key stakeholders including administrators and managers from within and outside of nursing, and individual learners (Abruzzese, 1996; Burk, 2008).

Institutional Economics and Resources for Staff Development Programs

An analysis of the institutional economics and financial health of the health care organization provides information on fiscal resources for curriculum development in staff development programs. A lack of resources for staff development is primary among the major issues faced by nursing educators in health care agencies. In lean financial times, the education function is often the first to be downsized. Staff development educators need to develop strong relationships with financial officers and agency administrators to build the case for financial investment in staff development programs. A description of budget planning and budget management appears later in this chapter.

Showing the relationship between educational programs and the achievement of organizational goals is an effective strategy for securing support and material resources for education, particularly if there is program evaluation and/or cost-effectiveness data to support the positive returns on investment in education. Existing resources for staff development programs include classrooms, laboratories for practicing clinical skills, a medical/nursing/health library, instructional technology for computer-assisted instruction and distance learning, and access to the intranet and Internet. Table 13.2 summarizes the guidelines for assessing the internal frame factors that influence the curriculum.

Analysis of the Needs Assessment Data and Program Decisions: Staff Development

Analyzing the data from the external and internal frame factors assessment often reveals multiple learning needs, more than can be addressed simultaneously. Reasoned choices will need to be made regarding the educational programs to be developed with the mission, philosophy, and goals of the institution serving as the foundation and rationale for decision making.

COMPONENTS OF CURRICULUM DEVELOPMENT IN STAFF DEVELOPMENT PROGRAMS

The same components of curriculum development discussed in Chapter 7 for schools of nursing apply to staff education. The following is a brief discussion of the adaptation of these components to the health care setting. Table 13.3 summarizes the questions for data collection and the desired outcomes that relate to each component for nurse educators to use in these settings when assessing, revising, or developing educational programs.

It is essential that the educational program's mission or vision, philosophy, and overall goals are congruent with those of the sponsoring agency. The overall goal(s) can be viewed as macro objectives and reflect the overall intent of the program. They are the expected outcomes of the staff education program. They should flow logically from the agency's mission, vision, and philosophy. Based on the overall purpose or goal of the staff development program, objectives are developed to provide the implementation plan for the program. Although there is a debate about the use of behaviorally stated goals and objectives, the overall goal and its objectives are usually stated in behavioral terms with measurable outcomes to facilitate the development of the instructional plan and the measurement of the success of the program. The use of behaviorally stated goals and objectives is especially relevant to nurse educators' practice where productivity, quality assurance, evidence-based practice, and cost-effectiveness can determine the continued existence of an educational program or initiation of a new program. Each goal or objective should explain what is to be learned, how the student will learn the material including an action verb that can be measured, when the objective is to be reached, what level of competency is expected, and it must be learner-centered. The reader is directed to Chapter 4 for a detailed discussion of educational taxonomies and the format for writing goals and objectives.

Individual class objectives flow from the program objectives and provide guidelines for the development of the instructional design for the class. The instructional design should include a brief description of the purpose of the class, characteristics and educational needs of the learner, teaching strategies, a content outline, the learning environment, teaching aids, necessary supplies and equipment, and an evaluation plan for measuring the success of the program.

CURRICULUM DEVELOPMENT APPLIED TO STAFF EDUCATION

Most health agencies have education departments for the purposes of staff orientation, employee training programs, new graduate programs, continuing education (in-service), competency assessment, and to prepare staff for specialty roles such as the operating room, emergency department, intensive care units, and so forth. The following are overviews of the essential curriculum components for each type of program, while recognizing at the same time that smaller agencies may not have the resources to support all of the programs mentioned.

Orientation, Employee Training Programs, and New Graduate Programs

Orientation, employee training, and new graduate programs have much in common with the development and evaluation of academic nursing education programs. The major differences are the characteristics of the target learning audiences and the

TABLE 13.3 Adaptation of the Components of the Curriculum to Staff Development and Patient and Family Education

Component of the Curriculum	Questions for Data Collection	Desired Outcomes
Agency Mission, Vision, and/ or Philosophy Statements	To what extent are the mission, vision, and/or philosophy statements visible to the agency's consumers? To what extent are the mission, vision, and/or philosophy statements of the agency congruent with its educational programs' missions?	The mission, vision, and/or philosophy statements are readily apparent and drive the type of health care services it provides to the community. All educational programs in the institution have mission, vision, and/or philosophy statements, and they are congruent with that of the agency.
Purpose or Overall Goal	To what extent does the overall goal or purpose of the agency flow from the mission, vision, and/or philosophy statements? To what extent does the overall goal or purpose of the agency imply the need for educational programs? What is the evidence of an overall goal or purpose for the agency's educational programs and is it congruent with the agency goal or purpose?	The agency's overall goal or purpose flows logically from the mission, vision, and/or philosophy statements. The overall goal or purpose of the agency explicitly or implicitly includes educational programs as part of its service. All educational programs within the agency have statements relating to their overall purpose and goals that are congruent with the agency's goal or purpose.
Organizing Framework	To what extent is the framework (if it exists) congruent with the mission, vision, philosophy, and/or overall goal or purpose? If the agency or service unit of the agency uses an organizing or conceptual framework for its educational program, to what extent do the programs' curricula reflect that framework?	The organizing or conceptual framework is congruent with agency's mission, vision, philosophy, and/or overall purpose or goal. Educational programs within the agency integrate its organizing or conceptual framework into curriculum plans.
Program Objectives	To what extent do the educational programs' objectives flow from the overall goal or purpose of the agency? To what extent are the educational objectives in a format that allows for measurement of the learners' success and evaluation of the teaching session(s)?	Educational programs within the agency have specific goal statements that are congruent with the agency's overall goal or purpose statements. Each objective is learner-centered and includes the content of the learning experience, how the learner will achieve the specified behavior, the knowledge or skill desired, at what level of competency, and when.
Implementation Plan	To what extent does the agency demonstrate support for its educational programs through staff, resources, facilities, and materials? Is there a dedicated budget for the educational program and under whose control is it? To what extent does each educational program include an overview, objectives, learner characteristics, content outline, teaching and learning methods, setting, and resources?	There is a central place for educational programs, staff, resources, learning environment facilities with available instructional support, and a listing of all educational offerings. There is a dedicated budget in place for educational programs and the budget is managed by the leader of the staff development department. The implementation plan for each educational program in the agency includes an overview, objectives, learner characteristics, content outline, teaching and learning methods, setting, and resources.

length of the programs according to the learning needs of the participants. Orientation programs are geared to new employees who have the educational and experiential qualifications to assume a specified position in the health care agency. These programs are often scheduled for an initial in-depth, intensive period, where critical pieces of information are presented such as the agency's mission, purpose, policies, procedures, and specific job functions and expectations. These sessions are followed up periodically to add important information and to answer any questions that arise as the new staff members adjust to the health care agency. The sessions also provide an opportunity for the agency to evaluate the new employee's performance within the introductory period.

New graduate orientation programs are usually at least 6 weeks long with periodic follow-up sessions to reinforce learning and introduce new knowledge. The content includes an in-depth orientation to the agency's mission, policies, procedures, and the physical plant, including the assigned unit(s). A core part of this orientation is assigning new graduates to experienced preceptors who guide them throughout their transition into clinical practice, mentor them throughout their orientation period, and continue to provide support as needed after the "official" orientation period has ended. Preceptorship is a vital component of the transition experience of newly graduated nurses into clinical practice. As stated by Nicol and Young (2007), "an empathetic preceptor who is aware of the graduate's needs can make the difference between the graduate nurse enjoying their professional role, surviving the first year, and leaving the profession" (p. 298). Research from the perspective of newly graduated nurses has illuminated the importance of the role of the nurse preceptor in orientation programs (Oermann & Moffitt-Wolf, 1997; Orsini, 2005; Schumacher, 2007). In addition to their teaching, supervising, and evaluating responsibilities, preceptors help newly graduated nurses socialize into their professional roles (Baltimore, 2004; Casey, Fink, Krugman, & Propst, 2004). Because of the significance of the role of the preceptor, it is to the advantage of the educational program and the new employees to include classes for preceptors on their role and functions in guiding new employees.

Employee technician training programs target new staff members in the health agency who may not have the education or experience for the positions for which they are hired. These include employees beginning positions in janitorial/environmental services, food services, plant maintenance, transportation, laboratories, and depending on state regulations and accreditation issues; some support staff including those under the supervision of nursing.

New employee education programs include orientation to the health care agency and content related to specific knowledge, skills, behaviors (professionalism), and attitudes (such as the importance of customer service) that accompany the positions they fill. The initial training programs vary in length, the length depending on the nature of the position and the material to be learned. The complexity of the programs will depend on the positions' job descriptions and performance expectations. It is important for the nurse educator to be aware of state regulations or accreditation standards that require approval of these types of programs or that provide standardized curriculum plans that can be tailored to the health care agency's education needs.

Each of these programs are developed according to their overall goal or purpose, application of learning and teaching theories that are appropriate to the target audience, specific behavioral learning objectives, the content and type of material to be taught, the strategies for teaching and learning, the specific length of the program and its sessions, the learning environment, necessary equipment and other resources, and an evaluation plan to measure the learning outcomes, learner and instructor satisfaction, cost analysis, and the program's contribution to the agency's mission.

Competency Assessment

Competency assessment programs are essential to the delivery of quality care and risk management in health care agencies. They are an integral part of new staff, employee training, and new graduate programs as well as other educational programs that prepare staff members for specialized tasks and the maintenance of skills in their health care provider roles. It is the staff development educator's role to identify the required skills for each specific job description and the level of competency expected for those skills.

Required by regulatory agencies and accrediting bodies, mandatory competencies are a part of most health care organizations. According to O'Hearne-Rebholz (2006), competency is validation that skills, processes, and concepts are completed or understood correctly as determined by an expert. Continuing competence mandates a commitment to lifelong learning activities for all professional nurses and is a "hallmark of professionalism and a means by which a profession is held accountable to society" (ANA, 2000, p.3). O'Hearne-Rebholz describes various methods that can be used to validate staff competency including paper and pen competencies, observation competencies, skills laboratory competencies, and scenario competencies. The paper and pen competency uses traditional testing techniques and although it is not the best method, it can be useful in situations that require a measurement of staff knowledge such as understanding of a policy or proper medication calculations. The observation competency allows the expert to actually watch the staff member performing in real time. Though difficult to carry out especially with large groups of staff, observation is an effective method to evaluate processes such as staff–patient interactions and pain assessment and reassessment. The skills laboratory competency takes a significant amount of time and planning to set up, however it is a valuable method to validate proper use of equipment and to test skills such as cardiopulmonary resuscitation and intravenous insertion. Finally, scenario competencies use a case study or storytelling approach to recreate a patient situation. Scenario competencies are useful in evaluating critical thinking and clinical judgment skills (O'Hearne-Rebholz, 2006).

A competent level of performance is expected for patient, health care provider, and agency safety. As skills become more complex, this expectation is maintained, however experience and additional education are necessary to reach the higher levels of performance. Most agencies have specific skills that are expected in their job descriptions and many times, these are part of clinical ladder programs or requirements for promotions. Education programs to promote competence should include an overall goal, specific behaviorally stated learning objectives, the competencies to be assessed, remediation plans to bring the learner up to competency, periodic recertification plans, and an evaluation plan to measure learning outcomes, satisfaction, and the success of the program in terms of its quality, cost-effectiveness, and contribution to the agency's mission.

BUDGET PLANNING FOR STAFF DEVELOPMENT

Staff development educators have a responsibility for planning, managing, and reporting budgets to the administration of the sponsoring health agency. It is an essential task to justify the existence of the educational program and its relevance to the mission of the agency and its service. It demonstrates cost-effectiveness as well as cost recovery over the long term. For example, well-oriented new staff members and well-prepared new graduates are more apt to become long-term employees rather than entering and exiting through a revolving door. Prior to developing a new business plan or revising an existing one, it is important to develop a business case. A *business case* is a document used to generate support from the agency leadership and other key stakeholders. It identifies the need, purpose, and the relationship of the program to the overall mission of the organization. It provides the context and content around the need and lists the desired objectives, outcomes, and its advantages to the health care organization.

When preparing a budget case and its related plan, the first item to assess is the source of revenues including the income generated by the health agency through general funds (if government sponsored), patient fees, insurance programs, and Medicare and Medicaid. Although historically these sources have been somewhat stable, recent changes in the national and international economy have made this income much less dependable while organizations continue to deal with changing patient care demands and ever-changing reimbursement and prospective pay systems. Thus, it is important for staff development educators to investigate other possible sources of income for the program such as grants from other health-related organizations, federal, state, or regional grants, benefactor gifts, and fees for educational programs. The type of revenue will determine how it will be spent. For example, established, long-term income and resources might be used to maintain ongoing programs whereas new program development, or one-time only programs, may be funded through short-term grants and other gift monies.

On the debit or cost side of the budget, the two largest items are capital expenditures and personnel. Capital expenditures include office, classroom, and laboratory facilities that are usually shared spaces and can be calculated according to the percentage of use by the educational program. Other capital expenditures include "big ticket items" such as instructional support systems (videoconferencing, telecommunications, and Web-based technology), computers, audiovisual hardware, mannequins, and large software teaching packages. Although they are usually considered on the debit side, their value can also be considered as assets with only their depreciation added to the costs each year. If the educational program expects to undergo accreditation or certification, the one-time expenses for preparing a readiness evaluation and site visits are included for that year.

Personnel expenses include the salaries and benefits of the educators, administrative support staff, administrators, and in some instances, the costs for released time of staff to attend educational programs. Each year, the budget must build in salary increases and concomitant benefit increases for the staff. The time of the staff members who precept new employees is an additional personnel cost to be calculated. Other expenses for the program include office supplies, books, journal subscriptions, teaching supplies, travel expenses for staff, continuing education and professional

TABLE 13.4 Educational Program Budgeting

Major Budget Item	Income or Debit	Items Included
Program Maintenance	Income	Agency funds from fees, insurance, reimbursements, and general revenues
Program Development or Enhancement	Income	Grants, contributions, gifts, endowments
Personnel	Debit	Salaries, benefits, released, and/or nonproductive time
Capital Expenditures	Assets and debit depreciation	Offices, labs, classrooms, conference rooms, furniture, equipment, utilities, contracts for maintenance of equipment, major software packages
Supplies and Services	Debit	Office and teaching supplies, texts, journal subscriptions, travel, food, and refreshments

meetings for the staff development educators, and meals or refreshments for class participants.

The budget is prepared several months in advance of its submission for approval by the administration. Health agency budgets run either on a fiscal year–basis (July to June) with quarterly reporting or on a calendar year–basis (January to December) with quarterly reporting. It is wise to build in a contingency fund to cover any unexpected costs that the program encounters during the year. When submitting the budget, it is advisable to include an attachment with sufficient justifications for each item.

In the ideal staff development setting, the manager or director of the education department manages the budget and has administrative assistance for tracking expenditures, preparing purchase orders, receiving, cataloging, and keeping inventory of equipment and supplies, and managing the payroll. Careful records are kept so that quarterly and end-of-year reports are easily assembled and provide the agency with the program's accountability as well as trends in income generation and expenditures for future planning. This discussion reviews the major items in budget preparation, management, and reporting. Although each agency has its own budget format, the items in the discussion can be adapted to the agency's specific format. Table 13.4 summarizes the discussion.

JUSTIFICATION AND FUNDING FOR EDUCATIONAL PROGRAMS IN HEALTH AGENCIES

It is not unusual for health agencies experiencing budget crises to think of cutting personnel and programs associated with "nonessential" services. Educational programs are frequently the targets of such cuts in spite of the impact they have on cost savings and the delivery of quality care to the agency's staff and its clients. In the previous discussion on the budget for education programs, there was a mention of the need to demonstrate cost-effectiveness and related cost savings from the educational program to the administration of the health agency as well as to the public or consumers of the program. For example, the nurse educator can compare the major costs of bringing in traveling registered nurses to staff the agency to the lesser cost of providing incentives for staff retention derived from the support of new graduates through preceptor and mentor programs, continuing education programs, and in-service opportunities for core staff. As to the value of the program, the health care agency that has a satisfied staff soon sees gains in the quality of the care delivered, which in turn, translates into patient or customer satisfaction. Magnet hospitals are excellent examples of quality care and part of their successes are staff development and educational program achievements that contribute to the overall retention of highly engaged employees. Information on Magnet hospitals can be found at http://www.nursecredentialing.org.

EVALUATION OF STAFF EDUCATION PROGRAMS

The principles of total quality management in staff development programs are the same as those applied to evaluation strategies in schools of nursing. The reader is directed to Section 5 and Chapter 14 of this text for an overview of definitions, concepts, theories, and models that are relevant to educational programs in health agencies and for an overview of total quality management applied to education. There are two major components of evaluation in staff development. On the micro level are the individual teaching and learning sessions provided to the target audience, and on the macro level is program evaluation to assess the effectiveness and worth of the total education program and its services for the health agency. A brief discussion follows that relates to each of these components of evaluation.

Evaluation of Individual Teaching and Learning Sessions

Developing and implementing individual teaching and learning sessions are ongoing processes and it is advised that plans for evaluation of the sessions occur during the initial development. Carefully stated learning objectives serve as one method for measuring the success of the session. If the objectives are learner-centered, include a time frame, how and what an action on the part of the learner that can be measured, and the level of competency expected; the evaluation becomes quite simple. As discussed previously, this validation can be accomplished through traditional testing methods such as the paper and pen or scenario techniques and/or through instructor observation in real time or in a skills lab setting.

In addition to learner achievement, there are other aspects of the educational session that the evaluator assesses. These include the effectiveness of the instructor and teaching strategies, the learning environment and materials, and learner and instructor satisfaction with the session. These latter assessments can be measured through surveys of the learners and instructors with rating-scale responses to questions or open-ended questions that are subject to content analysis.

Evaluation of Educational Programs

The evaluation of education programs in health agencies is an important activity on the part of nurse educators for several reasons. Positive evaluations provide justification for the education program's place and value of service in the agency. Evaluation activities such as continuous quality assessment lead to the improvement of the program and the achievement of excellence. Additionally, evaluation activities and reports contribute to the accreditation, licensure, or certification of the program and the health agency. The elements of program evaluation in staff education are similar to those found in schools of nursing. The first item to assess is the congruence of the health agency's mission and the mission of the education program. They should be in alignment and if not, a rationale for why there is a difference should be prominent in the description of the program, or the mission and purpose of the education program should be adjusted to the parent agency's mission and purpose.

The philosophy statements and conceptual frameworks of the agency and the education program should be compatible and the goals for each should flow from the philosophy, conceptual framework (if present), and the mission. Once the goal is assessed for its reflection of the intent of the program, the implementation of the program is assessed and evaluated for its consistency with the mission, purpose, philosophy, and framework. The next step is to determine to what extent the outcomes of the educational program are measured by its goals and objectives, its overall impact on the clients community served by the parent organization, its cost-effectiveness, its measure of quality compared to other staff development programs, its achievement of benchmarks that the agency and program set for it, and its accreditation, licensure, or certification status.

Table 13.5 summarizes these elements according to evaluation elements and the desired outcomes. As with nursing education programs, a master plan of evaluation is recommended so that evaluation becomes an ongoing process and guides the activities of the program for total quality management.

An excellent classic model for a comprehensive tool for the evaluation of education programs in health care agencies is the pyramid model of evaluation for continuing education programs described by Hawkins and Sherwood (1999). The model is based on Donabedian's (1966) structure, process, and outcome model of evaluation and the social science evaluation model developed by Rossi and Freeman (1993). It incorporates all of the elements of program and curriculum development discussed thus far in this chapter including a look at the internal and external frame factors that impact educational programs. In addition to assessing the program design, implementation, outcomes, and impact, it addresses cost-effectiveness issues. It is a highly recommended reading for nurse educators considering the use of a master plan of evaluation for staff education.

ISSUES AND TRENDS IN STAFF DEVELOPMENT

Issues of concern to staff development educators are in part related to the financial challenges faced by health care organizations today. Changes in our economy have resulted in decreased reimbursement to health care organizations while at the same time, increased levels of service are often needed. Organizations are faced with difficult decisions in terms of eliminating programs to remain financially solvent and often, funding for staff development programs is reduced or eliminated. Equally concerning is the continued nursing shortage that is only expected to worsen over the next several years. Certain areas of the country are impacted more drastically by this shortage in which newly graduated nurses have assumed an important role in the recruitment and

TABLE 13.5 The Elements of an Evaluation Plan for Staff Development

Evaluation Element	Questions for Data Collection	Desired Outcomes
Mission, Overall Purpose, and Philosophy	To what extent are the mission, overall purpose, and philosophy of the agency and its educational program congruent?	The mission, overall purpose, and philosophy of the educational program are congruent with that of the agency.
Goals (Long Term)	Is it evident that the overall or long-term goal(s) flow from the mission, purpose, and philosophy?	The overall or long-term goal(s) flow from the mission, purpose, and philosophy.
Objectives (Short Term) and Implementation Plan	Is it evident that the objectives for the program and each learning session flow from the overall goal(s) and are congruent with the mission and philosophy?	The objectives for the program and each learning session flow from the overall goal(s) and are congruent with the mission and philosophy.
	To what extent do the objectives include specification of the learner, the learning content, behavior of the learner, expected outcome, and time frame?	The objectives are stated in such a way that they can be measured for their outcomes.
	Is there evidence that the implementation plan flows from the mission, goal(s), and objectives?	The implementation plan flows from the mission, goal(s), and objectives.
Cost-effectiveness	What are the major sources of financial support for the program? To what extent is the education program self-sufficient?	The program is supported through multiple means such as organizational budget, fees for services, grants, and so forth. The education program is self-sufficient.
	Have other possible funding resources been identified and are they part of a plan to secure funds?	
	To what extent does the education program contribute to the financial stability of the agency? Is there a plan for either maintaining or reaching financial stability?	The education program contributes to the quality and financial stability of the agency.
Outcomes (Participants and Community)	To what extent do data from the assessment of the outcomes from the education program indicate achievement of its goal and objectives?	Outcomes from the education program indicate achievement of its goal and objectives.
	To what extent do participants report a high level of satisfaction from the program?	Participants (both learners and instructors) report a high level of satisfaction from the program.
	Is there a plan in place to either maintain or improve outcomes?	The community is aware of the agency's education program and holds it in high regard.
	To what extent is the community aware of the agency's education program?	
	Is there a plan in place for raising the public's awareness of the education program and its contributions to the community?	
Comparison to Similar Programs and Benchmarks	To what extent is the education program superior to or on a par with similar education programs?	The education program is superior to or on a par with similar education programs.
	Do the program costs meet budget limits?	The program costs meet budget limits.
	To what extent does the program meet its goals and objectives each year?	The program meets its goals and objectives each year and/or the program is re-evaluated and new benchmarks are set.
	Are there plans in place to improve the program or set higher benchmarks?	

(Continued)

TABLE 13.5 The Elements of an Evaluation Plan for Staff Development *Continued*

Evaluation Element	Questions for Data Collection	Desired Outcomes
Accreditation, Licensure, and Certification	Has the program received accreditation, licensure, or certification? If the program is an integral part of the health agency, to what extent does it contribute to accreditation, licensure, or certification? Is there a plan in place to continually assess the program for maintenance of accreditation, licensure, or certification? To what extent is there a record keeping system in place for accreditation, licensure, or certification?	Depending on the nature of the program, the education program has accreditation, licensure, or certification.

staffing strategies of hospitals. The transition experience of newly graduated nurses into the workforce is often fraught with stress and disillusionment resulting in a particularly alarming trend of new nurses leaving their first jobs within 2 years and many leaving the nursing profession altogether. The stress associated with this transition is compounded by the fact that it is no longer feasible to assign lower acuity patients to new graduates while they learn their roles in today's health care environment. These lower acuity patients simply do not receive care within the acute care setting. Furthermore, because of the dire need to fill vacant positions, employers are expecting newly graduated nurses to quickly function as competent professionals. A nurse who leaves an organization with less than 1 year of employment represents a loss of approximately $40,000 in hiring and orientation costs, further contributing to the financial constraints associated with staff development programs. (Bowles & Candela, 2005; Casey, Fink, Krugman & Propst, 2004; Grochow, 2008; Halfer & Graf, 2006).

MAINTAINING QUALITY PROGRAMS AND PLANNING FOR THE FUTURE

Heller, Oros, and Durney-Crowley (2000) discuss 10 trends in health care and nursing that have an impact on nursing education, including staff development. Although the article was published in 2000, it continues to be relevant to the current and future health care system and provides 10 major trends to watch as they influence education. The 10 trends they identify are as follows:

1. Changing demographics and increasing diversity
2. The technological explosion, globalization of world's economy and society
3. Educated consumers
4. Alternative therapies and genomics, and palliative care
5. Shift to population-based care and increasing complexity of patient care
6. Cost of health care and challenge of managed care
7. Impact of health policy and regulation
8. Growing need for interdisciplinary education for collaborative practice
9. Workforce development
10. Advances in nursing science and research

Their reflections on these trends are helpful in planning for the future and provide guidelines for factors to assess within each trend.

Consistent with the trends discussed by Heller, Oros, and Durney-Crowley, the task force commencing in March 2008 to lead the revision of the *Scope and Standards of Practice for Nursing Professional Development* identified the following education-specific issues that will need to be acknowledged and addressed moving forward: increased use of technology, global target audience, teaching/learning modalities, evidence-based practice, increased accountability, increased interdisciplinary involvement, fiscal management, need for complex implementation expertise, professional development metrics, decreasing time to achieve competency, generational differences, escalating competing priorities, knowledge management and succession planning, increased need for clinical affiliations and academic partnerships, move toward learning as an investment in human capital, cost avoidance versus expenditure, and focus on transition into practice (Benedict & Bradley, 2010). Careful attention to these issues and trends will serve staff development educators well as we move into a future filled with economic uncertainty and potentially, one of the worst nursing shortages our country has ever faced.

Though the discussion in this chapter focused on the role of the staff development educator working in a health care agency, nurse educators are found in a multitude of settings such as academia, public and private school systems, home care agencies, public health agencies, and industry. As our country continues to face significant economic challenges and we confront what will potentially be the worst nursing shortage our country has ever experienced, it is imperative that nurse educators in all of these settings join forces to promote their important role in shaping the future of nursing education and public policy to improve health care with the collective goal of reaching optimal health for our society.

DISCUSSION QUESTIONS

1. To what extent do you believe an assessment of the external and internal frame factors influences the development and evaluation of an educational program?

2. Give a rationale for applying the components of curriculum development and evaluation to staff education. Compare the components in the practice setting to those in the academic setting. What are the differences and similarities?

3. Identify an educational program and determine what learning theories, educational taxonomies, and teaching strategies apply to it. Give a rationale for your choices.

4. Why is it important for a staff development educator to be able to prepare, manage, and evaluate the budget of an education program? Explain your answer.

5. Discuss looming issues in the health care system that impact staff development. What strategies would you as a nurse educator take to help bring about solutions to these issues?

LEARNING ACTIVITIES

Select an education program in a health agency and assess it for its recognition of the impact of the external and internal frame factors on the program. Evaluate the program according to the classic components of curriculum development and evaluation. Include an analysis of the evaluation plan in place for individual sessions and the program as a whole. Is there evidence that the data collected for evaluation are used to revise the program and improve quality? Analyze the budget of the program for its relationship to the mission and goals of the agency and the education program.

REFERENCES

Abruzzese, R. S. (1996). *Nursing staff development: Strategies for success* (2nd ed.). St. Louis, MO: Mosby.

American Nurses Association. (2000). *Scope and standards of practice for nursing professional development.* Silver Springs, MD: Author.

American Nurses Credentialing Center. *Board certification of nurses makes a difference.* Retrieved from http://www.nursecredentialing.org

Bailey, K., Hoeppner, M., Jeska, S., Schneller, S., & Wolohan, C. (1995). The nurse as an educator. *Journal of Nursing Staff Development, 11*(4), 205–209.

Baltimore, J. (2004). The hospital clinical preceptor: Essential preparation for success. *Journal of Continuing Education in Nursing, 35*(3), 133–140.

Benedict, M.S. & Bradley, D. (2010). A peek at the revised nursing professional development: Scope and standards of practice. *The journal of Continuing Education in Nursing, 41*(5), 195–196.

Bowles, C., & Candela, L. (2005). First job experiences of recent graduates: Improving the work environment. *Journal of Nursing Administration, 35*(3), 130–137.

Burk, G. J. (2008). Forecasting instead of reacting to educational needs. *Journal for Nurses in Staff Development, 24*(5), 226–231.

Casey, K., Fink, R., Krugman, M., & Propst, J. (2004). The graduate nurse experience. *Journal of Nursing Administration, 34*(6), 303–311.

Donabedian, A. (1966). Evaluating the quality of medical care. *Milbank Memorial Fund Quarterly. 44*(3 Suppl.), 166–206.

Durham, C., & Sherwood, G. (2008). Education to bridge the quality gap: A case study approach. *Urologic Nursing, 28*(6), 431–453.

Gallagher, R. M. (2005). National quality efforts: What continuing and staff development educators need to know. *Journal of Continuing Education in Nursing, 36*(1), 39–45.

Grochow, D. (2008). From novice to expert: Transitioning graduate nurses. *Nursing Management, 39*(3), 10–12.

Halfer D., & Graf, E. (2006). Graduate nurse perceptions of the work experience. *Nursing Economics, 24*(3), 150–155.

Hawkins, V., & Sherwood, G. (1999). The Pyramid model: An integrated approach for evaluation continuing education programs and outcomes. *Journal of Continuing Education in Nursing, 30*(5), 203–212.

Health Leaders Media. (2009). *What the ANA's new professional development scope and standards mean for nursing staff.* Retrieved from http://www.healthleadersmedia.com/page-2/NRS-243558/What-the-ANAs-New-Professional-Development-Scope-and-Standards-Mean-for-Nursing-Staff

Healthy People. (2010). U.S. Department of Health and Human Services. Retrieved April 30, 2010, from http://www.healthypeople.gov

Heller, B. R., Oros, M. T., & Durney-Crowley, J. (2000). The future of nursing education: Ten trends to watch. *Nursing and Health Care Perspectives, 21*(1), 9–13.

Johnson, M. (1977). *Intentionality in education.* Albany, NY: Center for Curriculum Research and Services.

Knowles, M. S., Holton, E. F., & Swanson, R. A. (1998). *The adult learner: The definitive classic in adult education and human resource development* (5th ed.). Houston, TX: Gulf Publishing.

Krugman, M. (2003). Evidence-based practice: The role of staff development. *Journal for Nurses in Staff Development, 19*(6), 279–285.

Merriam-Webster Online Dictionary. (2010). Retrieved April 12, 2010, from http://www.merriam-webster.com

Nicol, P., & Young, M. (2007). Sail training: An innovative approach to graduate nurse preceptor development. *Journal for Nurses in Staff Development, 23*(6), 298–302.

Oermann, M. H., & Moffitt-Wolf, A. (1997). New graduates' perceptions of clinical practice. *Journal of Continuing Education in Nursing, 28*(1), 20–25.

O'Hearne-Rebholz, M. (2006). A review of methods to assess competency. *Journal for Nurses in Staff Development, 22*(5), 241–245.

Orsini, C. H. (2005). A nurse transition program for orthopaedics: Creating a new culture for nurturing graduate nurses. *Orthopaedic Nursing, 24*(4), 240–246.

Rossi, P. H., & Freeman, H. E. (1993). *Evaluation: A systematic approach.* Thousand Oaks, CA: Sage.

Schumacher, D. L. (2007). Caring behaviors of preceptors as perceived by new nursing graduate orientees. *Journal for Nurses in Staff Development, 23*(4), 186–192.

Smith, M. (2002). Malcolm Knowles, informal adult education, self-direction and andragogy. *The encyclopedia of informal education.* Retrieved, from www.infed.org/thinkers/et-knowl.htm

Strickland, R. J., & O'Leary-Kelley, C. (2009). Clinical nurse educators' perceptions of research utilization: Barriers and facilitators to change. *Journal for Nurses in Staff Development, 25*(4), 164–171.

U.S. Census Bureau. (2010). United States Department of Commerce. Retrieved, from http://www.census.gov

Program Evaluation and Accreditation

Sarah B. Keating

Section 5 analyzes theories, concepts, and models used to evaluate nursing education programs and curricula. Although it appears as the last step in curriculum development and evaluation, it occurs throughout the processes of curriculum development and its implementation. Evaluation activities are part of the accreditation processes that schools or health care agencies experience as part of their credibility for consumers of the programs and documentation of the institution's ability to meet professional and educational standards and criteria. Information from evaluation activities provides the impetus for major and minor changes that must take place to maintain an up-to-date and high-quality curriculum. Current economic and educational systems in the United States place an emphasis on outcomes and **total quality management** (i.e., continually assessing the program, correcting errors as they occur, and thus, improving the quality of the program). Earlier evaluation models in nursing focused on the process phases for delivering education. They spoke of student-centered teaching and learning processes. Faculty's role was to enable the learner to become actively involved and self-directing to acquire new knowledge, behaviors, attitudes, and skills. Outcomes were linked to and measured by the goals and objectives of the curriculum. These processes continue to be vital to evaluation; however, there is a demand for additional information that measures the outcomes in terms of graduates' performance and the quality of the program as compared to professional standards and its competitors.

Although evaluation theories, concepts, models, and processes apply to both the academic and practice settings, the discussion in Section 5 focuses on program evaluation in academe's and regional and professional accrediting bodies for nursing education. However, the information presented can be extrapolated from academe to the practice setting. Entities involved in the evaluation and accreditation of community-based education programs and staff development activities include the Joint Commission of Accreditation of Healthcare Organizations (Joint Commission) for accreditation of programs and the American Nurses Association that provides standards for nurse educators and professional practice.

The Role of Faculty, Students, Consumers, and Administrators in Evaluation

As is true for curriculum development, the faculty is key to the assessment of program outcomes and to the collection and analysis of the data. Students are an important part of the evaluation process as measured by their performance on tests and clinical skills, satisfaction with the program, and their assessment of teaching effectiveness and the quality of the courses in which they participate. Evaluation of the program must also come from the major consumers of the program, which include alumni, employers of the graduates, and the recipients of the graduates' nursing care. The program's success is assessed by the graduates' performance on licensure and certification exams, job skills, professional achievement, and promotion of the program to others. Employers of the graduates and the population receiving their services provide invaluable information and serve as a barometer of the program's match to the health care needs of the population and the system's demand for its graduates.

The role of administrators in education programs is to provide the leadership and financial resources necessary for evaluation processes and consultation services (internal or external expertise), if indicated. Administrators must see to it that there is adequate support staff for the ongoing collection of data and analyses and they have responsibility for assuring that the findings are disseminated in a timely fashion to stakeholders and for follow-up on the recommendations from the findings.

The Master Plan of Evaluation and Program Review

Chapter 14 focuses on major evaluation theories, concepts, and models related to program review and assessment. It describes the system of program approval and periodic review within the parent institution. Approval must be granted to initiate a program by peer and administrative review bodies, and traditionally, program review occurs every 5 years within the institution to ensure quality and, in some instances, justify the continuation of the program when enrollments decline or economic times require downsizing of academic programs.

With today's emphasis on outcomes, evaluation is essential for measuring success, establishing benchmarks, and continually improving the quality of the program. Because programs need to meet academic and accreditation standards, professional discipline expectations, and consumer demand, most institutions have a master plan of evaluation. The master plan may be organized around an evaluation model or theory or by criteria set by accrediting bodies, or it may choose to use both. The master plan provides the guidelines for collecting information to prepare required reports such as program approval or review, accreditation, and to demonstrate the worth of the program to the parent institution and the community. Institutions use the results of evaluation to continue and to improve the program, demonstrate excellence, and market their programs to the public.

Program Approval and Accreditation

Although assessment and evaluation activities for program approval and review and for accreditation often involve the collection and analysis of the same information, their purposes are quite different. Chapter 15 reviews regulatory program approval and accreditation activities for schools of nursing. The state board of nursing, in which the school of nursing is located, is a regulating agency and must approve the program initially and at periodic intervals. Although the board looks at quality, its primary charge is to view the program's performance in light of consumer protection. It also determines the program's eligibility for graduates to sit for RN licensure and in many states, approves nursing programs for advanced practice.

Accreditation is voluntary but at the same time, it gives credibility to the program on the regional, national, and professional levels. Its purpose is to ensure quality as measured by higher education and nursing education accrediting agencies' criteria set by professional peers. An accredited program provides advantages including its reputation for quality, eligibility for grants and other external funding, and for its graduates' eligibility for certification, admission into higher degree programs, and scholarships. Chapter 15 goes into detailed descriptions of the types of accreditation for higher education and nursing including regional, national, and specialty accreditation. It discusses the pros and cons of accreditation and provides educators with detailed guidelines for preparing for accreditation.

14

Program Evaluation

Sarah B. Keating

OBJECTIVES

Upon completion of Chapter 14, the reader will be able to:

1. Analyze common definitions, concepts, and theories of quality assurance and program evaluation.
2. Analyze several models of evaluation for their utility in nursing education.
3. Compare research to program evaluation processes.
4. Justify the rationale for strategic planning and developing a master plan of evaluation for educational programs.
5. Apply the guidelines and major components of a master plan of evaluation to a nursing education program.
6. Compare the roles of administrators and faculty in program evaluation.

INTRODUCTION

Chapter 14 reviews definitions, concepts, and theories related to evaluation and quality assurance as they apply to nursing education including the following:

- Conceptual models of evaluation;
- Utilization of standards, criteria, and benchmarks;
- Comparison of outcomes research and program evaluation; and
- Types of program evaluation and their purposes.

The chapter continues with a discussion of strategic planning, the development of master plans of evaluation, and the roles of administrators and faculty in evaluation.

As discussed in the section overview, educational evaluation occurs while assessing the program for its quality, currency, relevance, projections into the future, and the need for possible revisions in light of these factors. Although the administration usually assumes the leadership for strategic planning, faculty becomes part of the process, especially as it relates to responding to the information provided by the evaluation of the curriculum and the future plans for the institution. A master plan of evaluation provides the information necessary for curriculum revision and for program or institutional strategic planning.

COMMON DEFINITIONS, CONCEPTS, AND THEORIES RELATED TO EVALUATION AND QUALITY ASSURANCE

Although many of the terms, concepts, and theories of educational evaluation originated from business models, they have been adapted to education, especially in light of the recent emphasis on outcomes. The following definitions are commonly used terms in evaluation as they apply to nursing education. To initiate the discussion, the first term to consider is *evaluation* as compared to assessment. **Evaluation** is a process by which information about an entity is gathered to determine its worth. It differs from assessment in that the end product of evaluation is a judgment of its worth, whereas **assessment** is a process that gathers information that results in a conclusion such as a nursing diagnosis or problem identification. It does not end with a judgment but rather a conclusion. Weiner (2009) provides an overview of assessment processes and purposes in academe with descriptions of the roles of faculty and administrators in the establishment of a "culture of assessment." He lists some of the curricular and cocurricular activities that need to be part of assessment and that they must be included in the budgeting process. Student learning outcomes in courses and at the end of the program are essential elements in assessment and he provides samples of measurable student outcomes.

Quality is a term that takes on many meanings depending on the context in which it is used. For the purposes of this chapter and in the interest of simplicity, the Merriam-Webster's Online Dictionary's (2010) second definition of quality is used: "a degree of excellence." Examples of the context of quality include the standards by which an entity is measured, comparison to other like entities, and consumer expectations. **Quality control** is "an aggregate of activities designed to insure adequate quality in the product." **Quality assurance** is "the systematic monitoring and evaluation of the various aspects of a program to assure that standards of quality are being met" (Merriam-Webster). For the purposes of the evaluation of nursing education and this textbook, **total quality management** is defined as an educational program's commitment to and strategies for collecting comprehensive information on the program's effectiveness in meeting its goals and the management of its findings to ensure the continued quality of the program.

Formative and summative evaluation terms are used frequently when evaluating educational programs. The classic and still used definitions for the terms were developed by Scriven (1996). He describes **formative evaluation** as "intended—by the evaluator—as a basis for improvement" (p. 4). For example, in nursing, the faculty compares students' grades in prerequisites to their grades in nursing courses to determine if certain levels of achievement in prerequisites influence grades in nursing. Scriven describes **summative evaluation** as a holistic approach to the assessment of a program and it can use results from the formative evaluation. Continuing with the examples from nursing, faculty can evaluate the development of critical thinking skills in its graduates as a product of the educational program. In this instance, these skills would need to be measured both before and after the program to determine an increase in the skills. Both formative and summative types of evaluation "involve efforts to determine merit or worth, etc." (Scriven, p. 6). Scriven points out that summative evaluation can serve as formative evaluation. For example, if a nursing program finds that graduates' clinical decision-making skills are weak (summative evaluation), it can use that information to analyze the program (formative evaluation) for its strategies to promote these skills throughout the program and make improvements as necessary.

Additional definitions commonly used in evaluation are **goal-based evaluation** and **goal-free evaluation**. Scriven (1974) described goal-based program evaluation as that which focuses only on the examination of program goals and intended outcomes whereas an alternative method could be used to examine the actual effects of the program. These effects (goal-free evaluation) include not only the intended effects, but also the unintended effects, side effects, or secondary effects. An unintended effect in nursing might be an increase in the applicant pool owing to the community's interactions with students in a program-sponsored and nurse-managed clinic. Although this was not a stated goal of the program, it was a positive and an unintended outcome.

CONCEPTUAL MODELS OF EVALUATION

Conceptual Models

For years, nursing education programs used many of the models of evaluation developed in health care and education. Examples were Donabedian's (1996) structure, process, and outcome model for health care evaluation and Stufflebeam's (1971) context, input, process, and product (CIPP) educational model. These models served nursing well, but, as it developed, the uniqueness of the discipline, nursing began to use its own models for evaluation. Most of the models are based on accreditation or professional organizations' standards, essentials, or criteria to evaluate outcomes. For example, Kalb (2009) describes using the three C's model; that is, context, content, and conduct for a comprehensive evaluation of the curriculum and program. The author's school of nursing used the model to integrate its three nursing programs (Associate Degree in Nursing, Bachelor of Science in Nursing, and Master of Science Nursing) according to National League for Nursing Accrediting Commission's (NLNAC; 2008) accreditation standards and there were plans to use it for developing the Doctor of Nursing Practice as well. The evaluation processes in addition to the accreditation standards, included the organizational structure, the curriculum, courses, faculty, staff, students, and American Nurses Association's (ANA; 2004) professional standards.

DeSilets, Dickerson, & DeSilets (2010) describe the use of a hierarchical model, the Roberta Straessle Abruzzese model that moves evaluation from the simple to the complex and assesses the processes, content, outcomes, impact, and, finally, total program evaluation. The model is comprehensive and the author describes ways in which data are collected, analyzed, and used for programmatic decisions.

Benchmarking

More recently, programs are setting benchmarks to measure their own success and standards of excellence or to compare themselves to similar institutions. It can be used in competition with other programs for recruiting students or seeking financial support or, it can be used to motivate the members of the institution to strive toward excellence. Yet another function of benchmarking is the ability to collaborate with other institutions to share strengths with each other and to continually improve programs. Benchmarks can include the financial health of the institution, applicant pool, admission, retention and graduation rates, commitment to diversity, student, faculty, staff, and administrators' satisfaction rates, and so forth.

Evaluation Processes Models

In addition to using conceptual models for program and curriculum evaluation, some institutions choose to use process models for evaluation activities. Holden and Zimmerman (2009) describe the evaluation planning incorporating context (EPIC) model for the evaluation process. Included in their text are examples of the use of the model for assessing an educational program and a community-based service agency. These can apply to nursing as well. The EPIC model "assesses the context of the program, gathers reconnaissance, engages stakeholders, describes the program, and focuses the evaluation." The model is especially helpful in providing guidelines for conducting an evaluation.

The Centers for Disease Control and Prevention (CDC; 2010) developed a framework for program evaluation that is useful for education. Although it focuses on the processes for evaluation, it includes a framework for assigning value or worth to the findings from the evaluation process. The major steps of the process are:

1. Engage the stakeholders;
2. Describe the program;
3. Focus the evaluation plan;
4. Gather credible evidence;
5. Justify conclusions and recommendations; and
6. Ensure use and share lessons learned.

Finally, the cycle begins again with engaging the stakeholders. The steps of the model have at its core the standards against which the program is evaluated. For nursing programs, these are many and can include accreditation standards or criteria and professional/educational essentials or standards.

Formative Evaluation for Nursing Education

Formative and/or process evaluation strategies include course evaluations; student achievement measures; teaching effectiveness surveys; staff, student, administration, and faculty satisfaction measures; impressions of student and faculty performance by clinical agencies' personnel; assessment of student services and other support systems; students' critical thinking development and other standardized tests such as gains in knowledge and skills; National Council Licensure Examination (NCLEX) readiness; satisfaction surveys of families of students; retention/attrition rates; and cost-effectiveness of the program. Antecedent or input evaluation items include entering grade point averages (GPAs), Association of Classroom Teachers (ACT; 2010), Scholastic Achievement Test ([SAT], The College Board, 2010), Graduate Record Examination ([GRE], 2010) scores for applicants and accepted students; retention and/or attrition rates; scholarship, fellowship, and loan availability; and endowments and grants for program development and support.

Tools to measure input, support systems, processes, and outcomes are plentiful and it is strongly recommended that faculty and administrators review the literature for tools that demonstrate reliability and validity. Faculty should review the literature rather than developing new tools that have not been subjected to statistical analyses. Examples of instruments that exist are surveys, appraisal forms, interview schedules, videotaping formats, standardized tests, satisfaction measures, course evaluation forms, and student and faculty performance evaluation forms.

An example of utilization of both formative and summative evaluation tools comes from Graff, Russell, and Stegbauer (2007). They conducted an evaluation of a post-master's, nursing practice doctorate program by assessing students' progress during the program (formative evaluation) and a survey of graduates upon completion and 1 year following graduation (summative evaluation). The model they used for evaluation of the program presents ideas on the types of data to collect and the differences between formative and summative evaluation.

Summative Evaluation Using Standards, Essentials, and Criteria

Measures to determine outcomes of the program include follow-up surveys of the success rates of the graduates including their pass rates on licensure and certification exams; employers' and graduates' satisfaction with the program; graduates' performance, and alumni's accomplishments in leadership roles, as change agents, professional commitment, and continuing education rates. Additional outcome measures include graduation rates, accreditation, and program approval status, ratings of the program by external evaluators or agencies, faculty and student research productivity, community services, and public opinion surveys. Many of these outcome measures can be used to serve as benchmarks for setting achievement levels (e.g., 99% pass rates on NCLEX or for comparing the institution to other admired or similar institutions as a measure of quality). There is a plethora of instruments available for measuring graduates' performance and satisfaction as an indication of the success of the nursing educational program. Nurse educators are urged to review the latest literature in a search for the best tools for collecting and analyzing data to measure the outcomes and the processes used to reach the outcomes of the educational program.

TYPES OF PROGRAM EVALUATION

Basically there are two types of program approval evaluation in academe that differ from regulatory and accreditation processes. They are program approval and program review.

Program Approval

Before a new program is initiated, its parent institution must approve it. As reiterated throughout this text, it is the faculty who develop the curriculum for a new program and it should be based on a needs assessment that provides the rationale for why it is needed, how it meets the mission of the institution, and who the key stakeholders are. In addition to the curriculum plan, a budget should accompany it and it is expected that it projects the costs and income for at least the next 5 years to justify its start-up and maintenance.

In academe the usual rounds of approval are as follows. The first round is for the faculty within the originating department/school to approve the proposal; its next round depends on the hierarchal structure of the institution. The following levels of approval are based on a moderate to large-scale institution and it is understood that smaller institutions may not have as many approval rungs. After faculty approval within the originating program, the proposal may go to a curriculum or program approval committee within its college or division. Preliminary approval may have to be granted by administrators before it enters other formal approval levels to determine its economic feasibility and its fit to the mission and/or strategic plan.

After approval at the program's local level by committees and faculty, as a whole, it proceeds to the next level, which is usually a program or curriculum committee at the division or college level. With their approval, it goes to the overall university or college graduate or undergraduate committee for its review and approval. It then goes to a sub-committee of the senate that reviews program proposals. Upon their approval, the senate reviews it for their input and approval and then it goes to the chief executive for academic affairs such as a vice president or provost. Upon that person's approval, the president of the institution approves the program. The governing board such as a board of trustees or regents in the final rung of approval and it may have a subcommittee that reviews it with recommendations prior to its going to the full board. These levels of approval are for academic approval only and for professional programs such as nursing accreditation processes and state board of nursing approvals should be initiated along the way to reassure the academic entities that the program is qualified for professional approval and accreditation.

Program Review

Program review in academe occurs on average every 5 years within the parent institution. The purpose for program review is to ensure the quality and health of the program. Faculty prepares an overview of the program especially related to enrollments, the quality of the faculty, and student learning outcomes (Weiner, 2009), and enrollment and graduation projections. When economic times are tough, these reviews help to demonstrate the relationship of the program to the mission of the institution, its contributions to the community, and the quality of the program. Nursing often finds itself justifying its program owing to the relatively small faculty to student ratios when clinical supervision is factored in. Nursing programs need the data to support the program, its cost-effectiveness, its contributions to the core general education and prerequisite requirements.

The requirements and processes for program approval and review use the same data sets as many of the other assessment and evaluation activities related to professional accreditation and standards of excellence. Thus, it is not unusual for a parent institution to request copies of the most recent self-studies and accreditation reports that either substitute for program review criteria or supplement the requirements. Program approval and review should be integrated into the master plan of evaluation so that the data sets can serve all purposes for assessment.

RESEARCH AND PROGRAM EVALUATION

Sometimes there is confusion between what constitutes evaluation research versus the process of evaluation. The evaluation process starts with an identification of the program or entity that is to be evaluated, the purpose of the evaluation, and who the stakeholders are within the program. It requires many of the same steps of research including a review of the literature, identification of a theory or model of evaluation to guide the process, collection and analysis of credible data related to the program, synthesizing the analysis to come to a conclusion, and a judgment with recommendations for further assessment and strategies for improvement.

Research in evaluation, on the other hand, differs from the evaluation process. It begins with a description of a problem and a research question, its purpose for investigation, and follows with the usual steps of the research process (i.e., literature review, theoretical/conceptual framework, methodology, data collection and analysis, findings, and recommendations).

Research in evaluation is usually viewed as applied research and differs from basic research as it is searching for practical solutions to problems. Donaldson, Christie, and Mark (2009) describe applied research and evaluation processes and the continuing debates among the experts on the validity of quantitative and qualitative methodologies and their application to evaluation. They discuss current emphases in the disciplines on evidence-based practice, what constitutes credible evidence, evaluation theories, and these influences on applied research in evaluation. At the end, their text presents the latest in evaluation theories and their relevance to the search for evidence-based practice in education.

STRATEGIC PLANNING

Strategic planning for an institution provides the guidelines for carrying out the mission of the institution and at the same time, can be used to evaluate how well the institution is meeting its mission and goals. Strategic planning usually begins with the top executive and management team providing the leadership for its development. In academe, the parent institution's top administrators (president, vice presidents, provosts, deans, etc.) develop the plan that is in turn, implemented throughout the institution by the various academic divisions. Each division may choose to develop its own strategic plan; however, it should be congruent with that of its parent but unique to the program's mission and goals. The first step in strategic planning is to develop a vision statement. The vision statement presents a description of where the institution will be in the future, usually 3–5 years hence and incorporates the core values of the institution. The leadership team may wish to engage other stakeholders in the process and in the planning (strategic) to meet the vision.

Varkey and Bennett (2010) discuss the strategic planning process applied to health care agencies but the same processes can be adapted to educational milieus. They advise that the leadership team create a sense of urgency for developing the plan with the first session centered on developing a vision that is of the highest order and reflects the team's belief of where the organization needs to be in the future. Once the vision is developed through brainstorming and coming to consensus, the planning process commences. DeSilets (2008) uses the strengths, weaknesses, opportunities, and threats (SWOT) model of systems analysis for gathering data related to the vision and for developing possible strategies to meet the end goal or vision of the program. This analysis leads to action plans with deadlines set, people identified to carry out the content of the plans, and additional plans for checking periodically, on the progress of the plan toward meeting the goal.

Greene (2009) discusses the current situation in health care that is true of academe as well. Changes in systems and the economic times happen so quickly that decisions need to be made quickly, there is no longer the luxury of time to mull over options. That is why Greene says that the vision statement and strategic plans must include the core values of the institution/program and are key to making decisions that will benefit not only the program but also the people it serves (i.e., students, faculty, staff, and consumers of care).

Although nursing programs may not have a strategic plan per se, it is usually wise to have goals set for the future with action plans to carry them out. These goals and action plans are reviewed at least annually to assess the progress toward the goals and to adjust or develop new goals as the program and its needs and constituencies change. To avoid the pitfall of exquisite planning processes that fail to implement the plan, the use of a master plan of evaluation provides the structure and details for assessing and evaluating the progress that the program is making toward reaching its vision and short- and long-term goals.

MASTER PLAN OF EVALUATION

Rationale for a Master Plan of Evaluation

When developing a master plan of evaluation, one of the major tasks to integrate into the plan is to meet accreditation or program approval standards. These standards or criteria are the baseline requirements of the profession to ensure that programs are of sufficient quality to meet the expectations of the discipline. They also demonstrate to the public that a program is recognized by external reviewing bodies and, thus, the quality of its graduates meets educational and professional standards. Graduation from an accredited program is usually one of the admission standards for continued degree or education work. Many funding agencies for programs require accreditation because it indicates that the program is of high enough quality to assume the responsibility for the administration of grants and completion of projects. Most accrediting agencies require that a program have a master plan of evaluation and even if it is not required, a master plan helps to identify the components that need to be evaluated, who will do the data collection and when, what methods of analysis of the data will be employed, and the plans for responding to the findings for quality improvement. Having a master plan of evaluation in place greatly facilitates these processes when submitting accreditation self-study reports, program approval reports, or proposals for funding (Commission on Collegiate Nursing Education [CCNE], 2010; NLNAC, 2010).

With today's emphasis on outcomes, the evaluation process is essential to measuring success, establishing benchmarks, and continually improving the quality of the program. A master plan of evaluation is used to provide data for faculty's decision making as part of an internal review and for meeting external review standards. It is important to have a master plan that continually monitors the program so that adjustments can be made as the program is implemented and it is part of the total quality management process. It is equally important to measure outcomes in terms of meeting the vision, strategic plans, goals, and objectives of the program, and certain benchmarks that help to pinpoint the quality of the program.

Components of a Master Plan of Evaluation

The master plan must specify what is being evaluated and an organizing framework is useful so that, as nearly as possible, no crucial variable is omitted for review. Additionally, it is important to identify the persons who will:

- Collect the data;
- Analyze the findings;
- Prepare reports;
- Disseminate the reports to key people; and
- Set the timelines for collection, analysis, and reporting of the data.

Finally, there must be a feedback loop in place for recommendations and decision making. Reports from the evaluation should include:

- Identification of existing and potential problems
- Previously unidentification of new needs
- Successes and why
- Recommendations for improvement, discontinuance of a program, or proposals for new programs
- Action plans for changes that include the peoples' responsibility, and timelines
- A summary of the evaluation and judgment on the program's success or progress toward meeting its goals

Table 14.1 provides guidelines for developing a master plan of evaluation and the major components to be assessed for evaluation. In addition, including the curriculum and its components, it incorporates external and internal frame factors (Johnson, 1977), the infrastructure, the core curriculum, students, alumni, and human resources. As indicated in the table, these are only the major components. It is possible that as educational evaluation evolves, other components will emerge. The elements within each component are not listed. Each institution must determine which elements fall under the major components.

ROLES OF ADMINISTRATORS AND FACULTY IN PROGRAM EVALUATION

Administrators in academe provide the vision and leadership for the educational program. However, it is imperative for the administration and the major stakeholders of the institution to be in an agreement about its mission, vision, purpose, and goals. Stakeholders include the governing board, the chief executive officer, the administrators of the infrastructure and the academic programs, the faculty, students, and consumers served by the institution. These stakeholders make up the

TABLE 14.1 Major Components and Guidelines for Developing a Master Plan of Evaluation

Component	Action Plans						Follow-Up Plans	
	Responsible Party	When and How Often	Instruments and Tools for Data Collection	Data Findings and Analysis	Criteria, Outcomes or Benchmarks	Reports and Recommen- dations	Maintain and Monitor or Improve	By Whom, How, and When
External Frame Factors (Johnson, 1977)								
Internal Frame Factors (Johnson, 1977)								
Infrastructure Systems:								
Buildings								
Facilities								
Support systems								
Student services								
Financial								
Administration								
Technology								
Library								
Baccalaureate Curriculum:								
Prerequisites								
General education								
Electives								
Nursing major								
Graduate Curriculum								
Prerequisites								
Cognates								
Core nursing courses								
Specialty/functional Courses								
Curriculum Components								
Mission/vision								
Organizational Framework								
Philosophy								
Overall purpose/goal								
End of program (student learning outcomes) and level objectives								
Implementation plan								
Course objectives and content								
Learning activities								
Teaching effectiveness								
Students								
Admissions								
Enrollments								
Achievement								
Graduation								

(Continued)

TABLE 14.1 Major Components and Guidelines for Developing a Master Plan of Evaluation *Continued*

Component	Action Plans						Follow-Up Plans	
	Responsible Party	When and How Often	Instruments and Tools for Data Collection	Data Findings and Analysis	Criteria, Outcomes or Benchmarks	Reports and Recommendations	Maintain and Monitor or Improve	By Whom, How, and When
Alumni								
Licensure/certification								
Satisfaction								
Employment								
Achievements								
Human Resources:								
Milieu								
Administrators								
Faculty								
Staff								
Colleagues								

"personality" and body of the institution that marks it as unique in its contributions to society and they must be in agreement with the vision and purpose of the institution to maintain a strong educational program. Administration periodically reviews the mission and vision of the institution to match them to current needs and provides the leadership for revising them according to their needs. Additionally, administration monitors assessment and evaluation activities to ensure program quality and provides adequate resources in a timely manner for accreditation and program evaluation activities.

All faculty members participate in the evaluation of the curriculum and the program through their input into specific areas and needs for assessment, the collection of data, data analyses, and the formulation of recommendations for decision making regarding the program. In many schools of nursing, there are evaluation committees who lead the process or, in other cases, curriculum committees may be charged with the evaluation of the curriculum and program. As part of the parent institution, nursing representatives provide input into university/collegewide evaluation activities. As a professional program, nursing faculty has valuable input into evaluation processes owing to the necessity for meeting professional accreditation and organizations' standards and criteria.

SUMMARY

Chapter 14 reviews classic definitions, concepts, and models of evaluation with definitions of commonly used terms. The rationale for strategic planning and a master plan of evaluation is presented. Types of tools and instruments for data collection for evaluation of educational programs and the roles of administrators and faculty are reviewed.

DISCUSSION QUESTIONS

1. Explain the differences between conceptual models of evaluation and the use of benchmarks. Give examples of their application to the evaluation of an educational program.
2. To what extent do you believe faculty should be involved in a strategic planning process? Explain why.
3. Describe how a master plan of evaluation contributes to the external review of a nursing program.

LEARNING ACTIVITIES

Student learning activities

Using Table 14.1, develop a master plan of evaluation for the case study of a fictional school of nursing outreach program found in Chapters 5, 6, and 7.

Faculty development activities

Using Table 14.1, finds your school of nursing's or agency's evaluation plan and assesses it for any missing components or action plans.

REFERENCES

Association of Classroom Teachers. (2010). *Homepage.* Retrieved from ACT Assessment. http://www.act.org/aap

American Nurses Association. (2004). *Nursing: Scope and standards of practice.* Washington, DC: Author.

Centers for Disease Control and Prevention Working Group. (2010). Framework for program evaluation. Retrieved from http://www.cdc.gov/EVAL/framework.htm

The College Board. (2010). SAT Program. *Higher education.* Retrieved from http://www.collegeboard.com/highered/ra/sat/sat.html

Commission on Collegiate Nursing Education. (2010). *About CCNE.* Retrieved from http://www.aacn.nche.edu/accreditation/AboutCCNE.htm

DeSilets, L. D. (2008). SWOT is useful in your tool kit. *Journal of Continuing Education in Nursing, 39*(5), 196–197.

DeSilets, L. D., Dickerson, P. S., & DeSilets, L. D. (2010). Another look at evaluation models. *Journal of Continuing Education in Nursing, 41*(1), 12–13.

Donabedian, A. (1996). Quality management in nursing and health care. In J. A. Schemele (Ed.), *Models of quality assurance* (pp. 88–103). Albany, NY: Delmar Publishers.

Donaldson, S. I., Christie, C. A., & Mark, M. M. (2009). What counts as credible evidence in applied research and evaluation practice? Los Angeles: Sage.

Graduate Record Examination. (2010). *GRE Web site.* Retrieved from http://www.gre.org/splash.html

Graff, J. C., Russell, C. K., & Stegbauer, C. C. (2007). Formative and summative evaluation of a practice doctorate program. *Nurse Educator, 32*(4), 173–177.

Greene, J. (2009). The new pace of strategic planning. *Hospitals & Health Networks, 83*(11), 31–34.

Holden, D. J., & Zimmerman, M. A. (2009). *A Practice guide to program evaluation planning.* Los Angeles: Sage.

Johnson, M. (1977). *Intentionality in education.* (Distributed by the Center for Curriculum Research and Services, Albany, NY.). Troy, NY: Walter Snyder, Printer, Inc.

Kalb, K. (2009). The three Cs model: The context, content, and conduct of nursing education. *Nursing Education Perspectives, 30*(3), 176–180.

Merriam-Webster's Online Dictionary. (2010). Retrieved from: http://www.m-w.com

National League for Nursing Accrediting Commission. (2008). *NLNAC accreditation manual.* New York: Author.

National League for Nursing Accrediting Commission. (2010). *NLNAC Home Page.* Retrieved from http://www.nlnac.org/home.htm

Scriven, M. (1996). Types of evaluation and types of evaluator. *Evaluation Practice, 17*(2), 151–161.

Scriven, M. S. (1974). Evaluation perspectives and procedures. In J. W. Popham (Ed.), *Evaluation in education: Current applications.* Berkeley, CA: McCutchan Publishing Corporation.

Stufflebeam, D. L., Foley, W. J., Gephart, W. J., Guba, E. G., Hammond, R. L., Merriman, H. O., et al. (1971). *Educational evaluation and decision making.* Itasca, IL: Peacock.

Varkey, P., & Bennet, K. E. (2010). Practical techniques for strategic planning in health care organizations. *Physician Executive, 36*(2), 46–48.

Weiner, W. (2009). Establishing a culture of assessment. *Academe, 95*(4), 28–32.

Planning for Accreditation: Evaluating the Curriculum

Abby Heydman
Arlene Sargent

OBJECTIVES

Upon completion of Chapter 15, readers will be able to:

1. Analyze the various forms of accreditation and typical accreditation processes that are used to indicate a program that meets specific standards and criteria.
2. Outline a plan for accreditation, develop a timeline, and provide for involvement of faculty, students, and other stakeholders in the self-study and site visit.
3. Apply principles of continuous quality improvement (CQI) in accreditation activities.
4. Evaluate current issues in accreditation within higher education, particularly those related to the increasing role of federal agencies in establishing accreditation standards and policies, the impact of technology, and the development of a global marketplace in higher education.

INTRODUCTION

As noted in the overview to this section, accreditation is a process that educational programs and curricula undergo to receive recognition for meeting standards or criteria set by national, regional, or state organizations. Programs undergo accreditation to demonstrate their quality to the consumers of their products (students, alumni, and employers). Because programs such as nursing prepare students for the practice of a profession involving activities that have a direct impact on public health and safety, there are rigorous standards and more numerous types of accreditation reviews that are common for other academic programs. For this reason, it is important for faculty and program directors to have a broad understanding of accreditation and the significant role they play in evaluating the program and curriculum to meet accreditation standards.

Chapter 14 explored the broader areas of educational program evaluation and presents examples of models used in nursing education. Selecting a model for evaluation can assist faculty in focusing and organizing their work and in expressing their particular philosophy of education. Use of a particular model can provide a comprehensive framework to guide the work of faculty and staff in the evaluation process. Readers were introduced to the benefits of developing a master plan for program and curriculum evaluation. The development of a master plan for evaluation indicates that faculty thoughtfully considered key learning outcomes and the importance of determining the extent to which these outcomes were attained. Optimally, the master plan provides data that can be used for both formative and summative evaluation, with evidence being used for continuous improvement of the program.

Chapter 15 explores the world of accreditation and the external requirements that must be satisfied in order for a nursing program to operate successfully in the context of the state or province in which it exists, within its region, within the larger boundaries of the country, and within the special world of a profession. Trends toward globalization of accreditation are explored.

DEFINITION OF TERMS

1. **Institutional accreditation**—accreditation that provides a comprehensive review of the functioning and effectiveness of the entire college, university, or technical institute. The state mandate or particular institutional mission provides the lens used to guide the review.
2. **Programmatic or specialized accreditation**—accreditation that focuses on the functioning and effectiveness of a particular program or unit within the larger institution (e.g., nursing).
3. **Specialized or programmatic accreditation agencies**—accreditation agencies that focus on the functioning or effectiveness of a particular kind of program (e.g., nursing, nurse anesthesia) or that review a specialized, single-purpose college, or postsecondary school.
4. **Regulatory**—a form of approval, recognition, or accreditation required by a federal, state, or provincial government agency.
5. **Voluntary**—a form of accreditation not required by law or regulation. Voluntary accreditation processes are managed by private, voluntary organizations composed of peer member institutions or programs.
6. **National accreditation**—any accreditation agency that accredits colleges, universities, or technical institutes within an entire country.
7. **Regional accreditation agency**—one of six private, voluntary accreditation agencies within the United States, formed for the purpose of peer evaluation and setting of standards for higher education.
8. **State-regulatory agencies**—required to recognize or approve colleges, universities, or programs for operation with the state as governed by state statutes.
9. **CQI**—the implementation of a system designed to provide for ongoing evaluation, analysis of findings, and implementation of plans for improvement within an organization.

NATIONAL ACCREDITING BODIES

The United States is distinctive in that historically its accreditation efforts have been managed by private, voluntary organizations formed by peer institutions for the purpose of judging quality and setting standards to guide educational practice. Although the federal and state governments play a role, particularly as it relates to eligibility for licensure and state or federal financial aid, the independent accrediting agencies are key figures in quality assurance through accreditation of colleges, universities, and technical schools. In Canada, as is generally true in the international community, institutions are granted the right to operate within their respective province according to statutes established by provincial legislatures and the Ministry of Education (Ontario Ministry of Education, 2008). Since 1987, collegiate nursing programs in Canada that offer the baccalaureate degree in nursing may also apply for specialized accreditation from the Canadian Association of Schools of Nursing (CASN; 2010).

Although the structure of accreditation may differ from country to country, universities and nursing education programs are generally required to be accredited or approved by regulatory bodies within the country, state, or province in which they operate. Other forms of accreditation, even regional accreditation in the United States, are voluntary, that is, the institution or nursing program may choose to seek accreditation to demonstrate that it has a particular commitment to meeting high standards. Some would argue that it is a euphemism to say that regional accreditation and specialized accreditation are voluntary today, because eligibility for student financial aid in the United States is tied to these approvals, but technically, most forms of accreditation, except those that authorize a college or university to operate within a state, remain voluntary in the United States.

Depending on their purposes, accreditation agencies evaluate institutions or specialized units within an institution. Thus, colleges or universities have institutional accreditation, and programs, departments, or schools within larger institutions have specialized accreditation. Specialized accreditation is common among professional health science programs, as well as among other professions, and there are numerous specialized accrediting agencies. A few specialized accreditation agencies accredit single-purpose institutions of higher education, such as colleges of chiropractic medicine, acupuncture and oriental medicine, and colleges of nursing, some of which are hospital-based.

Over the years, as the number of students enrolled in postsecondary institutions increased dramatically, and as higher education received increased funding both for direct operations and for student financial aid, accreditation requirements and expectations for accountability have increased (Eaton, 2010). As a result, accreditation processes and standards continue to become more demanding and costly to address (Eaton, 2008b).

ROLE OF THE U.S. DEPARTMENT OF EDUCATION

Unlike many other countries, the United States does not have a central ministry of education that controls postsecondary institutions of higher education. States assume a role in the approval and control of colleges and universities within their boundaries and approval processes and regulations vary widely among them. Thus, American colleges and universities have operated with a great deal of autonomy and independence as reflected in their diverse missions and organizational structures. A distinctive feature of American higher education, and one that may be considered both a strength and a weakness, is the diversity in type and kind of institution operating with considerable variation in quality and reputation.

Although the states have primary jurisdiction over U.S. colleges and universities, the national government, through the U.S. Department of Education (USDE), has begun to play a larger role in higher education in the past decade. One of the USDE's primary roles is to ensure that federal student aid funds are used to provide access for students enrolling in academic programs and courses of high quality (Eaton, 2009; USDE, 2009). It does this by reviewing and approving both regional and specialized accrediting agencies. USDE's recognition process for accrediting agencies uses standards that address recruitment and admission practices, fiscal and administrative capacity and facilities, curricula, faculty, student support programs, records of student complaints, and success in student achievement. Only those colleges and universities accredited by a USDE-recognized accrediting agency are eligible to receive federal financial aid for students (Eaton, 2009).

Regional and specialized accrediting agencies are periodically reviewed by the USDE and/or a private organization, the Council for Higher Education Accreditation (CHEA). The recognition process for institutional and specialized accrediting agencies is a part of the federal regulatory mandate in the United States (Eaton, 2008a). Accreditation agencies are not only approved by the USDE and CHEA but their scope of authority is also determined. For example, an accreditation agency may be approved to accredit programs only at the certificate or baccalaureate level, but not at the master's or doctoral level. Approval may also be extended to include accreditation of programs offered through distance learning modalities. Abuses in federal financial aid have led to increasingly stringent oversight of all forms of accreditation that provide access to federal financial aid.

In the United States, six regional accreditation agencies accredit colleges and universities within defined geographic areas. For example, the Western Association of Schools and Colleges (WASC) accredits colleges and universities within California, Hawaii, Guam, and the Pacific Islands. Refer to Table 15.1 for a complete listing of the regional accrediting agencies and a description of the geographic areas they cover. In recent years, more colleges are establishing campuses across state lines from the original campus and more programs are being offered using technology that makes time and location unimportant. For this reason, among others, the regional accreditation agencies have formed the Council of Regional Accrediting Commissions (C-RAC). C-RAC develops policies on accrediting institutions that cross regional accrediting boundaries, and build consensus on accreditation policies and best practices on issues such as distance learning (New England Association of Schools and Colleges Commission on Institutions of Higher Education, 2010; WASC Senior Commission, 2009). In recent years, the USDE has become increasingly active in establishing rules and regulations to be followed by accreditation agencies. At regular intervals, the USDE appoints representatives from the various accrediting bodies to a negotiated rule-making team. Negotiated rule making is the process for developing recommendations for proposed regulations governing accrediting agencies. The proposed regulations, which reflect consensus of the team, are then considered by USDE. Recent topics considered in negotiated rule making included the definition of the credit hour, definition of a high school diploma, satisfactory academic progress, and state authorization, among others (National League for Nursing Accrediting Commission [NLNAC], 2009; USDE, 2009). USDE regulations have resulted in less flexibility for accrediting agencies, including definitive timelines by which institutions must come into compliance with accreditation standards. Colleges and universities are also monitored in regard to their financial performance each year and eligibility for financial aid is dependent on evidence of fiscal health. Fears of increasing oversight by the USDE had led to growing concern about the fate of historical autonomy of higher education in the United States (Fritschler, 2007).

THE COUNCIL FOR HIGHER EDUCATION ACCREDITATION

CHEA was formed in 1996 as a private, nonprofit, national organization designed to coordinate accreditation activities in the United States. CHEA accomplishes its purposes by providing formal recognition of regional, national, and specialized higher accreditation bodies. The Council's focus is on academic quality, whereas the USDE's concern is on quality and accountability as it relates to student financial aid. Accreditation agencies may be recognized (approved) by both the USDE and CHEA or by only one of these organizations depending on the accreditation agency's role and focus (Eaton, 2008a).

Various types of accreditation agencies have been developed to oversee the quality of more than 6,500 degree- and nondegree-granting postsecondary institutions in the United States. In all, there are 80 recognized institutional and specialized accrediting organizations operating in the United States (Eaton, 2009). Sixty-four accrediting agencies are recognized by CHEA (2010).

PURPOSES OF ACCREDITATION

The primary purpose of accreditation in general is to ensure that at least minimum standards of quality are met. Most voluntary accreditation agencies state that they aim to achieve higher than minimum standards as determined by peers in the field. A second purpose of accreditation is to provide recognition for funding and student financial aid. A third rationale for accreditation is to ensure consistency in quality across academic programs, thus facilitating transfer of academic credit from one institution to another and the acknowledgment of the comparability of one degree to another in the same field across institutions. Accreditation as well as licensure and certification are the various means used to regulate the professions (Barnum, 1997).

In the United States, where voluntary accreditation is the norm, accreditation is distinguished by emphasis on both self-regulation and peer evaluation. In this environment, accreditation processes tend to be both formative and summative, seeking continuous improvement rather than being oriented only to compliance. Accreditation standards typically require institutions or programs to develop evaluation plans and to write comprehensive self-studies to ensure that a system is in place to ensure CQI. These activities facilitate assessment and reflection on findings. Peer evaluation is also a core value in voluntary accreditation where peers work on setting standards, participating in site visits, and serve on review panels, appeal panels, and commissions.

In recent years, there has been some dissatisfaction with traditional accreditation processes and practices. Concern has been raised about whether quality is really assured by the current process of voluntary accreditation in the United States. For-profit postsecondary institutions of higher education and institutions offering degrees through distance learning modalities have proliferated and their students have participated heavily in federal financial aid. Some congressional leaders and educators have even recommended that eligibility to award financial aid should be separated from regional or professional accreditation (Guerard, 2002; Morgan, 2002). Increasingly, institutions of higher education are asked to demonstrate to the USDE (through regulations imposed on regional and professional accreditation agencies) that they are tracking trends in key performance indicators such as student graduation rates, graduates' loan default rates, and postgraduation employment (Bacon, 2003).

PROS AND CONS OF ACCREDITATION

Faculty will undoubtedly engage in discussions about the pros and cons of accreditation, such discussions being particularly common when in the midst of a self-study or a site visit. In addition to providing eligibility funding mechanisms, there are multiple other "pros" that accreditation offers to an institution or a program. Accreditation demonstrates to the public the program's quality and effectiveness. Accreditation can assist potential students to identify appropriate programs for their goals, assuring students that they have selected a college, university, or program that meets high standards in its operations. In addition, accreditation typically assures students that their course work will be acceptable for transfer credit to another institution of higher education. This is important for students who find they want to change colleges or universities (for whatever reason) or who want to go on to graduate school.

Accreditation indicates to employers that the employee graduated from a quality program with specific standards that were met. Qualified graduates of accredited programs also have ready access to graduate education. The biggest benefit to accreditation is the continuous emphasis it places on self-evaluation, reevaluation, and continuous improvement. In a recent article on accreditation, Nkongho (2006) indicates

> accreditation is important for nursing programs, their graduates, and for the profession of nursing. It indicates that a program has met certain predetermined criteria set by representatives of the profession. Achieving and maintaining accreditation provides recognition to society at large, employers, the nursing profession, and other health care professionals that a program's graduates are sufficiently prepared and qualified to compete in an ever-challenging environment. (p.70)

In terms of the "cons," accreditation certainly looms larger as a factor in faculty and staff workload than was the case some decades ago when accreditation was in its infancy. It should be remembered, however, that accreditation came about not just because of the public demand for accountability and quality, but because peers felt a responsibility to work collaboratively to establish standards that would guide their practice.

Perhaps the biggest complaint about accreditation is its cost. Staff and faculty time involved in planning for either institutional or specialized accreditation is significant and costly. Often, institutions or programs must postpone major initiatives while they are working on a major accreditation review. This highlights the "opportunity cost," which may be attendant to accreditation. In a time where resources are perceived to be scarce, institutions and programs sometimes feel these resources should be used for more important activities or initiatives (O'Neil, 1997). Duplication of effort with overlapping requirements in regional and specialized accreditation is yet another frequent complaint of current accreditation systems (The Center for Health Professions, 1999). Preparation of faculty for assessment of student learning, educating them about accreditation standards and policies, and involving them in the self-study and site visit present yet more challenges. Some see these as distractions from their primary role in teaching and research. Accreditation is also charged with being inflexible, parochial, failing to take institutional diversity into account, stifling innovation, and being too focused on inputs. Some critics have expressed the viewpoint that accreditation standards do not ensure quality (Morgan, 2002).

The use of technology in higher education and the overt development of higher education as a market commodity have also created new issues and criticism surrounding accreditation. Technology permits institutions to offer programs outside of their traditional state, provincial, or regional boundaries. More institutions are offering programs through distance learning strategies that provide global student access to degree programs. Thus, questions arise about which agency has jurisdiction in accreditation of these out-of-region programs. The entry of for-profit colleges and universities into the realm of higher education has also brought attention to the vast financial and economic enterprise of higher education. Consider the case of the University of Phoenix (UOP), the largest independent college in the United States. In 2010, UOP enrolled more than 450,000 students, operating campuses in 40 states plus Puerto Rico and Canada (Alberta and British Columbia). A large portion of its students are enrolled in programs that are offered totally online (UOP, 2010).

CONTINUOUS QUALITY IMPROVEMENT

In recent years, concerns about the deficiencies in accreditation and the very episodic nature of accreditation have led to consideration of alternative evaluation methods for educational programs. Higher education has begun to adopt concepts and processes of CQI from the corporate world in its evaluation systems. Building a culture in which CQI is a core value enables a college or department to create a system of evaluation, which is inclusive, systematic, and reliable (Suhayda & Miller, 2006). CQI calls on institutions or programs to identify customers clearly. Customers include students, alumni, clinical agencies, the profession, and consumers. Establishing key requirements for satisfaction of these stakeholders is an important step in the CQI process. Typically, evaluation strategies in CQI include evaluating satisfaction of students and other customers, as well as establishing whether key requirements have been met (i.e., benchmarks for graduates performance and learning outcomes). Cross-functional teams (staff and faculty) work to assess whether systems are optimal to produce best practices and results. A major advantage in the CQI process is that it is a continuous activity in which organizational data is evaluated regularly to target results needing improvement. Key performance indicators are established to provide a set of metrics that a program can monitor on a regular basis.

BALDRIGE EDUCATIONAL CRITERIA

The Malcom Baldrige National Quality Awards were established in 1987 by Congress to recognize U.S. businesses that have established outstanding programs of CQI. The award was named for former Secretary of Commerce, Malcolm Baldrige, who was responsible for encouraging U.S. businesses to begin a focused effort on improvement in quality to compete more effectively in world markets (National Institute for Standards and Technology, 2010). Baldrige principles focus on the development of effective systems that rely on data for decision making for quality improvement. Over time, this and other Baldrige principles have influenced quality improvement systems in hospitals and accreditation practices among accreditation agencies. Collin's (1997) captured the philosophy of continuous improvement that is just as essential today as it was when originally quoted in 1997:

> Accreditation is needed. However, accreditation must become an integral part of the daily functioning of the program or school, not an episodic event. It is justifiable use of resources when it leads to overall continuous program improvement. By incorporating quality standards of nursing education into ongoing activities, a seamless, continuous development of the program or school exists. (p. 6)

The challenge for academic leaders is to work with faculty and staff to create ongoing systems to ensure regular program improvement.

THE GLOBAL ENVIRONMENT

Developments in recent years have highlighted the growing competition for the international market of higher education as evidenced by universities offering high-demand programs around the world. Increasingly, higher education is becoming a "commodity" with value added because of the opportunities presented to those who receive credentials through higher education. These developments lead many to believe that current accreditation structures are antiquated and inadequate for dealing with new realities of the global marketplace for higher education (Van Damme, 2002).

POLITICAL REALITIES

A key question being asked today is whether all the money being spent on higher education is really worth the investment. Would this funding be better spent on health care, housing, or other pressing social needs? The accountability question is driving the federal appetite to become more directly involved in accreditation in the United States, particularly as it relates to an institution's eligibility to handle student financial aid awards. This debate is likely to become even more intense in the United States, given the reauthorization of the Higher Education Act of 1965 with the passing of the Higher Education Opportunity Act ([HEOA], Public Law 110-315) in 2008. This legislation includes many new provisions regarding student financial aid, along with new regulations for colleges and universities. Because of the growing importance of student financial aid, regional and specialized accreditation agencies feel a sense of urgency about demonstrating that voluntary accreditation processes are effective. Growing governmental intrusion is also viewed with some alarm (Eaton, 2008b). Regional accreditation agencies have been responding to this threat with several new initiatives that focus on evidence of quality (Gose, 2002; Higher Learning Commission, 2010).

ORGANIZATIONAL OVERVIEW OF THE STRUCTURE OF ACCREDITATION

As noted earlier in this chapter, legitimate accrediting agencies in the United States must be recognized by the USDE or CHEA. There are two major types of accreditation bodies, institutional and specialized or programmatic. Institutional accreditation agencies include six regional associations and their separate commissions that accredit senior colleges, community (junior) colleges, technical schools, and secondary (high) schools. A regional accreditation agency in the United States is a voluntary organization comprised of member schools from a defined geographic region of the country. These include the following regional accreditation agencies and the commissions that accredit postsecondary schools and colleges:

- Middle States Association of Colleges and Schools
    Commission on Higher Education
- New England Association of Schools and Colleges
    Commission on Institutions of Higher Education
    Commission on Technical and Career Institutions
- North Central Association of Colleges and Schools
    Commission on Institutions of Higher Education
- Northwest Association of Schools and Colleges
    Commission on Colleges
- Southwest Association of Colleges and Schools
    Commission on Colleges
- Western Association of Schools and Colleges
    Accrediting Commission for Community and Junior Colleges
    Accrediting Commission for Senior Colleges and Universities

Regional accreditation agencies offer institutional accreditation following a comprehensive review of the mission and goals, infrastructure, resources, and evidence of educational effectiveness of the institution seeking accreditation. Degree-granting institutions of postsecondary education are usually accredited by a regional accreditation body in the United States. However, some single-purpose professional schools and proprietary and/or technical schools are accredited by various national agencies that provide institutional accreditation. Nonetheless, regional accreditation is generally held to be the optimal standard required to ensure transferability of academic credit from one postsecondary institution of higher education to another in the United States.

TABLE 15.1 Regional Accrediting Agencies in the United States

Regional Accrediting Agency	Scope of Recognition
Western Association of Schools & Colleges	**Commission for Senior Colleges and Universities**—Accreditation and preaccreditation ("candidate for accreditation") of senior colleges and universities in California, Hawaii, the U.S. territories of Guam and American Samoa, the Republic of Palau, the Federated States of Micronesia, the Commonwealth of the Northern Mariana Islands, and the Republic of the Marshall Islands, including distance education programs.
	Accrediting Commission for Community and Junior Colleges— Accreditation and preaccreditation ("candidate for accreditation") of 2-year associate degree-granting institutions located in California, Hawaii, the U.S. territories of Guam and American Samoa, the Republic of Palau, the Federated States of Micronesia, the Commonwealth of the Northern Mariana Islands, and the Republic of the Marshall Islands, including the accreditation of such programs offered via distance education at these colleges.
Southern Association of Colleges & Schools, Commission on Colleges	Accreditation and preaccreditation ("candidate for accreditation") of degree-granting institutions of higher education in Alabama, Florida, Georgia, Kentucky, Louisiana, Mississippi, North Carolina, South Carolina, Tennessee, Texas, and Virginia, including distance education programs offered at those institutions.
Middle States Association of Colleges & Schools	Accreditation and preaccreditation ("candidacy status") of institutions of higher education in Delaware, the District of Columbia, Maryland, New Jersey, New York, Pennsylvania, Puerto Rico, and the U.S. Virgin Islands, including distance education programs offered at those institutions.
North Central Association of Colleges & Schools, The Higher Learning Commission	Accreditation and preaccreditation ("Candidate for Accreditation") of degree-granting institutions of higher education in Arizona, Arkansas, Colorado, Illinois, Indiana, Iowa, Kansas, Michigan, Minnesota, Missouri, Nebraska, New Mexico, North Dakota, Ohio, Oklahoma, South Dakota, West Virginia, Wisconsin, and Wyoming, including tribal institutions, and the accreditation of programs offered via distance education within these institutions.
Northwest Commission on Colleges & Universities	Accreditation and preaccreditation ("candidacy status") of postsecondary degree– granting educational institutions in Alaska, Idaho, Montana, Nevada, Oregon, Utah, and Washington, including the accreditation of programs offered via distance education within these institutions.
New England Association of Schools & Colleges	**Commission on Institutions of Higher Education**—Accreditation and preaccreditation ("candidacy status") of institutions of higher education in Connecticut, Maine, Massachusetts, New Hampshire, Rhode Island, and Vermont that award associate, bachelor, master's, and/or doctoral degrees, including the accreditation of programs offered via distance education.
	Commission on Technical and Career Institutions—Accreditation and preaccreditation ("candidate status") of secondary institutions with vocational-technical programs at the 13th- and 14th-grade level, postsecondary institutions, and institutions of higher education that provide primarily vocational/technical education at the certificate, associate, and baccalaureate degree levels in Connecticut, Maine, Massachusetts, New Hampshire, Rhode Island, and Vermont. Recognition extends to the Board of Trustees of the Association jointly with the Commission for decisions involving preaccreditation, initial accreditation, and adverse actions.

Source: U.S. Department of Education Web site: Regional and National Institutional Accrediting Agencies.

INTERNATIONAL ACCREDITATION

In many countries, a centralized ministry of education governs postsecondary education, including quality standards and quality assurance. In Canada, the Constitution Act provides authority to each province to make laws and statutes governing education, including higher education. Each of the provinces typically has its own minister of education or a comparable official who is charged with the oversight of universities and degree programs within the province. Institutions may not operate without the approval of the provincial ministry or some other authority such as an agency authorized to accredit independent colleges or universities. An example of this type of agency in Canada is the Campus Alberta Quality Council (CAQC) to which the provincial government has delegated accreditation authority. The CAQC reviews all proposals for new degree programs from both public and private institutions to ensure they are of high quality before they are approved. The Council also conducts periodic evaluations of approved degree programs to ensure that quality standards continue to be met (Government of Alberta, 2009).

Accrediting agencies in the United States are also involved in international accreditation. In many cases, this involves U.S. programs that are being offered overseas but in some cases, agencies actually accredit programs from other countries upon request (Eaton, 2008a). Cooperation between and among accreditation agencies is also occurring globally as is evident in the mutual agreement on accreditation between the CASN and the Commission on Collegiate Nursing Education (CCNE; 2009a) in the United States.

SPECIALIZED ACCREDITING AGENCIES

Accreditation of nursing education programs in the United States began in 1893 with the founding of the American Society of Superintendents of Training Schools of Nurses whose purpose was to establish universal standards for training nurses (Kalisch & Kalisch, 1995). In 1912, this organization became the National League for Nursing Education and in 1917, it published *Standard of Curricula for Schools of Nursing*. In 1952, the National League for Nursing (NLN) was established and assumed responsibility for accrediting nursing education programs (NLNAC, 2008).

From 1952–1998, the NLN was the only professional accrediting agency for nursing. The NLN operated its accreditation functions through four councils that established criteria for programs at various levels (practical, diploma, associate, and baccalaureate and higher degree). Subsequently, the NLN reorganized its accreditation structures, founding the independent NLNAC (Bellack, O'Neil, & Thomsen, 1999). In 1996, however, the American Association of Colleges of Nursing (AACN) announced its intention to establish an accreditation body, the CCNE, which would accredit only baccalaureate and higher degree programs. Both the NLNAC and CCNE are approved by the DOE and CHEA. It is important to note that only those programs whose institutions are not part of a regionally accredited college or university may use NLNAC accreditation to establish eligibility for federal student financial aid assistance. Overbay and Aaltonen (2001) have provided an interesting comparison of NLNAC and CCNE accreditation criteria and commissions for those considering which agency to choose for accreditation (see Table 15.2).

TABLE 15.2 National Nursing Accreditation Agencies in the United States and Canada

Agency Name	Scope of Accreditation	Year Accreditation of Schools Initiated	Last Approved by Department of Education CHEA
National League for Nursing Accrediting Commission (NLNAC) Sharon J. Tanner, Executive Director 3343 Peachtree Road NE, Suite 500 Atlanta, GA 30326 Tel: (404) 975-5000 Fax: (404) 975-5020 E-mail address: stanner@nlnac.org Web address: www.nlnac.org	Accreditation in the United States of programs in practical nursing, and diploma, associate, baccalaureate, and higher degree nurse education programs, including those offered via distance education *Title IV note: Only diploma programs and practical nursing programs not located in a regionally accredited college or university may use accreditation by this agency to establish eligibility to participate in Title IV programs.*	1998*	2007 2001
Commission on Collegiate Nursing Education (CCNE) Jennifer L. Butlin, Director One Dupont Circle NW, Suite 530 Washington, DC 20036-1120 Tel: (202) 887-6791 Fax: (202) 887-8476 E-mail address: jbutlin@aacn.nche.edu Web address: www.aacn.nche.edu/accreditation/index.htm	Accreditation of nursing education programs in the United States, at the baccalaureate and graduate degree levels, including programs offering distance education *Title IV note: Accreditation by this agency does not enable the entities it accredits to establish eligibility to participate in Title IV programs.*	2000	2006 2002
Canadian Association of Schools of Nursing (CASN) 99 Fifth Avenue, Suite 15 Ottawa, ON K1S 5K4 Tel: (613) 235-3150 Fax: (613) 235-4476 Lise Talbot Director of Accreditation Tel: (613) 235-3150 Extension 24 E-mail address: ltalbot@casn.ca	Accreditation of undergraduate nursing programs *CASN. accreditation is a combination of institutional and specialized accreditation in which educational units and nursing education programs are assessed against predetermined standards.*	1987	Not applicable

*The National League for Nursing originally engaged in accreditation in 1952. The independent NLNAC was established in 1998.

Both NLNAC and CCNE have established accreditation criteria that programs must meet to become accredited. These criteria are reviewed and revised on a regular basis by the respective constituencies. Both accrediting bodies operate through a peer review system whereby accreditation site visitors from comparable educational institutions serve as the on-site evaluators. In addition to peer educators, CCNE also includes a practicing nurse whose experience is congruent with the program as part of the evaluation team. The site visitors, upon completion of the site visit, provide a written report to the Board of Review of the respective accrediting agency. In recent years, both nursing accrediting agencies have developed criteria for the clinical doctorate, as well as for programs at other levels. However, only the NLNAC accredits practical, diploma, and associate degree nursing programs.

There are a few additional specialized nursing accreditation agencies for advanced practice nursing programs in the United States. These include the nurse anesthesia and nurse-midwifery. Additional information on these agencies is provided in Table 15.3 that follows. Information on eligibility, standards, and policies for accreditation for these agencies are available on the Web. New programs in nurse-midwifery and nurse anesthesia now require a preapproval process prior to enrolling students (Van Ort, 2009).

In 2006, the Alliance of Advanced Practice Registered Nurse (APRN) Credentialing was established because of concerns that the accreditation of multiple specialties was costly and duplicative for programs. The Alliance, comprised of numerous advanced nursing specialties, has worked toward common processes, common data sets, and commonly accepted standards and norms to reduce duplication of efforts. Because of the rapid expansion of some advanced practice nursing programs, there has been growing concern about the quality of advanced nursing education. Culminating in 2009, a new consensus model for the regulation, licensure, accreditation, certification, and education of advanced practice registered nurses was published. The consensus model was completed through

TABLE 15.3 Specialized Nursing Accreditation Agencies in the United States

Agency Name	Scope of Recognition	Year Established
Council on Accreditation of Nurse Anesthesia Educational Programs Francis Gerbasi Director of Accreditation and Education 222 South Prospect, Suite 304 Park Ridge, IL 60068-4010 Tel: (847) 692-7050 Fax: (847) 692-7137 E-mail address: fgerbasi@aana.com Web address: www.aana.com	Scope of recognition: The accreditation of institutions and programs of nurse anesthesia within the United States at the post-master's, certificate, master's, or doctoral degree levels, including programs offering distance education. *Title IV note:* Only hospital-based nurse anesthesia programs and freestanding nurse anesthesia institutions may use accreditation by this agency to establish eligibility to participate in Title IV programs.	1952
American College of Nurse-Midwives (ACNM), Accreditation Commission for Midwifery Education (ACME) Mary C. Brucker Chair, ACNM Accreditation Commission Nurse-Midwifery Program 8403 Colesville Road, Suite 1550 Silver Spring, MD 20910 Tel: (240) 485-1802 Fax: (240) 485-1818 E-mail address: Mary_Brucker@Baylor.edu Web address: www.midwife.org	Scope of recognition: The accreditation and preaccreditation of basic certificate, basic graduate nurse-midwifery, direct entry midwifery, and precertification nurse-midwifery education programs. The accreditation and preaccreditation of freestanding institutions of midwifery education that may offer other related health care programs to include nurse practitioner programs, and including those institutions and programs that offer distance education. *Title IV note:* Only freestanding institutions of midwifery education may use accreditation by this agency to establish eligibility to participate in Title IV programs.	1982

the work of the APRN Consensus Work Group and the National Council of State Boards of Nursing APRN Advisory Committee. Efforts to move forward on this model continue through these organizations (APRN Joint Dialogue Group, 2008).

ACCREDITATION OF SCHOOLS OF NURSING IN CANADA

Specialized accreditation for nursing in Canada is under the auspices of the CASN. The CASN Board of Accreditation is authorized to review and approve policies. It makes decisions on candidacy and accreditation reviews within established policies and procedures. CASN accreditation is conducted according to guiding principles of the Association of Accrediting Agencies of Canada (AAAC) of which it is a founding member. Accreditation policies were last revised in 2005 and are available online (CASN, 2010).

THE COMMISSION ON GRADUATES OF FOREIGN NURSING SCHOOLS

The Commission on Graduates of Foreign Nursing Schools (CGFNS) is not an accreditation agency per se. However, this independent, nonprofit organization plays a key role in the certification of nursing credentials of nurses migrating into the United States. Faced with a growing rate of migration, and significant complexity in evaluating the educational preparation of nurses educated in foreign countries, several national and state nursing and professional associations held a conference in 1975 to address the problem of foreign nurse credentials. CGFNS was formed as an outgrowth of this conference, and today the organization operates to ensure that nurses educated in countries other than the United States are eligible and qualified to meet state licensure requirements. Eighty-five percent of state boards of nursing require foreign nurses to be screened through the CGFNS process. CGFNS offers a certification program in which a nurse must meet three requirements to be considered for licensure. These include a credentials review, successful passing of a standardized examination, and an English language proficiency examination. Nurses eligible for this program include those who are graduates of first-level general nursing education programs as defined by the International Council of Nurses. General nursing education includes didactic and clinical instruction across a broad spectrum of nursing practice. The Commission provides both a credential evaluation service and a certification program (CGFNS, 2010).

THE ACCREDITATION PROCESS

The accreditation process typically involves five major elements. These include an institutional self-study, peer review, site visit, action by the accrediting association, and periodic monitoring and oversight (Eaton, 2009). The self-study is a self-analysis of performance completed by the school based on the standards of the accrediting association. Peer review occurs because of the broad involvement of the various stakeholders in the educational environment: faculty, administrators, key partners, and the public. Site visits are typically conducted to verify the results of the self-study and to provide additional clarification to the accrediting agency. The action of the accrediting agency occurs after the submission of the self-study and the site visit with consideration of the entire body of evidence by the review panel for the accrediting agency. Programs or schools are normally reviewed in a cycle of 5–10 years, with monitoring and oversight occurring through the submission of annual reports by the schools and substantive change reports to the agency when major change occurs.

Curriculum Planning and Accreditation

Curriculum planning should take accreditation requirements and statements of essential competencies into account from the onset (AACN, 2008, 2010; CCNE, 2009b, 2009c; NLNAC, 2008). A basic understanding of accreditation requirements enables faculty to develop a program that complies with key requirements established by accreditation agencies. Although such agencies generally attempt to avoid being overly prescriptive, there may be specific criteria or standards that must be met by a program to be approved. Accreditation standards for professional programs, for example, will often outline a minimum set of academic and clinical requirements that must be included in the program. Thus, the minimum number of credits for the entire professional component of the program may be prescribed and even the minimum number of credits or hours of clinical practice within a specialized clinical area may be indicated. These requirements have been established by the accreditation agency or regulatory board based on broad input from the profession as well as other constituents including public consumers. Among the many considerations in developing a new or revised curriculum are the standards and criteria established by those agencies that accredit the college or university as well as those required by nursing accrediting bodies (CCNE, 2009c; NLNAC, 2008).

The development of the organizing curriculum framework warrants consideration of accreditation standards. Daggett, Butts, and Smith (2002) describe the development of an updated organizing framework by one faculty in its long-term preparation for accreditation. Seager and Anema (2003) and Heinrich et al. (2002) describe the benefits of using a matrix or audit process to ensure curriculum integrity in preparation for accreditation and as a part of continuous improvement efforts.

Planning for Accreditation

Developing an Evaluation Plan

The previous chapters provided guidance on the development of a school or program evaluation plan. It is a good idea to formulate this plan early on to begin collecting baseline data when students first begin a nursing program. Thompson and Bartels (1999) review the literature on assessment and describe one school's response to the development of a systematic plan for outcomes assessment. Similarly, Davenport and coauthors offer a step-by-step process for curriculum review to aid in preparation for accreditation (Davenport, Spath, & Bauvelt, 2009). It is also important that this plan focus on learning outcomes and not just program outputs. Ewell (2001) describes this shift in emphasis to learning outcomes in a CHEA publication on accreditation and student learning outcomes. Ingersoll and Sauter (1998) also describe how accreditation criteria can be integrated effectively into the evaluation plan. Accreditation standards, criteria, procedures, and policies are readily available from the accrediting associations and their Web sites.

Theoretical Framework for Evaluation

Several evaluation theories are available to provide a framework for the evaluation plan. The use of a theoretical approach helps provide an organizing lens for identification and analysis of data. Refer to theories described in the previous chapter for guidance in this area.

Developing a Timeline

Accreditation is like any major project. The scope and size of the work can be overwhelming. A way to deal with this effectively is to break this task up into manageable bits that can be delegated and timed over a lengthy preparation period. Often, the accrediting agency will provide some useful direction about possible key dates in a planning timeline. Preparation time may need to be extended if it must include faculty development for the director and/or faculty who do not have prior experience with the accreditation process.

Role of Administrators, Faculty, Students, and Consumers

Everyone has a role in the accreditation process. Administrators provide leadership and direction, supporting the efforts of the task force or faculty committee assigned to conduct the self-study. The members of the faculty aid the work of the team by becoming familiar with the accreditation standards, providing timely information needed for the self-study, providing critical feedback on the draft of the report, and preparing to participate in the site visit. Students participate by learning about accreditation, cooperating with the site visitors during visits to classes and clinical sites, and by participating in school committees engaged in CQI. Other stakeholders include clinical partners and consumers who participate by responding to evaluation surveys and serving on advisory committees. One of the major recommendations of a national task force on accreditation of health professions (and a key principle in CQI) is that programs should be required to establish effective linkages with their stakeholders, including the public, students, and professional organizations (The Center for Health Professions University of California, San Francisco, 1999). When developing the evaluation plan, faculty should consider how these linkages can be effectively established. As the focus of accreditation has shifted to evaluation of evidence of achievement of program outcomes rather than inputs, linkages with alumni and employers has become increasingly important, as these groups are often a key source for evaluation evidence.

Preparing the Accreditation Report

Assignments should be given to teams or individuals to prepare drafts of the various sections of the self-study report. The drafts should be widely circulated for discussion among faculty members. An open forum for faculty, students, and other stakeholders may be offered to provide maximum opportunity for constructive criticism and shaping of final recommendations. This process provides the opportunity for faculty members to refocus on the accreditation criteria and analyze how their respective courses reflect the accreditation criteria and fit into the overall curriculum plan. One person should do the final writing of the report to provide a coherent and consistent voice to the document.

It is also recommended that someone be asked to do a final editing of the report before printing. The report should be candid and accurate. You do not want the site visitors to find that the report glossed over major issues or controversies.

Preparing for the Site Visit

The purpose of the site visit is to provide an opportunity for external reviewers (site visitors) to verify the information provided in the self-study and to provide supplemental information to aid the review panel in making the accreditation decision. Thus, planning for the site visit is a key part of the accreditation process. Faculty, students, and staff will need to be oriented to the site-visit process and procedures and careful attention to this aspect of the process can make a major difference in the success of the visit (Davidhizar & Vance, 1998).

Approximately 2–3 months before the site visit, planning begins to shift to the site-visit phase of accreditation. The designated chair of the institution's accreditation process should follow the guidelines of the accreditation agency in making hotel accommodations for site visitors. This information may be available on the agency's Web site.

Faculty and support staff members who have not been involved in the self-study process should be oriented to the accreditation process and procedures prior to the site visit. Davidhizar and Vance (1998) suggest that such sessions provide an opportunity to review the organizing framework of a curriculum and key policies (e.g., grievance procedures), with both students and faculty. It is also advisable to make an appointment with administrators such as the president, academic vice president, and dean of the division, if nursing is a part of a larger academic unit, to familiarize them with the date and purpose of the visit, providing a context for their involvement and likely interviews by the site visitors. It is very important to provide significant advanced notice of the site visit to these individuals to ensure they will be available at some point during the visit if requested by the site visitors.

Some programs find that arranging a mock site visit a month or so before the actual site visit can be a valuable exercise if most of the faculty members have never experienced an accreditation visit previously. A mock site visit can be arranged by having one or two peers, who have accreditation experience, visit the institution to conduct interviews and to make class and clinical visits just like the official site visitors will do. A mock visit is like a dress rehearsal and can be a real learning experience for less seasoned faculty as well as for students. Often, this experience motivates faculty to read the self-study with more care than they might otherwise exercise.

It is highly recommended that accommodations be provided, which are not too distant from the campus to save travel time. Depending on the size of the team, it is often feasible that the chair of the team be provided with a larger hotel room or suite to accommodate team conferences and writing of the summative report. A meeting space at the hotel is important as the team will often spend long evening hours discussing the materials and interviews scheduled for each day and writing the report.

An exhibit room on campus should provide for displays of evidence and supplemental materials that the site visitors can use to verify information presented in the self-study report. It is helpful to provide a matrix of the display materials according to the standards and criteria so that the visitors can quickly find them (Flannigan, Cluskey, & Gard, 2002). Typically, the materials in the exhibit room are those materials that are too large or too numerous to be included in the self-study report. These include the faculty handbook, samples of examinations or of student work, institutional data such as fact books, institutional and departmental strategic plans, recruitment materials, departmental newsletters, university publications, and so on. Careful attention to the selection and organization of materials can be important in highlighting program strengths and creating a favorable impression (McDaniel, 2010). The exhibit room should provide a computer and printer for the site visitors' use on campus. A conference table for meetings of the team is also recommended to be available in the exhibit room.

Site visitors themselves usually make travel arrangements. Institutions and programs are discouraged from entertaining or providing gifts to site visitors other than some small token such as items with the institution's logo (e.g., a mug or portfolio). Sometimes even this type of courtesy is prohibited and site visitors may even be required by the agency to pay for their own meals to ensure that there is no perception of conflict of interest. It is important to remember that site visitors do not make the accreditation decision themselves. Typically, the site visitor describes findings and may note strengths or weaknesses in the program, but the review panel of the accrediting body will be the actual decision maker. For this reason, site visitors may recommend that supplemental materials be sent to the review panel if they find information that has not been included in the self-study but which may be important to demonstrating that an institution or program is meeting accreditation standards.

Typically, the board or designated review panel of the accrediting agency or regulatory body meets at regular intervals to review the entire body of evidence provided by the institution and the site visitors. A few members of the review panel may be assigned as primary readers and reviewers of the materials. Following a summation of evidence, the review panel will make its decision. Review panels usually only meet a few times a year so programs may not learn about the outcomes of their accreditation report and site visit until several months after the team has left campus. Normally programs will be given some indication by the site visitors on whether there are any major deficiencies or recommendations to address. It is often advantageous to begin work on these items shortly after the visit because these items are very salient to faculty who are motivated to respond to the recommendations. It should be remembered, however, that the review panel makes the final recommendations and may not come to the exact same conclusions as the site visitors.

Once the accreditation commission reviews the program, a formal decision and set of recommendations will be received from the accrediting agency. A copy of this report is usually sent to the president or chancellor of the institution as well as to the dean or director of the school. Follow-up activities may include a progress report after a defined period if deficiencies have been noted or if institutional capacity to sustain its present positive state is not clearly demonstrated.

Once initial accreditation is achieved, faculty and administration will benefit from viewing accreditation as an ongoing process. Faculty has the responsibility to evaluate the curriculum in light of the accreditation standards on a regular basis. Administration and faculty share the responsibility of evaluating data related to student outcomes as well as other survey data that reflect the achievement of program goals and adherence to accreditation standards. Documentation of evaluation activities, including decisions made to improve program quality is essential. Minutes of committee and departmental meetings should reflect the fact that data on program outcomes has been analyzed regularly and that an action plan for improvement has been implemented.

SUMMARY

Preparation for accreditation is a core activity for the current generation of nursing faculty. An effective way to build the collective expertise of faculty in accreditation is to plan for orientation and faculty development on this topic on a regular basis. Engagement in regular activities that demonstrate the principles of CQI are recommended to ensure faculty and student appreciation and cooperation in accreditation activities. Development of an evaluation plan, which uses selected tools such as a curriculum matrix or audit, is identified as a best practice in preparation for accreditation. Student, alumni, and employer surveys to assess stakeholder key requirements and satisfaction are other elements that should be used regularly rather than episodically to enhance program improvement. Data on program outcomes such as comprehensive exams, licensure results, analyses of capstone projects, and employer evaluations are a few examples of evidence of educational effectiveness, which should be gathered and analyzed over time. Development of an accreditation timeline with definitive deadlines is strongly recommended as a tool to manage the accreditation process.

DISCUSSION QUESTIONS

1. What are ways in which students and faculty can be motivated to participate actively in preparation for accreditation?
2. What strategies can be used to begin to imbed a culture of CQI within a school of nursing?
3. What data would provide credible evidence that a nursing program is being successful in achieving its mission and stated learning outcomes?

LEARNING ACTIVITIES

Student Learning Activities

1. In a small group, explore the implications of accreditation for you as a student nurse. What difference would it make if your nursing school does not have accreditation?
2. Go to a Web site for specialized nursing accreditation and review the standards for accreditation. Describe how these standards focus on achievement of learning outcomes and educational effectiveness.
3. Pick one standard and write a draft report on how your program meets that standard. Indicate what information you would have to collect to provide evidence that your program meets that standard.

Faculty Development Activities

1. Take the evaluation plan for your nursing program or school and develop a timeline for the next accreditation visit.
2. Develop an orientation program about accreditation and the accreditation process for a new faculty.

3. Describe the two issues and challenges facing accreditation in the rapidly changing environment of higher education today.
4. Describe three strategies that a faculty can engage in each semester/term to verify continued compliance with accreditation criteria.

REFERENCES

Advanced Practice Registered Nurse Joint Dialogue Group. (2008). *Consensus model for APRN regulation: Licensure, accreditation, certification & education.* Retrieved July 7, 2008, from http://www.aacn.nche.edu/Education/pdf/**APRN**Report.pdf

American Association of Colleges of Nursing. (2008). *The essentials of baccalaureate education for professional nursing practice.* Washington, DC: Author.

American Association of Colleges of Nursing. (2010). *The essentials of master's education in nursing (draft).* Washington, DC: Author.

Bacon, P. (2003). Do not know much about history: Congress debates bringing colleges to bear with academic standards. *Time Magazine.* Retrieved May 12, 2003, from http://www.time.com.time/archive/preview

Barnum, B. S. (1997). Licensure, certification, and accreditation. *Online Journal of Issues in Nursing.* Retrieved August 13, 1997, from http://www.nursingworld.org/ojin/tpc4/ptc4-w.htm

Bellack, J., O'Neil, E., & Thomsen, C.(1999). Responses of baccalaureate and graduate programs to the emergence of choice in nursing accreditation. *Journal of Nursing Education, 38*(2), 53–61.

Canadian Association of Schools of Nursing. (2010). *CASN Accreditation: Recognition of excellence.* Retrieved, from htpp://www.casn.ca/Accreditation

The Center for Health Professions University of California, San Francisco. (1999). *Strategies for change and improvement: Taskforce on accreditation of health professions education working papers.* San Francisco: Author. Retrieved, from http://futurehealth.ucsf.edu/pubs.html

Collins, M. S. (1997). Issues of accreditation: A dean's perspective. *Online Journal of Issues in Nursing.* Retrieved, from http://www.nursingworld.org/ojin/tpc4/tpc4-1.htm

Commission on Collegiate Nursing Education. (2009a). *Mutual recognition agreement on accreditation between the Canadian Association of Schools of Nursing (CASN/ACESI) and the Commission on Collegiate Nursing Education 2009–2012.* Retrieved, from http://ccne.org

Commission on Collegiate Nursing Education (2009b). *Procedures for accreditation of baccalaureate and graduate degree nursing programs.*Washington, DC. Retrieved, from http://acne/nche.edu/accreditation

Commission on Collegiate Nursing Education (2009c). *Standards for accreditation of baccalaureate and graduate nursing education programs.* Washington, DC. Retrieved, from http://aacn/nche.edu/accreditation

Commission on Graduates of Foreign Nursing Schools. (2010). *General frequently asked questions.* Retrieved, from http://www.cgfns.org/sections/tools/faq

Council for Higher Education Accreditation. (2010). *Directory of CHEA Recognized Organizations.* Retrieved from http://www.chea.org/pdf/2010_2011_Directory_of_CHEA_Recognized_Organizations.pdf

Daggett, L. M., Butts, J. B., & Smith, K. K. (2002). The development of an organizing framework to implement AACN guidelines for nursing education. *Journal of Nursing Education, 41*(1), 34–37.

Davenport, N. C., Spath, M. L., & Bauvelt, M. J. (2009). A step-by-step approach to curriculum review. *Nursing Education, 34*(4), 181–185.

Davidhizar, R., & Vance, A. R. (1998). Preparing for a National League for Nursing Accreditation Commission site visit. *Association of Black Nursing Faculty Journal, 9*(3), 65–8.

Eaton, J. S. (2008a). *Accreditation and recognition in the U.S. council for higher education accreditation.* Washington, DC: Council for Higher Education Accreditation. Retrieved, from http://www.chea.org

Eaton, J. S. (2008b) *The higher education opportunity act of 2008: What does it mean and what does it do? Inside higher education*. Washington, DC: Council for Higher Education Accreditation. Retrieved October 30, 2008, from http://www.chea.org

Eaton, J. S. (2009). *An overview of U.S. accreditation*. Washington, DC: Council for Higher Education Accreditation. Retrieved, from http://www.chea.org

Eaton, J. S. (2010). *Accreditation 2.0. Inside higher education*. Washington, DC: Council for Higher Education Accreditation. Retrieved January 18, 2010, from http:// www.chea.org

Ewell, P. T. (2001). *Accreditation and student learning outcomes: A proposed point of departure*. Washington, DC: Council for Higher Education Accreditation Occasional Paper.

Flannigan, P., Cluskey, M., & Gard, C. (2002). Accreditation strategies: Planning for an accreditation visit. *Nurse Educator, 27*(4), 157–158.

Fritschler, A. L. (2007). Government should stay out of accreditation. *Chronicle of Higher Education*, B-20.

Gose, B. (2002). A radical approach to accreditation. *The Chronicle of Higher Education*, A25–A27.

Government of Alberta. (2009). Education in Alberta—Types of institutions. *Alberta Learning Information Service*. Retrieved, from http://alis.alberta.ca/et/studyinalberta/institutions.html

Guerard, E. B. (2002). Lawmakers question role of college accrediting agencies. *Education Daily, 35*(i187), *8*(2).

Heinrich, C. R., Karner, K. J., Gaglione, B. H., & Lambert, L. J. (2002). Order out of chaos: The use of a matrix to validate curriculum integrity. *Nurse Educator, 27*(3), 136–140.

Higher Learning Commission. (2010). HLC pathways construction project: A proposed new model for continued accreditation (Draft Version 6, January 31, 2010). Retrieved, from http://www.ncahlc.org

Ingersoll, G. L., & Sauter, M. (1998). Integrating accreditation criteria into educational program evaluation. *Nursing and Health Care Perspectives, 19*(5), 224–229.

Kalisch, P. A., & Kalisch, B. J. (1995). *The advance of American nursing*. Philadelphia: J. B. Lippincott.

McDaniel, T. R. (2010). Five tips for surviving accreditation: A tongue-in cheek reflection. *Faculty Focus*. Retrieved March 28, 2010, from http//:facultyfocus.com/?p511956

Morgan, R. (2002). Lawmakers at hearing on college-accreditation system call for more accountability. *The Chronicle of Higher Education*. Retrieved, from http://chronicle.com/daily/2002/10/2002100204n.htm

National Institute for Standards and Technology. (2010). Education criteria for performance excellence. *The Baldrige National QualityProgram*. Retrieved, from http://www.nist.gov/baldrige/publications

National League for Nursing Accrediting Commission. (2008). *National league for nursing accrediting commission accreditation manual*. Retrieved, from http://www.nlnac.org

National League for Nursing Accrediting Commission. (2009). *Executive director appointed to a second U.S. DOE negotiated rule-making team*. Retrieved, from http://nlnac.org/home.htm

New England Association of Schools and Colleges Commission on Institutions of Higher Education. (2010). *U.S. Regional Accreditation: An Overview*. Retrieved from http://cihe.neasc.org/about_accreditation/regional_accreditation_overview

Nkongho, N. (2006). The NLNAC mentoring program: Demystifying the accreditation process. *Nursing Education Perspectives, 27*(2), 70–71.

O'Neil, E. (1997). Using accreditation for your purposes. *AAHE Bulletin*. Retrieved June 1997, from http://aahebulletin.com/public/archive

Ontario Ministry of Education. (2008). Degree authority in Ontario. *Ontario Ministry of Training, Colleges, and Universities*. Retrieved, from http://www.edu.gov.on.ca/eng/general/postsedc/degreegauth.html

Overbay, J. D., & Aaltonen, P. M. (2001). A comparison of NLNAC and CCNE accreditation. *Nurse Educator, 26*(1), 17–27.

Seager, S. R., & Anema, M. G. (2003). A process for conducting a curriculum audit. *Nurse Educator, 28*(1), 5–6.

Suhayda, R., & Miller, J. M. (2006). Optimizing evaluation of nursing education programs. *Nurse Educator. 31*(5), 200–206.

Thompson, C., & Bartels, J. E. (1999). Outcomes assessment: Implications for nursing education. *Journal of Professional Nursing, 15*(3), 170–178.

University of Phoenix. (2010). *Just the Facts*. Retrieved, from http://phoenix.edu/about_us/media_relations/just-the-facts.html

U.S. Department of Education. (2009). *An overview of the U.S. Department of Education*. Retrieved from http://www2.ed.gov/about/overview/whattoc.html?src=In

Van Damme, D. (2002). Quality assurance in an international environment: National and international interests and tensions. In *International quality review: Values, opportunities, and issues*. Washington, DC: Council for Higher Education Accreditation Occasional Paper.

Van Ort, S. (2009). *Overview of accreditation in achieving excellence in accreditation: The first 10 years of CCNE*. Retrieved, from http://ccne.org

Western Association of Schools & Colleges Senior Commission. (2009). Guidelines for the evaluation of distance education (On-line Learning, C-RAC). Retrieved, from http://www:wascsenior.org

VI Issues and Trends in Curriculum Development and Evaluation

Sarah B. Keating

Section 6 reviews current trends and issues in nursing education for their effect on curricula and the imperatives derived from them that influence curriculum development and evaluation activities now and in the future. This section of the text addresses specific trends in nursing education related to the growth of technology-driven distance education programs and the utilization of clinical simulations and other high-technology devices for the acquisition of nursing knowledge and skills. These phenomena had a dramatic effect on the delivery of nursing education and raise issues related to quality, cost-effectiveness, and competitiveness of programs in the marketplace.

Chapter 16 examines informatics and technology and their influence on nursing education. It traces the history of distance education from the early home study programs to today's high technology–based programs delivered from home campuses to distant satellite campuses as well as virtual campuses in cyberspace. The chapter goes on to examine realistic clinical simulation programs that allow students to acquire basic, advanced, and critical-thinking nursing skills in a safe environment prior to actual clinical practice. Other high-technology devices and systems such as personal digital assistants (PDAs), electronic record systems, and advanced communication systems add to the rapid changes in the delivery of education and the need for students and faculty to keep abreast of the newer innovations.

Chapter 17 reexamines some of the issues raised in the text and offers possible solutions that could affect the future of nursing education. A look at nursing education in hindsight leads to a forecast of the future including several scenarios for education and their impact on the profession. Members of the nursing profession are asked to discard old prohibitive ways of thinking about nursing education and its mandate to provide knowledgeable, competent, and caring professionals and move into the future with innovative and creative nursing programs that continue to educate nurses ready for the challenges of the health care system. Several curricula are proposed with new ways to embrace the traditional career ladder feature of nursing and, at the same time, facilitate a nonstop quality education ending in a doctorate that produces nurse researchers, theorists, educators, advanced practice nurses, and leaders. The proposed curricula are not meant as templates but rather as stimulants for discussion among nurse educators and those in practice to bring about needed changes now and in the future.

The issues and challenges raised throughout the text can change the face of nursing education and the profession. They cannot be ignored. Unfortunately, if changes are not made, the profession may find itself outdated and unable to keep up with changes in the health care system to meet the needs of the populations it purports to serve. With other health care disciplines moving rapidly toward entry-level doctorates, nursing must continue to move its trajectory for higher education or find itself out-of-sync with other professionals and the health care system. Chapters 16 and 17 begin the discussion for nurse educators and their role in meeting the challenges and their plans for the future.

Effects of Informatics and Technology on Curriculum Development and Evaluation

Sarah B. Keating

OBJECTIVES

Upon completion of Chapter 16, the reader will be able to:

1. Analyze the various types of distance education programs that are utilized in the delivery of nursing education programs.
2. Analyze the application of technology and informatics and their effectiveness in the implementation of the nursing curriculum.
3. Review the literature related to the efficacy of distance education programs.
4. Examine the issues facing nurse educators that relate to the application of informatics and technology in nursing education.

INTRODUCTION

Chapter 16 discusses the effects of informatics and technology on curriculum development and evaluation. Distance education formats are reviewed including land-based satellites, broadcasting by teleconferences and videoconferences, and Web-based platforms. Other technological advances such as patient simulations, electronic record systems, and information systems applied to education and health care are analyzed. A brief review of the research findings on the efficacy of these programs and student satisfaction are presented and issues related to distance education and technology are introduced.

DISTANCE EDUCATION PROGRAMS

Distance education is defined as any learning experience that takes place a distance away from the parent educational institution's home campus. It can be as close as a few blocks away in an urban center to as far away as another nation(s). It implements the curriculum through a planned strategy for the delivery of courses or classes that include off-site satellite classes managed by the home faculty or credentialed off-site faculty, broadcast of classes through videoconferencing, and teleconferencing to off-campus sites, Web-based instruction, and faculty-supervised clinical experiences including preceptorships and internships. Distance education offers continuing education programs, degree programs, single academic courses, or a mixture of on-campus and off-campus course offerings.

The following discussion reviews off-site satellite programs with land-based facilities and programs that use videoconferencing and teleconferencing to broadcast the program. Distance education formats through cyberspace follow the discussion on videoconferencing and teleconferencing.

Needs Assessment and Compatibility With the Components of the Curriculum

When planning for a distance education program, nurse educators must have supporting data from an assessment of the external and internal frame factors that document the need for a distance education program. It should include the projected success of the program based on a business case, cost analysis, assured applicant pool, and a business plan. Once the needs assessment is completed and a time frame is in place, planners review all of the components of the curriculum to ensure congruence with the originating educational program. For details on curriculum components, see Chapters 5, 6, and 7. In addition, an evaluation plan is developed to ensure the quality of the program.

External Frame Factors

Using the components of assessment from the internal and external frame factors, a needs assessment reveals the feasibility of mounting a distance education program. If the program plans an off-campus but on-land satellite program, the external frame factors include an assessment of the community where the program is to take place with such factors as community location and receptivity to distance education, the population's characteristics and its sophistication in technology, the delivery of education afar from the home campus, and the ability to create an academic setting away from the home campus. Additional external frame factor considerations include the political climate and body politic (i.e., the openness to off-site educational programs and possible competitive issues from vendors of distance education programs and other nursing education programs that serve the region). The health care system and health needs of the populace have an influence on the program as to how the graduates of the program can serve them. It is necessary to learn if there are potential collaborative opportunities to supply the program with students who are staff in the off-site health care agencies and who are interested in furthering their education for career opportunities.

A demonstrated need for a distance education program includes an adequate student body that will continue for at least 5–10 years, support from members of the nursing profession in the region that is to be served, and national, regional, and state regulations and accreditation agencies' approvals. Usually, the sponsoring program must notify all accrediting and approval agencies of its plans to offer the distance education program with each of these agencies requiring specific descriptions of the program including the potential student body, faculty, curriculum plan, academic and capital infrastructure support systems, timelines, plans for evaluation, and most importantly, financial feasibility with a business plan.

Internal Frame Factors

Much like the external frame factors, a review of the internal frame factors provides additional information in the planning for a distance education program. Of prime concern is the support of the parent academic institution and its experience with distance education programs. If it has a history of managing these types of programs, it is more apt to be supportive of the nursing program. Even more advantageous is an established distance education program from the parent institution that exists in the proposed delivery site. A check with the mission and purpose, philosophy, and goals of the parent institution and the nursing program is in order to ensure the distance education's program's congruence with those of the parent. The internal economic situation and its influence on distance education programs are critical to the financial feasibility of the program.

Cost Issues

If the recommendations from the needs assessment demonstrate that the distance education program is viable, the school of nursing administration prepares a business case to present to the parent institution. The purpose for a business case is to persuade key administrators and stakeholders that establishing a distance education program meets the mission of the institution, has a substantial potential student body, and adapts the existing accredited program to a satellite format without compromising its quality. The business case describes the program in detail and demonstrates that it is economically feasible. If prior distance education programs have demonstrated success in bringing revenues to the program or are indeed successful, at the least self-sufficient, it is more likely that new programs will be supported. After presentation to and approval by the administration, the business case is developed into a detailed business plan.

The first and foremost cost issue to address in the business plan is the economic feasibility of the distance education program based on an analysis of expected start-up costs, administrative costs, required number of faculty and staff, capital expenses (on-site facilities and technology support systems), and academic support (recruitment, admission, records, library access, and student support systems). Many times, the needs assessment becomes a write-off at the expense of the nursing program and is financed through contingency funds or program development funds generated from grant overhead costs. The plan should include possible initial grant support for start-up funds and plans for eventual self-sufficiency. The resources that are required from the parent institution are listed and include any off-site offices, laboratories, and classrooms; clinical experience facilities; technological support systems for videoconferencing, teleconferencing, and/or Web-based instruction; administrative, faculty, and staff expenses; and academic support systems such as library, academic, and student services. Included in the assessment is a list of potential administrators, staff, faculty, and the proposed program's student body characteristics.

The administration's role and costs include supervisory or management functions to implement the program such as budget and personnel management, liaison activities with regional stakeholders, public relations, coordination, marketing plans, and preparation of reports to seek approval and accreditation of the distance education program from relevant agencies. Some of the staff and/or faculty cost considerations are the required full-time and part-time equivalents, benefits, travel and other expenses, supplies, and equipment.

These expenses vary according to the selected method of delivery of the educational program. For example, off-site offices, classrooms, and laboratory facilities are necessary for satellite courses or classes conducted by on-site faculty or traveling faculty from the home campus. Expenses for this type of program are rent, telephones, computer support for faculty, staff, and students, and the usual office and classroom teaching supplies, hardware, and software such as computers, printers, audiovisual hardware and software, laboratory supplies, paper, correspondence materials, desks, chairs, laboratory clinical equipment and supplies, and so forth.

Curriculum and Evaluation Plans

In addition to the economic feasibility for the program, an analysis of the curriculum is in order to ensure that the proposed distant program is congruent with the mission, goals, organizational framework, and student learning outcomes of the parent program. Although the format and delivery of the curriculum may differ from the original, it must meet the same goals and objectives of the program. Administrators and faculty must make decisions regarding the format and have a rationale for why certain formats are chosen (e.g., on-land satellites, videoconferencing and/or teleconferencing, Web-based platforms).

The new program should be integrated into the master plan of evaluation of the parent program to ensure its quality. Additionally, it should have its own evaluation plan for monitoring the program because it is implemented for corrections along the way (formative evaluation), and to have summative evaluation plans in place that measure the success of the program is terms of student learning outcomes and success, satisfaction of the stakeholders, and its continued congruence with the components of the parent program's curriculum. See Table 16.1 for guidelines for the development of distance education programs.

TYPES OF DISTANCE EDUCATION PROGRAMS

The following is a description of the major types of distance education program. Some of the pros and cons for them are listed.

Satellite Campuses

For the purposes of this discussion, **satellite campuses** are defined as those programs that offer the curriculum in whole or in part on off-campus sites from the parent institution. Although they can incorporate technology methods such as videoconferencing and Web-based instruction, the majority of the teaching and learning takes place in classrooms and involves in-person interactions between the faculty and students. Faculty members who teach in the parent institution serve as on-site faculty or act as consultants to off-site faculty who teach the same curriculum. For those faculty members on the home campus who actually teach in the satellite, travel costs and the related time

TABLE 16.1 Guidelines for the Development of a Distance Education Program

Guideline Topic	Questions for Data Collection and Analysis	Desired Outcome
Needs assessment: External Frame Factors	To what extent are the distant sites supportive of the program and sophisticated in the use of technology?	The community is receptive to distance education programs, sophisticated or open to the technology of distance education, and has a health care system supportive of the program, the nursing profession, and student clinical experiences, if indicated.
	To what extent has the health care system demonstrated support for the program and the nursing profession?	
	To what extent is the health care system open to student clinical experiences and what resources do they have available for the experiences?	The program is competitive with other programs.
	To what extent is the program competitive with other educational program at the site(s)?	There is a potential student body that will continue at least 5–10 years.
	To what extent is there a potential student body at the site(s) and is there an indication that it will continue for at least 5–10 years?	
External Frame Factors	Have program approval and accreditation bodies been notified of the program and do they approve or is there an indication that they will approve the program in the future?	Relevant program approval and accrediting agencies have been notified and approve the program or there are indications for approval in the future.
Needs assessment: Internal Frame Factors	To what extent does the distance education program's mission, philosophy, organizing framework, goals, & objectives reflect those of the parent institution?	The mission, purpose, philosophy, organizing framework, goals, and objectives of the distance education program are congruent with the parent institution.
	To what extent does the parent institution have experience in the selected modality(ies) of distance education and/or have the resources to support it?	The parent institution has experience with and/or the resources to support the program.
	Are there plans in place that indicate adequate resources for the program including infrastructure, human resources, and academic program support?	Plans are in place and resources are adequate for academic infrastructure, human resources, and academic program support.
Economic feasibility	To what extent will the parent institution support a needs assessment for the distance education program? If there are no funds from the institution, are there other possible resources?	There is support from the parent institution or other sources for a needs assessment.
	Are there start-up funds available from the institution or are there other sources such as funds from partner health care or educational institutions?	There are start-up funds from the parent institution or other sources.
	Does the business case justify the need for the program including its congruence with the mission of the institution, a demonstrated need for the program in the community, an adequate potential student body, and assurance of the maintenance of its quality?	The business case is persuasive and includes justification for the development of the program, (i.e., meets mission, meets a need, has an adequate potential student boy, maintains quality).
		The business plan includes funds for the required personnel, administrative costs, facilities (if indicated), academic support systems, and the required technology system.

(Continued)

TABLE 16.1 Guidelines for the Development of a Distance Education Program *Continued*

Guideline Topic	Questions for Data Collection and Analysis	Desired Outcome
	Has the business plan accounted for personnel costs (staff, technicians, and faculty); administrative costs; facilities (if indicated); academic support systems, (e.g. library, enrollment services, financial aid, etc.); and the required technology system(s)?	There are financial plans in place for self-sufficiency and maintenance of the program.
	To what extent are there plans for self-sufficiency? Are there projections for the size of the student body and other resources necessary to maintain the program?	
Congruence with the components of the curriculum	To what extent does the curriculum plan for the distance education program reflect that of the parent institution, (e.g. course descriptions, credits, objectives, and content)?	The distance education program's curriculum plan is congruent with that of the parent institution.
Delivery model options: Options	Have all modalities been considered including off-site, on-land satellite campuses, video-conferencing and/or teleconferencing, and online or Web-based methods?	All modalities for the delivery method are reviewed to lead to a rationale for the selected model or combination of several.
Delivery model options: Selection and its rationale	To what extent does the selected model fit the learning needs of the students?	The selected model fits the learning needs of the students.
	To what extent are there faculty who can utilize the model(s)? If not are there faculty development plans and technical support in place?	The selected model is within the scope of the faculty's expertise or there are faculty development plans in place.
	To what extent is the selected model "user-friendly" for students and faculty?	The selected model is "user-friendly" for students and faculty.
Delivery model: Implementation plan	To what extent is the selected model(s) congruent with the curriculum plan?	The selected model is congruent with the curriculum plan.
	Does the selected model fit the implementation plan of the curriculum (i.e. is it possible to deliver theory, lab, and clinical experiences)?	The curriculum plan can be implemented through utilization of the selected model(s).
Delivery Model: Evaluation	Is there an evaluation plan in place and to what extent is it congruent with the master plan of the parent institution?	There is an evaluation plan in place and it is congruent with the master plan of evaluation for the parent institution.
	Does the evaluation plan include both formative and summative evaluation measures?	The evaluation plan includes both formative and summative measures.
	To what extent does the evaluation plan include strategies for follow-up and revisions if necessary based on the data analyses and recommendations from the evaluation plan?	The evaluation plan has mechanisms in place to revise the program according to data analyses and recommendations from evaluation activities.
	Is the selected delivery model(s) relevant to current education practices?	The selected delivery model is relevant to current education practices and adaptable to future changes in the education, profession, and health care systems.
	To what extent is the selected model adaptable to future changes in the profession and education and health care systems?	

it takes for travel are included in the costs of implementing the program. These costs are weighed against the cost of the salary and benefits for hiring on-site faculty.

There are added challenges for finding off-site faculty who are qualified to teach the subject matter and they must be oriented to the curriculum to ensure its integrity. Thus, it is not unusual for the parent institution to have an academic manager for the satellite program(s) who can serve as the curriculum and academic services coordinator. In the instances of off-site satellite campuses, the course content and materials for both theory and clinical are identical to that of the home campus. Special events to link the off-site and home campuses are often planned to foster the socialization process for students and faculty so that there is a milieu of all people belonging to the same institution.

Additional resources are needed to implement the distant satellite campus such as students' access to texts through either the home bookstore or other resources such as online book companies, library access, online access if it is part of the curriculum, and student services including academic, financial aid, and personal counseling usually through the on-site coordinator and his or her staff. Recruitment, admission, and enrollment services are additional resources that can be served by on-site personnel if the program is large or by home-campus staff who travel periodically to the satellite campus.

Some of the arguments against these types of program are the loss of students on the home campus, possible incongruence between the implementation of the courses in the curriculum owing to a loss of interactions among students and faculty with the home campus, a danger that the majority of the faculty and staff are part time and therefore some of the commitment to the institution is lost, and the possibility that the program is too costly and cannot become self-sufficient. Some of the arguments for these types of distance education programs include the interpersonal communications and relationships between faculty and students and a sense of belonging to the parent institution through face-to-face encounters on campus or other on-land locations. If there is a careful plan for implementing the curriculum, there is an assurance that the curriculum remains intact. Some cost savings for students and the institution can be realized in travel and personnel expenses if some of the faculty and staff are part time.

Videoconferencing and Teleconferencing

Some distance education programs are delivered to off-campus sites through videoconferencing and/or telecommunications. Videoconferencing requires dedicated classrooms that can send and receive satellite broadcasting both on-site at the home campus and off-site at the distant campus(es). The ideal videoconferencing system has classrooms located on all sites with the ability to send and receive thus facilitating live interactive teaching and learning experiences among students and faculty. However, some off-site campuses might have only reception ability, thus limiting live interactions with other students and faculty except, perhaps, by telephone to facilitate audio communication or communicating by computer using chat rooms, e-mail messages, or electronic mailing list (LISTSERV) systems.

Although the videoconferencing method of distance education is expensive, the rate of success is high for state- and regionally supported academic programs with satellite capabilities among the various levels of higher education; for example, community colleges and state university systems. Additionally, partnerships between educational institutions and health care organizations that use satellite videoconferencing for staff development and patient and family education services are of benefit to both partners. The advantage to academic nursing programs for entering into these types of arrangements with established health care systems is the tremendous cost savings for mounting and maintaining the program. The disadvantage is that, unless nursing was an early pioneer in the delivery system and has a major role in it, it may face implementation problems such as least desirable times for broadcasting and possible displacement of class times owing to the priority rights of the sponsoring agency.

Videoconferencing and teleconferencing require an infrastructure for cable television or closed-circuit television, dedicated classrooms that can both broadcast and receive communications, and technological support staff who manage the broadcasting, hardware, and software for instructional support purposes. Unless the sessions are taped and can be shown after the session for independent viewing, the scheduling of the classes is time certain and cannot be changed owing to the demand for the services by other entities.

As with all delivery modes, the courses and/or classes offered through videoconferencing must be congruent with the curriculum and follow its goals and objectives. Videoconferencing includes all of the usual teaching methods and resources such as lectures, the use of overhead projectors, slides, videotapes, movies, and Power-Point (PPT) presentations. Students and faculty can interact in real time through exchanges on camera, telephone, or Web-based live chat rooms. These types of interactions require telecommunication and Web-based systems as well as satellite broadcasting systems. Negative aspects to this type of delivery of distance education programs are the expenses related to it such as the hardware and technical staffing, inflexible time frames (although they are no different than traditional scheduled classes on the home campus), and the need for faculty expertise in various teaching media. Positive aspects include real-time, live interactions between faculty and students; the wide array of available resources; the delivery of the same subject matter to more than one audience and therefore, more students; and the likelihood that the integrity of the curriculum is maintained.

Hartland, Biddle, and Fallacaro (2008) describe the use of videotapes that depicted simulated patient situations for assessing the medical and nursing students' development of clinical judgment skills. They compared the recall of students exposed to videotapes of patient situations vignettes to the recall of students assigned to only reading the same situations. They found the videotapes far more effective for student learning and retention. The authors liked the advantage of using videotapes because they could be transmitted electronically to distant students.

Clinical Courses and Distance Education

It is possible to provide quality clinical experiences for students through distance education modalities. For example, the off-site satellite campus with on-site faculty usually provides clinical experiences in the "traditional" mode. Faculty develops the clinical courses (including skills laboratory courses), according to the implementation plan of the curriculum. Students are assigned to clinical laboratories for the acquisition of assessment and clinical skills as well as to health care agencies for supervised clinical experiences. The latter are under the supervision of faculty who either directly supervise a group of students in the clinical setting or coordinate student preceptorships with students assigned to qualified staff nurse preceptors.

With careful planning, it is possible to provide clinical experiences for students enrolled in courses through videoconferencing or teleconferencing and Web-based instruction. Keeping in mind that course objectives must remain the same to ensure the integrity of the curriculum, faculty responsible for clinical courses can design the course so that the didactic and discussion components of the course are delivered through the selected distance education technology. Assignments, logs, or journals describing the clinical experiences, examinations, and pre- and post-conferences can also take place through technology and can be **asynchronous** (occurring at various times) or **synchronous** (simultaneous). The actual clinical experiences occur through faculty-coordinated preceptorships, local faculty hired by the institution for clinical supervision of students, or by faculty traveling to the clinical site to supervise a group of students.

If faculty serve as coordinators for clinical experiences with off-site preceptors and students, they must secure agreements between the educational program and the health care agency and preceptor; set standards for the qualifications of the preceptors; orient the preceptors to the curriculum, the course, and the role of preceptors; provide guidance throughout the experience to the preceptors and students; develop a communications network for all participants; supervise preceptors and students; assign the grades with input from the preceptors; and evaluate and revise the program based on feedback.

A review of the literature provided a few articles that discuss distance education and clinical experiences. Vandenhouten and Block (2005) describe a community health nursing course for RN students earning a bachelor of science in nursing. The clinical course was part of a distance education program with students enrolled across the country. The authors describe in detail the finite arrangements necessary to gain the experiences for students in community and public health agencies. Some of the challenges confronting them included regulatory issues such as faculty qualifications requirements by individual states, legal contracts, liability issues, and so forth. Vandenhouten and Block identify the need for a coordinator for these types of arrangements and the need to have the same person that arranges for the experience as the faculty member for the course. A benefit from the program was the ability of the students to compare community and public health nursing services across different regions of the nation.

Beason (2005) describes a collaborative program between the Veterans Administration (VA) and Department of Defense, Uniformed Services University of the Health Sciences Graduate School of Nursing to prepare adult nurse practitioners. Preceptors for the students in VA facilities were oriented to the program and served as mentors. Through careful planning between the two institutions, the program was a success. The program facilitated the preparation of nurse practitioners located throughout the country. Evaluations from graduates and other stakeholders demonstrated that students in the program performed better than traditional nurse practitioner students from other schools. The program was carefully planned and coordinated with open communication lines between the two agencies' students and preceptors as the program developed.

Servonsky, Daniels, and Davis (2005) describe in detail their use of the Blackboard WebCT-base platform for their Pediatric Nurse Practitioner Program. The article is useful as an overview of this specific system and what the faculty, using the system and transforming courses into this format, can expect. They list recommendations for improvements of the platform such as security of the examinations and ways in which to download batches of student papers rather than individually.

THE GROWTH OF INFORMATICS AND TECHNOLOGY

Technology in the Classroom

The utilization of technology in the classroom and through distance education guides the implementation of the curriculum by determining the format for delivery of its courses. Technology applied to the classroom and distance education programs have grown exponentially over the past few decades. It moved from teacher-centered lectures to movies and slide shows to illustrate concepts. Videotapes, compact disks (CDs), PPT presentations, and voice-over PPTs are added to the multiple devices available for teaching on campus and also delivered through Web-based platforms. Additional student-centered devices include electronic clickers for classroom participation and electronic note-taking software that links to course syllabi, materials, and lectures. The development of these multimedia teaching/learning aids promote active student participation in the learning process and facilitate the change from teacher-focused strategies to student-centered learning processes.

Day-Black and Watties-Daniels (2006) describe the application of technology to contemporary classrooms including Smart Classrooms (in-class computers, overhead projectors, access to the Web, and electronic software programs that allow students to re-visit lectures and take electronic notes). The authors liken the early days of technology to Socrates' concerns shared with Plato when the first written words were recorded and taking the place of oral communication and the sharing of knowledge. They voiced concern that students would come to rely on the written word rather than using their intellectual skills. This concern echoed through the ages as calculators began to replace hand written mathematics, computers replaced the typewritten word, and smart phones provided access to all sorts of communications and systems. One can only imagine the future as technology continues to expand.

Online/Web-Based Programs

Online and Web-based instruction had its beginnings through faculty and student use of communication tools such as LISTSERVS, e-mail, and access to resources and references on the World Wide Web. In the 1990s and early 21st century, the use of Web-based instruction through learning management systems became more prevalent. They proved so popular with students that some courses are mounted as a combination of Web-based and on-campus instruction classes for home campus students as well as off-campus students. Web-based instruction is usually delivered through the use of learning management systems for which the institution has a contract. As the popularity of this method of teaching and learning increased, the systems grew in complexity and at the same time, became user-friendly. Delivery of Web-based programs and courses grew to the extent that in 2006–2007 over two thirds of higher education programs including community colleges and baccalaureate programs offer such programs.

According to the Institute of Education Sciences (IES; 2008) survey of post-secondary schools:

> 66 percent of 2-year and 4-year degree-granting institutions reported offering online, hybrid/blended online, or other distance education courses for any level or audience. Sixty-five percent of the institutions reported college-level credit-granting distance education courses, and 23 percent of the institutions reported noncredit distance education courses. Sixty-one percent of 2-year and 4-year institutions reported offering online courses, 35 percent reported hybrid/blended courses, and 26 percent reported other types of college-level credit-granting distance education courses.

There were 12.2 million students enrolled in distance education programs. Asynchronous learning was reported as the most frequent instructional strategy used in the courses. The respondents reported that the leading reason for offering online education was to accommodate students' schedules, opening access to those who would otherwise not have access, and increasing enrollments.

Development of Online Programs

The American Distance Education Consortium (ADEC; 2010) provides classic teaching and learning principles applied to distance and Web-based education. It is an overview of what should be considered as part of distance education and online programs. Web-based teaching and learning requires a learning management system, computer access to the Web by faculty and students, technological support through the use of instructional support staff, and training sessions for faculty and students who are not familiar with the system. Some institutions of higher learning use experienced instructional technology staff and faculty who mount and manage courses for teachers whose only responsibility is for the actual teaching of the course. This method provides technical support for teaching faculty; however, it may remove some of the academic freedom from the teacher-of-record. For example, the teacher does not have the ability to change course assignments or formats without going through the support staff to make the changes. It can also prove to be expensive since the institution is paying for several staff members when only one may be required.

The initial time spent in converting a traditional course to a Web-based course is great and as with all courses, it requires updating and revisions each subsequent time that it is taught. Multiple learning activities are available through the Internet such as synchronous real-time chat rooms and live-classrooms where students and faculty meet at a prearranged time and discuss topics or review questions about course assignments. Asynchronous entries (occurring at various times and also labeled as threaded discussions) about selected topics provide the students and faculty with opportunities to discuss topics and present their ideas and views on them. The assignments related to these usually require reading assignments and/or a review of the literature so that the discussions are scholarly treatises on the subject at hand. Faculty can post a lecture through an essay or PowerPoint presentation that includes notes, illustrations, references to URLs, videotapes, movies, and other audiovisual media and pose thought questions for discussions related to the "lecture." Group work assignments are possible through the use of chat rooms, live classrooms, threaded discussions, and e-mail communications. Many of the learning management systems have programs that allow the faculty to develop surveys and examinations that are secure and provide statistical analyses of the results. A few examples of Web-based educational and live-time platforms are Blackboard (2010), Moodle (2010), Skype (2010), and Wimba (2010).

Learning Theories for Online Formats

Most distance education programs employ **andragogy** (adult learning) strategies for the delivery of courses and classes through off-campus satellite sites, videoconferencing, telecommunications, online, and Web-based technology. The majority of teaching and learning strategies offered in these formats is learner centered and facilitates active student participation in the process rather than the traditional pedagogical methods for presenting information to the student. See Chapter 3 for learning theories that apply to online educational formats and for ideas for research on the utilization of learning theories for online instruction.

Legg, Adelman, Mueller, and Levitt (2009) conducted an extensive review of the literature related to learning theories and online education. Their premise is that there are many studies in the literature that validate online teaching as effective, if not more effective as on-campus, in-person learning environments. They propose that the constructivist learning theory is appropriate for and can be applied to online learning.

By using the theory, courses can be designed to enable students to build on previous knowledge with the course providing the scaffolding for building new knowledge and opening new horizons. They present ideas for research needed to study the effects of various learning theories for online presentations and to investigate further the efficacy of online learning.

Research Findings on the Efficacy of Online Formats

The U.S. Department of Education (2009) in a meta-analysis of the literature related to online education found that online delivery of content results in better student learning outcomes than traditional classroom instruction. In addition, the blending of the online format with face-to-face meetings was even more effective; although, it was pointed out that in those instances, additional materials may have enriched the learning experience. The meta-analysis of the literature applied mostly to programs in higher education, thus the authors warned that these findings cannot be applied to K through 12 education.

Huckstadt and Hayes (2005) described the evaluation of the effectiveness of online interactive case studies. The two case studies developed by the authors for nurse practitioner students promoted independent study and student interaction with the information in the case studies. After completion of the case studies, students took a posttest on the material. The authors found that the case study format was effective for students' learning and in addition, the students reported that they enjoyed the experience. The students suggested the need for follow-up on the items that they missed on the test and the authors reported that this feature was added to the modules to enable students to have immediate access to the instructors once the grades were posted on the text.

Disadvantages and Advantages of Web-Based Education

Some of the disadvantages of online systems are the need for technological support; initial and on-going costs related to contracts for learning management systems and computers; the lack of face-to-face encounters between faculty and students; the large amount of faculty time consumed in mounting the course; the possible loss of nursing values such as visible and tactile communications; and a minimal sense of belonging to the home campus. Advantages include flexible times for students and faculty, multiple learning and teaching strategies, active participation on the part of all students, moderate maintenance times for managing and updating the course once it is mounted, and relative assurance of curriculum integrity.

APPLICATION OF TECHNOLOGY TO EDUCATION

Patient Simulations

The application of technology occurs in the implementation of the curriculum both on-campus and through distance education delivery systems. An example is the use of realistic interactive patient simulations in the laboratory setting for students to practice skills in a safe environment prior to providing nursing care in the clinical setting. Patient simulators come with ready-made case scenarios or faculty can develop their own scenarios that can be programmed into the simulators. Some examples of simulators are the Human Patient Simulator (METI, 2010), SimMan (Laerdal, 2010), and VA/Stanford Simulation Center (2010). Many schools of nursing located on multidisciplinary health sciences campuses pool resources with other disciplines that result in shared state-of-the-art facilities to practice skills and foster interprofessional education opportunities.

Waxman (2010) describes a collaborative effort on the part of the Bay Area Simulation Collaborative (BASC) to develop guidelines for the development of scenarios. After a review of the literature that failed to identify a template for developing scenarios, the BASC group identified principles for developing scenarios with a conceptual model and guidelines for creating scenarios. The author argues that learning objectives should guide the scenario not the technology. Listed among the guidelines are overall broad objectives to set the purpose, specific objectives with application of the usual educational domains of knowledge, and the integration of evidence-based clinical practice. It was recommended that faculty who facilitate scenarios be familiar with the case study in order to act as monitors and facilitators in the learning process and to anticipate student-learning processes. It was further recommended that case scenarios be shared among the various health disciplines to foster inteprofessional collaboration. Guimond and Salas (2009) provide an overview of simulators by describing differences among high- and low-fidelity mannequins. They promote the application of training theories to the use of simulators.

Research Findings on the Efficacy of Case Scenario Simulations

Grady, Kehrer, Trusty, Entin, and Brunye (2008) conducted a study on the learning outcomes for nasogastric tube insertion and urinary catheterization using high-fidelity mannequins. Students reported their satisfaction with the experience for preparing for real-life clinical situations. The authors found that male students were more comfortable with the high-fidelity aspects of the mannequin than female students. However, the authors pointed out the need in today's high-tech environment for all nursing students to become comfortable with high technology-supported educational and practice experiences.

Reese, Jeffries, and Engum (2010) measured multidisciplinary (medical and nursing) students' learning outcomes when interacting with a simulated postsurgical patient that was experiencing cardiac arrhythmias. The simulation case study was based on the Jeffries (2005) Nursing Education Simulation Framework (NESF). Reese et al. found that students reported increased confidence in the care of patients with these problems when transferred to reality and they had positive experiences in working with another discipline. Furthermore, the simulated experiences assisted their learning in a safe environment.

Leski (2009) interviewed faculty and students on the use of Computer-Based Instruction (CBI) for transferring knowledge and skills in a community college nursing program. She found that students reported that CBI was especially helpful in theory course, especially in having the ability to review the material in the course. However, students believed that in-person sessions are necessary for acquiring hands-on skills. At the same time, CBI helps to demonstrate the skills but actual practice is necessary.

Electronic Records and Information Systems

As electronic patient records and information systems become more prevalent in the health care system, it becomes necessary for schools of nursing to provide the theoretical and technical knowledge related to these systems for nursing students. Skiba (2009) provides an overview of the integration of informatics and technology into specific nursing curricula. She provides ideas and resources for faculty development for schools to provide learning experiences for students such as simulated patient information systems, electronic documentation, and patient records. She promotes the need for faculty development workshops for instructors to gain the expertise to integrate these concepts and experiences into the curriculum.

Flood, Gasiewicz, and Delpier (2010) provide an example of a baccalaureate program that integrated informatics throughout the curriculum. After a review of the literature, the authors found scanty information on the integration of informatics into the curriculum in spite of the growing need for it and recommendations from the report of the summit on Technology Informatics Guiding Education Reform (TIGER; 2006). The authors describe the introduction of informatics in the baccalaureate program by assignments that have students interact with electronic reference databases. Later in the curriculum, they have access to complex patient clinical records and if possible, meet with an informatics manager to see the influence of this technology in the health care system.

Issues in the Utilization of Informatics and Technology

Schutt and Hightower (2009) in an extensive review of the literature found that in spite of the profession's and health care system's urgent recommendations and newer accreditation standards from National League for Nursing Accrediting Commission (NLNAC; 2008) and the "Essentials" from American Association of Colleges of Nursing (AACN; 2010), the faculty and the curriculum are lacking in the integration of informatics into the curriculum. Nurses in the practice setting urge nurse educators to include informatics especially regarding patient safety and quality care. The authors provide an update on the TIGER Initiative (TIGER, 2006). TIGER is a coalition aiming to advance informatics and technology into nursing education. It cites benchmarking and sharing best practices as key to achieving its goals. Schutt and Hightower urge nurse educators to provide faculty development for instructors to upgrade their skills in informatics and promote student knowledge, skills, and readiness for practice in a health care system that functions in a high tech informatics world.

TRENDS, ISSUES, AND CHALLENGES FOR THE FUTURE

To remain competitive and current in the higher education market, nursing programs need to determine how they will expand their programs to meet the needs of students who may live and work some distance away from the home campus. Although entry-level programs, especially undergraduate programs will continue to take place on traditional home campuses supplements by technology; there is a need to offer higher education programs for licensed personnel and other experienced learners afar from home campuses. Distance learning through technology offers the best opportunity for working nurses to continue their education and, as described earlier in the chapter, has been successful. Through consortia of varying levels of education, regional collaborative, and the health care industry, these programs can be cost-effective and reach many more nurses than ever imagined.

The increasing market for learning management systems provides cost-effective, quality educational delivery programs through Web-based technology and in many ways, is proving to be an effective modality for engaging students in transformative learning experiences. These types of programs are far less expensive than videoconferencing and telecommunications; however, they require the technology, staffing, and faculty development programs to realize their full potential.

No matter the modality, the program must be within the context of the program's mission, philosophy, organizational framework, and goals and objectives. As with all curriculum development projects, faculty must examine the purpose of the distance education program in light of these components. In some cases, the program may not be compatible with the mission and therefore, not an option. For those programs that are compatible, the usual formative evaluation strategies must take place to ensure that the planning and implementation phases of the program are congruent with the overall curriculum plan. An evaluation plan to measure outcomes must be in place to maintain quality, meet program approval and accreditation standards, and ensure a quality program for its stakeholders such as students, consumers, and faculty.

The majority of distance education programs have copyright and intellectual property policies in place that are congruent with the parent institution. For new programs, along with faculty development and implementation support, it is advised that these policies are developed early in the process. The ideal policy is one that gives the individual faculty member the rights to the course syllabus and learning activities; however, the course description and objectives remain the property of the institution.

Privacy issues are addressed through the maintenance of the same policies of the parent institution. For Web-based courses, owing to identification theft and computer hackers, many institutions issue identification numbers for students, staff, and faculty rather than social security numbers. Most learning management systems have built-in privacy safety mechanisms allowing only students and faculty access to courses through personal identification numbers.

Often, videoconferencing is delivered through closed-circuit television or public broadcasting system and thus, open to public access. However, only students officially enrolled in the courses can receive academic credit and have access to supplemental material necessary for the course such as library services, course resources, e-mail, list serves, and chat rooms.

An issue not addressed frequently in the literature, is the matter of faculty to student ratios in distance education programs and their effect on quality education, faculty workload, and method of instruction. Videoconferencing leads other technologies in reaching the greatest numbers of students while Web-based courses are limited in size per faculty member; usually to a maximum of 20–25 students. Web-based instruction requires high-intensity interactions among students and faculty for effective learning to take place. Videoconferencing can reach many students in multiple sites, but as with all lecture-type classes, fosters minimal student participation unless active learning assignments are included. All of these factors must be taken into consideration when planning the delivery choice.

As distance education programs increase in the future, new issues and challenges face faculty and institutions of higher learning. Less attention will be needed on the actual technology of the delivery systems and more attention will be necessary on the quality of the programs as they match the mission and purposes of the educational programs. Outcomes from distance education programs will be measured by increased opportunities for nurses to continue their education and the continued partnerships between education and service that result in a nursing workforce ready to meet the challenges of an ever-changing health care system and the health promotion and disease prevention needs of the populace.

SUMMARY

Chapter 16 reviewed the various types of distance education programs and their relationship to curriculum development and evaluation. The influence of informatics and technology on nursing education was discussed. Some of the issues facing these types of programs were reviewed including cost-effectiveness, faculty workload, the application of teaching and learning principles, and student learning outcomes.

DISCUSSION QUESTIONS

1. To what extent do you believe that technology-supported distance education programs changed nursing education for the 21st century?
2. Of the multiple technology-supported distance education programs, which do you believe:
   a. Is most cost-effective?
   b. Meets desired outcomes?
   c. Reaches the highest number of students?
   d. Fosters faculty development?
   Explain your rationale.
3. Discuss the pros and cons for the delivery of clinical courses through distance education strategies.

LEARNING ACTIVITIES

Student Learning Activities

Search the current literature (last 5 years) for at least three research articles on distance education programs, Web-based education, or the application of informatics and technology on nursing education. Analyze them for a description of the outcomes for specific distance education modalities. Compare the modalities according to the outcomes that relate to teaching and learning effectiveness and student and faculty satisfaction.

Faculty Development Activities

Select one course that you teach and adapt it to either videoconferencing or Web-based technology. Explain your rationale for selecting one or the other as it applies to the course.

If you teach a course(s) online, evaluate it for its student learning outcomes and other measures of its effectiveness. Compare it to the program mission and program goals/objectives. Develop a plan for revising the course based on your evaluation.

REFERENCES, RESOURCES, AND WEB SITES

American Association of Colleges of Nursing. (2010). *"Essentials" Series*. Retrieved from http://www .nlnac.org/manuals/SC2008.htm

American Distance Education Consortium. (2010). *ADEC Guiding principles for distance teaching and learning*. Retrieved from http://www.adec.edu/admin/papers/distance-teaching_principles.html

Beason, C. (2005). Lessons learned: a successful distance learning collaborative between the Department of Veterans Affairs and the Department of Defense. *Military Medicine, 170*(5), 395–399.

Blackboard. (2010). *Blackboard. Higher education.* Retrieved from http://www.blackboard.com/Solutions-by-Market/Higher-Education.aspx

Day-Black, C., & Watties-Daniels, A. (2006). Cutting edge technology to enhance nursing classroom instruction at Coppin State University. *ABNF Journal, 17*(3), 103–106.

Flood, L., Gasiewicz, N., & Delpier, T. (2010). Integrating information literacy across a BSN curriculum. *Journal of Nursing Education, 49*(2), 101–104.

Grady, J. L., Kehrer, R. G., Trusty, C. E., Entin, E. B., Entin, E. E., & Brunye, T. T. (2008). Learning nursing procedures: the influence of simulator fidelity and student gender on teaching effectiveness. *Journal of Nursing Education, 47*(9), 403–408.

Guimond, M., & Salas, E. (2009). Linking the science of training to nursing simulation. *Nurse Educator, 34*(3), 105–106.

Hartland, W., Biddle, C., & Fallacaro, M. (2008). Audiovisual facilitation of clinical knowledge: a paradigm for dispersed student education based on Paivio's Dual Coding Theory. *AANA Journal, 76*(3), 194–198.

Huckstadt, A., & Hayes, K. (2005). Evaluation of interactive online courses for advanced practice nurses. *Journal of the American Academy of Nurse Practitioners, 17*(3), 85–89.

Institute of Education Sciences (2008). *Distance education at degree-granting postsecondary institutions: 2006–07.* Retrieved from http://nces.ed.gov/pubsearch/index.asp?HasSearched=1&searchcat2=subjectindx&L1=137&L2=1

METI. (2010). *Human Patient Simulator.* Retrieved from http://www.meti.com/products_ps_hps.htm

Jeffries, P. R. (2005). A framework for designing, implementing, and evaluating simulations used as teaching strategies in nursing. *Nursing Education Perspectives, 26*(2), 96–103.

Laerdal. (2010). *SimMan.* Retrieved from http://www.laerdal.com/essential

Legg, T. J., Adelman, D., Mueller, D., & Levitt, C. (2009). Constructivist strategies in online distance education in nursing. *Journal of Nursing Education, 48*(2), 64–69.

Leski, J. (2009). Nursing student and faculty perceptions of computer-based instruction at a 2-year college. *Journal of Nursing Education, 48*(2), 91–95

Moodle. (2010). *Moodle home.* Retrieved from http://moodle.org/about

National League for Nursing Accrediting Commission. (2008). *NLNAC 2008 standards and criteria.* Retrieved from http://www.nlnac.org/manuals/SC2008.htm

Reese, C. E., Jeffries, P. R,, & Engum, S. A. (2010). Learning together: Using simulations to develop nursing and medical student collaboration. *Nursing Education Perspectives, 31*(1), 33–37.

Schutt, M. A., & Hightower, B. (2009). Enhancing RN-to-BSN students' information literacy skills through the use of instructional technology [corrected] [published erratum appears in J NURS EDUC 2009 May;48(5):248]. *Journal of Nursing Education, 48*(2), 101–105.

Servonsky, E. J., Daniels, W. L., & Davis, B. L. (2005). Evaluation of Blackboard as a platform for distance education delivery. *ABNF Journal, 16*(6), 132–135.

Skiba, D. J. (2009). Emerging technologies center: Teaching with and about technology: providing resources for nurse educators worldwide. *Nursing Education Perspectives, 30*(4), 255–256.

Skype. (2010). *About Skype.* Retrieved from http://about.skype.com

Technology Informatics Guiding Education Reform (2006). TIGER summit report. Retrieved from http://www.nursingsociety.org/aboutus/PositionPapers/Documents/TIGER_Final_Summit_Report.pdf

U.S. Department of Education. (2009) Evaluation of evidence-based practices in online learning: A meta-analysis and review of online learning studies. Washington, D.C.: Author.

VA/Stanford Simulation Center. (2010). *The MedSim-Eagle Patient Simulator.* Retrieved from http://med.stanford.edu/VAsimulator/medsim.html

Vandenhouten, C., & Block, D. (2005). A case study of a distance-based public health nursing/community health nursing practicum. *Public Health Nursing, 22*(2), 166–171.

Waxman, K.T. (2010). The Development of Evidence-Based Clinical Simulation Scenarios: Guidelines for Nurse Educators. *Journal of Nursing Education. 49*(1), 29–35.

Wimba. (2009). *Solutions for higher and further education.* Retrieved from http://www.wimba.com/solutions/higher-education

Issues and Challenges for Nurse Educators

Sarah B. Keating

OBJECTIVES

Upon completion of Chapter 17, the reader will be able to:

1. Analyze the issues and challenges raised throughout the text that apply to curriculum development and evaluation.
2. Consider some strategies for resolution of the issues raised and ways to meet the challenges with an eye to the future.
3. Review the need for evidence-based research in nursing education to develop a personal agenda for conducting research in curriculum development and evaluation.
4. Study the proposed parallel career ladder steps and the entry-level doctorate curricula for their application to current and future unified nursing education programs.

INTRODUCTION

Chapter 17 summarizes the text and discusses trends, issues, and challenges raised throughout the text. It ends with a sample curriculum that progresses from the lower division level of higher education to the doctorate and features step out points along the way for nurses wishing to enter the workforce at various levels. It integrates some newer prerequisite courses from other disciplines to support the knowledge base for nursing in a complex, and ever changing health care system. It continues the career ladder concept of nursing education so that its practitioners can enter subsequent levels of education without repeating previously learned knowledge and skills. At the same time, it promotes a nonstop, progressive curriculum for those who wish to enter at the doctorate level.

Following the sample curriculum that builds upon current curricula in nursing found in Table 17.1, Table 17.2 proposes an entry-level doctorate program for the future. It is a blueprint for an 8-year prenursing and nursing curriculum that graduates the student in 8 years with either a Doctor of Nursing Practice (DNP) or a research and theory–building doctorate, that is, the PhD or Doctor of Nursing Science (DNSc). The author is the first to admit that it is not perfect. Its intent is to raise issues, provoke thought, and generate discussion for future planning.

CHAPTER 1: HISTORY OF NURSING EDUCATION AND FACULTY ROLE

Chapter 1 describes the history of nursing education and raises many of the issues related to it and its impact on the profession. The explosion of DNP programs across the nation, the recognition of PhD and DNSc degree programs as the discipline's research and theory–building degrees, and the impact of technology and health care legislation on the profession will be the major forces that influence the history of nursing in the early 21st century.

CHAPTER 2: CURRICULUM DEVELOPMENT AND APPROVAL PROCESSES IN CHANGING EDUCATIONAL ENVIRONMENTS

When joining the faculty of a school of nursing, a person should orient himself/herself to the curriculum's, mission, philosophy, goals, organizing framework, and objectives to ascertain if they are in congruence with one's own conceptual base of nursing education. If there is a major lack of compatibility, then it is advised that the person seek a faculty role in another school that corresponds with the individual's philosophies and beliefs about nursing education.

As a member of the faculty, a person should continually monitor the curriculum to maintain its integrity as it is implemented through instructional processes. This includes theory classes, laboratory practice, and clinical experiences. If incongruence occurs, the faculty member who identifies the problem has a responsibility to work with other members of the faculty to bring the course(s) into line or to consider and implement changes in the curriculum through the appropriate channels.

It is the responsibility of nursing faculty to continually assess the components of the curriculum, its processes, and outcomes to ensure quality education in nursing. Ways in which faculty can participate in this process are to join committees that pertain to the curriculum, collaborate with other faculty members at various levels to observe the curriculum plan in action, identify problems or potential problems, and offer ideas for improving the program. At the same time, faculty must be willing to compromise and give up unnecessary content to make room for newer concepts that prepare nurses for the evolving health care system.

Nursing faculty must know the health care system and changes that occur to prepare graduates to meet the needs of the system and the people they serve. This requires looking into the future and collaborating with nurses and other health care providers to obtain an overall picture of the current and future health needs of the populace and how the system will meet the needs. The most efficient method for accomplishing this mandate is to invite consumers and members of the health care system as well as students to curriculum planning meetings and for them to participate in the evaluation of educational programs and their products.

Nursing faculty must collaborate with other disciplines to provide interdisciplinary education to imbue in their graduates a sense of teamwork in meeting the needs of the people whom they serve. The knowledge base and clinical experiences for students should include in-depth experiences in a variety of health care settings to prepare nurses who can provide interprofessional as well as nursing services to clients who move in and out of various levels of care.

CHAPTERS 3 AND 4: LEARNING THEORIES, EDUCATIONAL TAXONOMIES, AND CRITICAL THINKING

Chapter 3 reviews six major categories of learning theories commonly accepted in today's education system and provides subsets and examples of each and their application to nursing education. Familiarity with the major categories of learning theories and philosophical discussions among faculty members are essential parts of curriculum development early in the process. The theories set the stage for how the curriculum will be organized and how its students will achieve program goals in preparing for the profession. In addition to describing the importance of learning theories to curriculum building, the chapter raises issues relative to the application of learning theories in the current milieu of high technology and the use of informatics for teaching and application to the health care system.

Chapter 4 reviews the traditional educational taxonomies and domains of learning as they apply to nursing education. Although nursing adopted and continues to use modified models based on Tyler (1949) and Bloom, Engelhart, Furst, Hill, and Krathwahl (1956) for organizing the curriculum, there is a need to examine newer taxonomies that integrate the domains of learning and foster students' dispositions toward the development of critical and creative thinking. The newer taxonomies lift objectives from previous expectations related to rote or recall memorization to higher orders of understanding and conceptualization. The modalities of problem solving, critical and creative thinking, and decision making are suited to today's changing health care system. There is a need for professionals who can respond to health care needs with strategies that utilize evidence-based and innovative solutions to health care problems and that foster health promotion and prevention of disease.

CHAPTERS 5 AND 6: A NEEDS ASSESSMENT MODEL FOR CURRICULUM DEVELOPMENT

Section III of this text introduced a conceptual model for conducting a needs assessment for curriculum development and evaluation in nursing. Chapters 5 and 6 reviewed the major components of a needs assessment that include the external and internal frame factors that influence, facilitate, or impinge upon the curriculum. Although the principal activities of faculty in curriculum development and evaluation is on the curriculum plan itself and the need for improvement based on evaluation of the processes of implementation and the program outcomes, the needs assessment should become part of the education repertoire of the faculty. Even if faculty is not involved in the details of the needs assessment, it should be aware of all of the factors that have an influence on the curriculum. These factors can mean the life or death of an education program and thus, faculty members sophisticated in the assessment of external and internal frame factors have an advantage in viewing the curriculum and its place in the scheme of financial security, position within the health care system and the profession, role in meeting the health care needs of the community and industry, and significance to the parent institution.

It is recommended that nurse educators in both the academic and practice settings use this model when evaluating education programs, considering revisions of existing programs, or initiating new programs. Although administrators may take the leadership role in conducting needs assessments, faculty should participate in the decisions for what type and how much data to collect and what decisions are made that affect the curriculum and are based on the analysis of the needs assessment.

CHAPTER 7: COMPONENTS OF THE CURRICULUM AND ISSUES ARISING FROM TODAY'S NURSING CURRICULA

Chapter 7 organizes the components of the curriculum in the traditional way, that is, mission, philosophy, goal, organizational framework, student learning outcomes (objectives), and implementation plan. The components of the curriculum provide an organizing framework for initiating or revising an educational program. Major concepts related to the underlying philosophy and the beliefs faculty hold about nursing and education are examined in light of their contribution to and place in the curriculum. Examples include, evidence-based practice, quality of care and patient safety, cultural competence, and the like. When revising the curriculum or developing new programs, faculty should initiate the change processes by discussing these concepts and how they apply to the level of nursing education in their program. Most faculty members will agree that these concepts are fundamental to nursing education. The challenge occurs when deciding at what level of competency for each concept/essential they expect of their graduates, that is, undergraduate and/or graduate levels.

Although it may seem cumbersome at times, in the long run, examining the curriculum by its major components results in a logical order for planning and evaluation. When faculty members are contemplating change in response to assessment of the curriculum, evaluating the outcomes of the program, and reviewing changes in the health care system, each component of the curriculum is examined for its congruence with the proposed changes. This may lead to a radical revamping of the curriculum for it may be discovered that the demands for graduates or from the health care system have so dramatically changed that the mission, philosophy, and goals of the program are outdated or irrelevant.

Approaching the curriculum holistically by viewing all of its components leads to orderly revisions rather than the "band-aid" approach that attempts to mend one portion of the program without considering its effects on the other components. Nurse educators are frequently guilty of this maneuver to respond to obvious need for changes. The problems associated with this method are their impact on other parts of the program to their detriment or adding to an already overloaded curriculum.

Another issue related to the totality of the curriculum and its components is the need for faculty members to become familiar with them. The membership of the faculty is constantly in a state of flux. When curricula are revised or created, all members of the faculty are involved; however, teachers retire or move to another institution and new members come to the program. It is at this point that orientation to the curriculum must take place. Usually the curriculum committee chair is the most logical person to initially orient new faculty members. The orientation continues through other faculty members such as level and/or specialty coordinators and faculty of record for specific courses. Part-time and clinical faculty members are often neglected owing to time constraints and frequent changes of personnel that can result in divergence from the curriculum's intent. Faculty who coordinate courses in which part-time or clinical faculty teach, have the responsibility to share the curriculum with them to preserve its integrity and to provide an overview of the rationale and place in the curriculum for the courses in which they teach.

CHAPTERS 8 THROUGH 13

Chapters 8 and 9 discuss the two current, major curricula for entry into practice, that is, the associate degree (ADN) and the baccalaureate/Bachelor of Science in Nursing (BSN). Both of these programs have been in existence since the mid-20th century, replacing the hospital-based diploma programs that continue to exist, but are decreasing in numbers. Chapter 9 describes generic (entry-level) baccalaureate programs as well as fast-track baccalaureate programs for college graduates and RN to BSN programs. The old issue of entry into practice rears its ugly head as the ADN and baccalaureate are examined; however, with the need to produce more nurses as rapidly as possible to meet health care demands and the need for additional education beyond the ADN, the authors of Chapters 8 and 9 describe curricula that embrace both programs and foster career ladder opportunities. Each chapter provides excellent examples of curricula for preparing nurses for the current health care system and can serve in the interim as nursing meets the challenge to educate clinicians, educators, practitioners, scientists, and researchers for the future who are prepared at even higher levels of education.

Chapter 10 examines graduate education at the master's level including entry-level master's programs for nonnursing college graduates. The traditional place for advanced practice roles such as the nurse practitioner, nurse anesthetist, nurse midwife, and clinical specialist has been at the master's level. However, the DNP degree is replacing the master's, and the American Association of Colleges of Nursing (AACN) has a position paper recommending the DNP as the terminal practice degree by 2015 (AACN, 2004). This position paper led to an explosive growth of DNP programs across the nation, starting first with a post-master's degree and moving toward the BSN to DNP program to prepare advanced nurse clinicians and nurse administrators/executives. Many issues arise from this situation with the profession struggling with where case managers, clinical nurse leaders, nurse managers and administrators, and community health nursing fall into these changes. Chapter 11 raises these issues as graduate/doctorate levels of nursing education continue to evolve.

Graduate programs are particularly hard hit by the looming shortage of doctorate-prepared teachers as the faculty members age and retire and the numbers of new graduates from doctoral programs do not meet the demand. This situation provides the impetus for accelerating access to graduate education for both new entrants into the discipline and practicing nurses and educators who have an interest in teaching. Additional incentives for the faculty role need to be in place to make the educator role competitive with that of practice, administration, and research. Chapter 12 discusses research-focused degree programs and their role as "Stewards of the Discipline" by their research and leadership activities and as faculty members in schools of nursing.

An issue related to doctoral-prepared faculty is the debate that continues about the practice doctorate (DNP) versus the research-focused degrees, that is, the DNSc/DNS and the PhD and their place in nursing education. It is posed that PhD and DNSc-prepared educators are suitable for tenure-track positions in schools of nursing, whereas DNP graduates are meant for clinically focused teaching positions. However, a counterargument is that the DNP prepares nurses for applied research and evidence-based practice and could compete in tenure-track roles. It is also argued that DNP graduates understand the role better than research-focused faculty and can be role models for the students. There are persuasive arguments on both sides, but the majority of opinions agree that for either degree, nurses planning to teach in schools of nursing need additional knowledge and skills (courses) in education, for example, curriculum, instructional strategies, and student and program evaluation.

Chapter 13 applies the principles of curriculum development and evaluation to staff development in the practice setting. Nurse educators in academe and in the practice setting have much to offer each other. Nurse educators who focus on staff development can provide nurse faculties with their perspectives on the competencies and knowledge base of students and graduates of the programs. Their wisdom is valuable in helping faculty prepare new graduates for practice in the reality setting. Nursing faculty on the other hand, has expertise in andragogy and can share these strategies with nurse educators in the practice settings. They also have clinical specialty knowledge and skills that can be offered as in-service opportunities for nursing staff in health agencies in addition to educating nurse preceptors and mentors for students and new graduates.

Research partnerships between nursing service and education benefit nursing faculty members as they earn promotion and tenure and keep abreast of changes in health care, while students can carry out their graduate theses or dissertations in the practice arena. All levels of students can apply the newest knowledge from research to evidence-based practice. This in turn is shared with nursing staff members who can reciprocate with their knowledge and clinical skills in the latest advances in health care.

There are increasing instances of industry and education partnerships with industry assisting schools of nursing with the costs for additional faculty members to help increase enrollments. Qualified staff members from the agencies serve as instructors while continuing in their practice roles in the agencies. It is imperative that the integrity of the curriculum be protected by ensuring that faculty from the service area is well oriented to the curriculum and its goals and objectives. There must be opportunities for new members' participation in faculty and curriculum meetings as well as for their responsibilities to the curriculum. Experienced faculty must act as mentors to impart the curriculum plan and the knowledge and skills necessary to the teaching and learning role. It is possible in these types of arrangements that the result is recruitment of clinical personnel into full-time faculty roles, a great advantage to schools of nursing and the profession.

CHAPTERS 14 AND 15: PROGRAM EVALUATION AND ACCREDITATION

Nursing education program and curriculum evaluation is evolving from an emphasis in the past on the use of models of evaluation in education to the adaptation of business models to measure productivity, outcomes, cost effectiveness, and quality. Issues that are raised relate to the increasing emphasis on outcomes and benchmarks to measure quality and the possible loss of equal attention to the processes that lead to the outcomes. Owing to many accreditation standards, educational programs usually have master plans of evaluation in place to facilitate the process of collecting and analyzing data. These data relate to the standards expected for accreditation and the goals and objectives of the program. One flaw in many of the master plans is the lack of specific plans to follow up on the analyses and their recommendations. Implementing strategies to follow up on the recommendations closes the loop between data collection and actions for change in the curriculum; thus, maintaining an up-to-date and vibrant program.

Chapter 14 of this text describes common definitions of terms used in evaluation program for a nurse practitioner program. The latter is an illustration of the use of formative and summative evaluation strategies. Chapter 15 discusses in detail accreditation agencies, their purpose, and their role in total quality management. Included in the chapter is a description of the process for undergoing accreditation. Although accreditation is voluntary, it carries certain advantages for the institution and its students and graduates. For example, an accredited institution demonstrates to the public that it meets quality standards or criteria set by education and the profession, and therefore increases its marketability. For students and graduates, an accredited program signifies that they are eligible for certain financial aid programs and in most cases, admission to an institution of higher education for the next degree level(s).

Two major issues are raised regarding accreditation. The first is the question of these agencies keeping their standards and criteria up-to-date. With the expansion of technology-driven distance education programs and rapid changes in the health care system, it becomes difficult to make changes in the curriculum in response to the changes and at the same time, ensure that the program continues to meet program approval standards and accreditation criteria. Many state boards of nursing and accreditation agencies require notification of any major (or even minor) changes in the existing program. Although this ensures quality and maintenance of approval or accreditation, it can hamper creativity and a speedy response to external changes and demands on the program.

The advantage of notifying program approval and accreditation agencies of pending changes is the preservation of quality, whereas the disadvantage is a lowered motivation for creating change. In these cases, the wise strategy is to consult with the agencies when the idea for change begins to form and to continue the consultation throughout the planning stages so that the appropriate paper work and visits, if necessary, are ready for timely approval processes. In addition, educators have a responsibility to participate in accreditation processes including review of standards and criteria, becoming site visitors, and becoming members on review boards and committees of the agencies. These kinds of activities contribute to faculty's professional development and the ability of the approval and accrediting agencies to keep abreast of changes occurring in education and the profession that call for modifications of standards and criteria.

CHAPTER 16: EFFECTS OF INFORMATICS AND TECHNOLOGY ON CURRICULUM DEVELOPMENT AND EVALUATION

The growth of technology and informatics and their impact on nursing education are explored in Chapter 16. From the time of offering courses off-campus at a remote (satellite) place to today's complete degree programs totally online/Web-based has been tremendous. Chapter 16 reviews the types of programs that utilize current technology including videocasting and Web-based formats. Outcome studies demonstrate the effectiveness of these formats in realizing student learning outcomes, and it is expected that these programs will continue to grow. Schools of nursing find that to remain competitive and to serve the needs of adult learners, it is time to create programs that embrace the use of technology.

The information age and high technology require that faculty keeps abreast of changes and gains the knowledge and skills required for facilitating learning, conducting research and other scholarly activities, and transmitting new knowledge and theories to students. The majority of today's students has technological savvy and can work collaboratively with faculty to integrate technology and informatics into the curriculum and its application to nursing practice. Faculty should view students as partners in the teaching and learning processes and ensure their participation in the evaluation of the curriculum and program outcomes.

The application of technology and informatics to the classroom and learning laboratory is reviewed. In some cases, faculty preparation has not kept pace with the rapid growth of the utilization of technology and studies demonstrate the need for faculty development in this area to meet the needs of today's health care system that is rapidly adapting informatics and technology to the delivery of care. High-fidelity mannequins that provide realistic case scenarios for student training in the laboratory setting help to increase their confidence and competency prior to experiences in the clinical setting. Research opportunities abound in measuring the effectiveness of these tools in achieving learning outcomes. To look into the future for additional innovations that will occur is unimaginable but extraordinarily exciting.

FROM WHENCE WE CAME AND WHERE TO GO?

Chapter 1 reviews the history of nursing education from the mid- to late 1800s to the 21st century. It is interesting to see the visions of nurse leader educators over the centuries who called for a unified approach to curriculum development in nursing and the falling by the wayside of some of these approaches resulting in the "Nursing Education Civil War" as the author of Chapter 1 so aptly puts. The "Civil War" alludes to the conflict over "entry into professional practice." It is equally interesting to see the influence that international wars and the major changes in the health care system and society had on nursing education. Nursing education programs found that with government help, they could accelerate nursing programs in institutions of higher learning and produce graduates for high demand eras. Advanced practice roles at the master's level came about as high technology and managed care systems began to change the health care delivery system and doctoral programs came about as nursing sought its professional identity and began to build the scientific body of knowledge through research. The explosive growth of the DNP since AACN's 2004 position paper of the DNP as the terminal degree in nursing for practice has been remarkable in less than a decade. As the graduates of these programs increase and impact the health care system at the same time that federal legislation for reform takes place, the role of nursing become even more crucial.

The growth of technology-driven distance education programs is an example of one response to the latter 20th and early 21st centuries' health care needs and the demand for nurses with baccalaureate and graduate education by the health care industry. However, the history of nursing's responses to shortages in the workforce seems to repeat itself. Nursing needs to take advantage of its successful recruitment activities with an emphasis on enrolling the best and the brightest of the youth interested in nursing and assuring that it is diverse in gender and ethnic and cultural attributes. To accomplish this objective, nursing must become an attractive profession as a career option. This places the responsibility on every nurse to become an advocate for the profession by publicizing its vital role in the health care delivery system, providing high-quality nursing care services in collaboration with other disciplines, shaping public policy as it applies to health disparities and services for the unserved and underserved, and advocating for compensation that is appropriate to the professional services rendered.

Nursing curricula are changing rapidly to keep abreast of changes in society and the health care system. Technology contributed to improved access to continuing education for nurses with online programs for RNs to BSNs and for graduate education. Low-fidelity and high-fidelity simulated mannequins provide a safe practice arena for students to gain competency and confidence in skills prior to their real-life experiences in the clinical setting. Smart classrooms support interactive learning so that the focus on the learner becomes the modus operandi and formal lectures with no learner participation are becoming a thing of the past. What does the future hold, what are the challenges facing nursing education, and how can these challenges best be met in a timely manner?

CHALLENGES FOR NURSING EDUCATION IN THE FUTURE

Trends in Undergraduate Nursing Education

Speziale and Jacobson (2005) reported on a survey conducted on baccalaureate, associate degree, and diploma nursing programs for their perspectives on changes occurring in curriculum, teaching, evaluation, faculty, and students from 1998 to 2008. The Connecticut Colleagues in Caring group supported the study and the NLN provided a list of schools nationwide. Relative to the curriculum, the researchers found an increasing emphasis on evidence-based practice in diploma and baccalaureate programs. For all programs, diversity in response to the growing diversity of the populations served, health care costs and the economics of health care, management/delegation, patient care outcomes, health promotion, critical thinking, and informatics were viewed as concepts that are increasing in the curriculum. The survey confirmed what the profession recommends for entry-level nursing preparation. However, several major concepts are not mentioned and include genetics, patient safety, and quality of care. The Speziale and Jacobson study states that it is a pilot study and it is recommended that similar studies take place at least every 10 years to measure changes, analyze trends, and forecast for the future.

Interdisciplinary and Specialty Education

Interdisciplinary education. For years in education, there has been discussion for the need for **multidisciplinary** and **interprofessional** education and practice to better serve clients in the health care system. Even the terms become topics of debate with multidisciplinary insinuating the use of broader disciplines and interprofessional teams composed of health-related professionals. There is also the notion of multidisciplinary meaning parallel services from several disciplines whereas interdisciplinary is an integration of services among the disciplines. Another term used in this realm is **cross-disciplinary** that implies parallel, yet coordinated services rendered to clients from single disciplines. In this environment, the task for accomplishing interprofessional education and services is difficult as single professions struggle for their individual identity and turf issues rise when services overlap among professions.

Oliver (2008) discusses one university in England who developed an interdisciplinary program for the education of professionals to meet the agenda set by the government for *Every Child Matters*. The disciplines included adult nursing, children's nursing, diagnostic imaging, learning disabilities nursing, mental health nursing, midwifery, occupational therapy, physiotherapy, radiotherapy, and social work. Modules were developed for student learning that required cross-discipline experiences not only for students but also for faculty. It was found that agencies serving children were inflexible in adjusting to cross-trained professionals and reverted back to preferring traditional single professionals for services. Many issues came out of the program including the need for continuing dialogue among professionals in the practice setting, faculty, and students to accomplish true interprofessional practice.

Public Health Nursing. Ervin (2008) in an editorial examines the current trends in nursing practice and education and the place of community/public health nursing. She iterates the specialty in terms of generalist (undergraduate) to specialist (graduate) levels and analyzes where research and applied practice will take place through doctoral studies, both research-focused and applied practice. It is her belief that collaboration between practice and education can result in the best preparation of clinicians for the specialty, and she urges the specialty organization to examine these issues for recommendations for the future. Although her observations specify community/public health nursing, the same types of discussions apply to other specialties in nursing.

Cultural Diversity

Core values. Shaw and Degazon (2008) discuss the need for recruiting and retaining culturally diverse students into nursing education and thereby, increasing the diversity of the nursing workforce that aligns with that of the general population. They define *diversity* as representative of ethnicity, culture, gender, age, sexual orientation, and national origin. It is their belief that education and inculcating students of varying backgrounds into the core professional values of nursing will engender a cadre of nurses who practice competently but also have a common set of values that imbue profession. The core professional values that they identify come from the AACN and include human dignity, integrity, altruism, autonomy, and social justice (AACN, 1998). Although these values/essentials come from a decade ago and AACN updated the *Essentials* (AACN, 2010), these values still ring true. Shaw and Degazon point out the fact that nursing has its own culture and that as a profession, common core values help its members who differ in backgrounds to deliver quality care for the equally diverse people they serve.

LVN to BSN. Porter-Wenzlaff and Froman (2008) describe a baccalaureate program developed for moving LVNs (LPNs) to the baccalaureate level of nursing. The undergraduate program was adapted to the needs of LVNs who bring life and nursing experiences to the program along with a need to change their perceptions of professional practice and their belief to accomplish collegiate work. Supportive faculty and one person designated as advocate and coordinator of the program were key to the success of the program. It is posited that LVNs come from diverse backgrounds and are an excellent resource for diversifying the nursing workforce.

Successful recruitment strategies. Edwards et al. (2009) describe a project in Oklahoma to recruit and retain underrepresented minorities into their BSN nursing program. The program included mentors from faculty and elders from the specific ethnic groups that the students represented. The retention and pass rates on NCLEX were excellent and in addition to nurturing the underrepresented students through the program, the development of cultural competence was improved for all nursing students. The project led to the establishment of a Center for Cultural Competency and Health Care Excellence, which is a clearinghouse for information and resources and consultation for students and faculty.

Technology

Emerging technologies. Technology, as would be expected, takes a major role in forecasting trends in nursing education. Skiba (2008) lists three major trends in technology that will have an effect on education. They include social networking such as Facebook, Twitter, Smilebox, Skype (video and audio–real-time communications), and computer gaming. She mentions the iPhone with its touch-screen capabilities, and more recently is the advent of electronic readers and the iPad that has all computer capabilities except the telephone and a touch screen to boot. It is not beyond reality to forecast that these devices will be required for access to online courses and that hard-copied textbooks will rapidly become a thing of the past as texts are delivered electronically.

    Clinical simulation. Jeffries (2009) in an editorial discusses the growing use of clinical simulations for clinical learning and with many state boards of nursing allowing up to 25% of clinical practice to occur in a simulated laboratory setting, additional nursing education programs will be adding and/or expanding on these experiences for students. She mentions the Web site Simulation Innovation Resource Center (SIRC, 2010; http://sirc.nln.org/) as a resource for faculty who wish to learn more about simulated learning experiences.

    Legality issues. Haigh (2009) provides an extensive list of newer technologies, their terms, definitions, and application to nursing education. In addition, she raises copyright and other legal issues as to ownership of electronic and other high technology tools for education. While she speaks about these issues in nursing education in Britain, many of these same concepts apply to U.S. nursing education.

EVIDENCE-BASED EDUCATION

Although there are many studies in the literature examining the effectiveness of teaching/learning strategies, there are few on curriculum development and evaluation. Types of curricula and comparing programs delivered online to mixed-format and traditional curricula on-campus are called for. Questions to evaluate and compare programs should be posed such as, to what extent do:

- Student learning outcomes differ among Web-based, hybrid, and traditional curricula differ?
- Entry-level undergraduate and graduate level programs differ on NCLEX and certification results, program satisfaction, and socialization into the professional role?
- Curricula at the ADN, BSN, MSN, and doctorate levels differ in breadth and depth for certain core nursing values/essentials, for example, caring, social justice, evidence-based practice, cultural competence, and so forth?
- Employers of nurses differentiate practice, roles, and compensation according to level of education and experience?

The National League for Nursing (NLN) recommended research on innovations in nursing education to create reform including the following:

- New pedagogies
- Use of instructional technology, including new approaches to laboratory/simulated learning
- *Flexible curriculum designs
- *Community-driven models for curriculum development
- *Process for reforming nursing education
- *Educational systems and infrastructures
- Student–teacher learning partnerships
- Community-based nursing and service learning strategies
- Clinical teaching models
- New models for teacher preparation and faculty development, particularly as they relate to minority faculty and preparation for teaching diverse student populations (NLN, 2008)

These are laudable ideas and need to be studied and implemented, especially the four that relate specifically to curriculum development as marked by the asterisks. Additional recommendations from NLN for research and the development of nursing science that apply directly to curriculum development and evaluation are the following:

Evaluation Research in Nursing Education: Evaluating Reform

- Economics of and productivity in nursing education
- Quality-improvement processes
- Program evaluation models
- Student and teacher experiences in schools of nursing
- Evaluating the success of diverse student populations
- Nursing education innovations, including facilitators and barriers to innovation and reform
- Best practices in schooling, teaching, and learning
- Grading, testing, and evaluation of students, faculty, and curricula

Development of the Science of Nursing Education: Evidence-Based Reform

- Best practices in schooling, teaching, and learning
- Nursing education database development
- Strategies supportive of nursing education researchers
- Validation of key concepts and keywords related to evidence-based teaching practices
- Meta-analysis related to innovation or evaluation in nursing education
- Concept analysis related to innovation or evaluation in nursing education (NLN, 2008)

CAREER PATHWAYS AND PROMOTING PROFESSIONAL DEVELOPMENT

Donley and Flaherty (2008) conducted an extensive review of the development of nursing "career ladder evolution" and describe it in three phases including the "spiral staircase, career ladders, and professional advancement" stages. Although they discuss entry-level and career ladder opportunities in nursing over the year, they do not discuss entry-level programs at the graduate level (i.e., entry-level master's or doctorate programs). Those programs have been in existence for some time and are increasing in some states, such as California (Board of Registered Nursing [BRN], 2010). Donley and Flaherty discuss the ongoing debate in nursing, which includes clinical experiences within the educational program and the issues of whether experience is required before moving on to the next phase of higher education. Their review describes the complexity of nursing education over the years and the arduous path it takes in reaching professionalism.

Present-day entries into nursing and professional practice are discussed by Raines and Taglaireni (2008). They include entry-level master's programs with the various pathways into nursing. Nursing continues with a plethora of tracks into practice. All types of nursing programs need to work with the next level of education to develop programs that reflect uniformity of credits, courses, and requirements across all schools of nursing, if not for the logic of it, at least for the marketability of schools to potential students wishing to continue their education. Until professional nursing education transforms into doctoral education, the career stepladder curriculum is essential for the majority of nurses who are educated at the diploma, associate degree, and baccalaureate levels to continue their education and at the same time, increase the number of entry-level doctorates in nursing that model nursing education.

Associate Degree: Lower Division Programs

Table 17.1 provides parallel career stepladder and entry-level graduate curricula that propose a unified approach to nursing education allowing for entry into practice at several points, maintaining the career ladder option for persons wishing to enter the workforce in a short time with re-entry later, and a nonstop option to facilitate persons completing a doctorate in nursing much like other professions. The proposed curriculum is not revolutionary; there are no new concepts that have not been discussed in the past, instead traditional courses in nursing are included and the prerequisites and corequisites are much the same as current curricula, except for the addition of proficiency in a language other than the student's primary one, genetics, economics, and computer science. These latter additions should be self-explanatory for their relevance to the nursing curriculum, that is, the multicultural and ethnic world population for whom nursing cares, the breakthroughs in genetic research, the major role of health care economics in the delivery systems, and the ever-expanding world of technology-driven communications.

Baccalaureate: Upper Division Programs

The two parallel curricula in Table 17.2 are much the same as that presented in Table 17.1 although the order may be varied according to the student's place in the respective programs, (i.e., undergraduate or graduate levels). As much as possible, generic labels are assigned to courses to indicate the core content and concepts in courses recognizing that each institution has different titles for courses that contain the same or similar content. The lower and upper division level courses are prescriptive; however, the choices at the

TABLE 17.1 Sample Career Stepladder and Nonstop Graduate Entry-Level Curricula (with options)

Career Stepladder Program Lower Division Associate Degree				Nonstop Graduate Entry-Level Program (With Step-Out Options) Lower Division			
Prerequisites and corequisites	*Semester units*	*Nursing courses**	*Semester units*	*Prerequisites and corequisites*	*Semester units*	*Nursing courses**	*Semester units*
Verbal and Written Communications	6	Introduction to Nursing and Health Care	3	Verbal and Written Communications	6	Introduction to Nursing and Health Care	3
Anatomy and Physiology	8	Basic Health Assessment and Skills	2	Anatomy and Physiology	8	Basic Health Assessment and Skills	2
Microbiology	4	Nursing Process with Skills	2	Microbiology	4	Nursing Process with Skills	2
Pharmacology	3	Geriatric Nursing and Clinical	4	Pharmacology	3	Geriatric Nursing and Clinical	4
Nutrition	3	Parent–Child Nursing and Clinical	6	Nutrition	3	Parent–Child Nursing and Clinical	6
Human Growth and Development	3	Adult Nursing and Clinical	6	Human Growth and Development	3	Adult Nursing and Clinical	6
Introduction to Computer Science	3	Psychiatric/ Mental Health Nursing and Clinical	6	Introduction to Computer Science	3	Psychiatric/ Mental Health Nursing and Clinical	6
Competency in a language other than the student's primary language; otherwise, 2 liberal arts electives	6	12-Week Internship* (RN licensure eligibility upon completion of ADN and internship)		Competency in a language other than the student's primary language; otherwise, 2 liberal arts electives	6		
Total	36	Total ADN units = 65 + Internship	29	Total	36	Total lower division units = 65	29

*Student and faculty choose a mutually agreed upon area of a clinical specialty for a 12-week 35 hours/week internship prior to taking NCLEX.

graduate levels are flexible, allowing for each institution to determine the prerequisites, corequisites, and nursing courses for preparing nurse leaders and educators at the master's level (functional roles versus advanced practice roles). The most frequent functional roles at this point in time include administration, case management, clinical nurse leader, and nurse educator. Advanced practice, nurse executive, and research roles are assumed at the doctorate level.

The major argument for or against professional education becomes apparent in the undergraduate programs. If the curriculum is maintained at 65 units for completion of the lower division, a total of 125 units for the lower and upper divisions, and the necessary prerequisite and corequisite knowledge for nursing are retained, there is no room for electives. Adding electives or prerequisites to nursing prerequisites or corequisites

TABLE 17.2 Sample Baccalaureate and Nonstop Graduate Entry-Level Programs

Career Stepladder Program Upper Division Baccalaureate				Nonstop Graduate Entry-Level Program (With Step-Out Options) Upper Division Courses: Baccalaureate Equivalent			
Prerequisites and corequisites	Semester units	Nursing courses	Semester units	Prerequisites and corequisites	Semester units	Nursing courses	Semester units
Lower Division Associate Degree	65 + RN	Introduction to Research	3	Lower Division	65	Introduction to Research	3
Anthropology (Sociology)	3	The Nursing Profession	3	Anthropology (Sociology)	3	The Nursing Profession	3
Chemistry	4	Acute Care with Clinical**	6	Chemistry	4	Acute Care with Clinical**	6
Economics	3	Nursing Leadership	3	Economics	3	Nursing Leadership	3
Ethics	3	Transcultural Nursing	3	Ethics	3	Transcultural Nursing	3
Genetics	4	Interprofessional Health Care Practice in the Community with Clinical	4	Genetics	4	Interprofessional Health Care Practice in the Community with Clinical	4
						Optional 12-week Internship* (RN licensure upon completion of degree and internship)	Step-out
36 lower division + 24 upper division prerequisites or corequisites	60	29 lower division and 36 upper division nursing courses Total BSN degree units: = 125	65	36 lower division + 24 upper division prerequisites or corequisites	60	29 lower division and 36 upper division nursing courses Total baccalaureate units: = 125	65

*Student and faculty choose a mutually agreed upon area of a clinical specialty for a 12-week 35 hours/week internship prior to taking NCLEX.
**Student chooses area of a clinical specialty with 1 hour seminar and 7 hours clinical preceptorship (total 30 hours/week for 15 weeks or the equivalent).

adds to the length of the program and thereby, the time for students to enter the workforce and to meet health care demands. An analysis of the prescribed curriculum reveals that the nursing major has a total of 65 nursing units (a little over half of the total 125) with the remaining in the arts and sciences. Nor is there room for the institutions' general education requirements that might or might not allow for double counting from the requirements prescribed for the nursing major.

For too long, nursing has been dominated by other disciplines in the academe that have a major influence on the length, composition, and type of degree nursing will have. Convincing other disciplines in higher education institutions of the need to educate nurses with a strong foundation in the arts and sciences and at the same time, prescribing the nursing curriculum that remains within the usual number of units for associate (65 to 70) and bachelor's degrees is difficult (120 to 125). There are numerous courses that nurses value as foundations for practice such as history, the arts, political science, and business as it applies to health care. And yet, there is no room for courses in these disciplines in the 125-unit nursing degree program.

The proposed unified curriculum in Table 17.2 is ideal, but unrealistic owing to the aforementioned issues. Yet, nurse educators should strive to revise or build curricula that are close to the unit requirements rather than continuing to require excess units in undergraduate degrees. At the same time, uniform curricula for both levels that allow seamless entry into the next level are necessary to provide the existing nurse workforce with career ladder opportunities and options for the current applicants to nursing programs.

These issues related to undergraduate education elucidate the need for nursing to move into graduate education. If nurse educators try to integrate the missing arts and sciences components into the curriculum, they add units far exceeding the usual 120 to 125 for the baccalaureate. One needs only to interview nurses with baccalaureates in the 40+ years of age to discover the excess number of credits in their degree work to realize the enormity of the problem and the injustices nurses suffered in gaining education beyond the diploma and associate degree with no academic recognition of their additional work. Going one step further, nurses in that age group or older who hold master's and/or doctorate's suffer the same overabundance of credits, earning far more than their colleagues in medicine, pharmacology, education, engineering, religion, and law. Table 17.2 summarizes current requirements for nursing degrees and can serve in the interim while schools of nursing with bravado develop doctoral programs that accommodate the foundations of a liberal, scientific, and professional education that serve as models for the future.

Based on the curricula in Table 17.2, the argument for "entry into practice" ends with the idea that a candidate is eligible for licensure at various points of the education track commencing with the completion of the associate degree (lower division) and 3-month internship, or completion of the bachelor of science with an internship, or a master's with an internship, or finally, a doctorate upon completion of a clinical residency. Thus, students have a choice for entering practice through licensure at the associate, bachelor's, master's, or doctorate degree levels. At the same time, the curricula contain the same courses or content, thus allowing nurses to enter at the next step of their education to continue their career opportunities. If these generic curricula were adapted by schools of nursing, there would be no need for challenge examinations and repetition of knowledge and skills already assimilated.

Schools of nursing bear the responsibility for evaluating the credentials of applicants with prior education or degrees not in nursing. There is a need for flexibility in granting credit for courses equivalent to those prerequisites and corequisites in nursing and nursing courses (for registered nurses [RNs] with degrees not in nursing) to enter into the curricula and to complete the next academic level. Examples are RNs with baccalaureates in other disciplines and nonnurses with baccalaureates or higher degrees who matriculate directly into master's programs rather than repeating the baccalaureate. Of course, RNs need upper division level nursing courses or their equivalent and nonnurses need nursing courses equivalent to the baccalaureate but offered at the graduate level prior to entering master's- or doctorate-level nursing courses.

Master's Degree Programs

Table 17.3 presents a curriculum at the graduate level for the preparation of nurses for leadership/administrative, case management/clinical nurse leader, and nurse educator roles. It moves advanced practice roles such as nurse practitioners, midwives, anesthetists, and clinical specialists to the doctoral level. (Community/public health nursing is considered a clinical specialty in this model.) Based on AACN's Position Paper (2004) on the DNP as the final degree for advanced practice, it is apparent that a majority of nursing programs is transitioning advanced practice programs at the master's level into the doctorate.

Doctorate Degree Programs

Table 17.4 continues the step-career ladder and entry-level graduate programs very similar to what happens today in nursing as nurses seek higher degrees, having initiated practice at the diploma, associate degree, or baccalaureate levels. The difference in the sample curriculum from existing programs is that it provides an articulated curriculum among the various levels and thus, provides easy transfer of credit between programs and savings of time. At the same time, the curriculum on the right side of the table provides for a nonstop program to allow students to accelerate through the various levels toward a doctorate.

Entry-Level Doctorate Programs

Nursing needs to expand entry-level doctorate programs to accommodate the vast body of knowledge and skills expected of the professional nurse today and in the future. It has been more than 60 years since baccalaureate and associate degree programs began to flourish. In that time, major revolutions in technology and health-related sciences have taken place. It is no wonder that the undergraduate programs can no longer accommodate all of the new knowledge and skills that must be included in a nursing curriculum. Table 17.5 introduces an 8-year entry-level doctorate curriculum with a ninth year for a PhD option. The program is divided into a 4-year prenursing program ending with a baccalaureate and continuing into a 4-year school of nursing. See Table 17.5 for an outline of the program.

The development of entry-level doctoral programs should not disenfranchise education programs that prepare nurses at the undergraduate and master's levels. In fact, as increasing numbers of programs become graduate programs, the need for foundation courses will still exist at the lower and upper division levels of undergraduate education. A prenursing curriculum in the undergraduate program should contain introductory courses to nursing and health care and require faculty at that level. Nursing courses in graduate level programs require nursing faculty who are expert in the specialties to facilitate students' assimilation of the knowledge and skills required for the specialties.

Table 17.5 outlines a prenursing and nursing school curriculum plan that should be considered for the future. It is dangerous to set a deadline, but ideally, the mid 21st century is a desirable target. To accomplish the task, existing and new programs could begin to initiate these programs and eventually phase out the old plans. Although it is difficult

TABLE 17.3 Sample Master's and Nonstop Graduate Entry-Level Programs

	Career Stepladder Program Graduate-Level Master of Science in Nursing			Nonstop Entry-level Graduate Program (With Step-Out Options) Graduate-level Postbaccalaureate		
Prerequisites and corequisites	Semester units	Nursing courses	Semester units	Prerequisites and corequisites	Semester units	Nursing courses	Semester units
Baccalaureate with RN and 36 units in upper division nursing or equivalent	125	Nursing Research	3	Baccalaureate with selected prerequisites and 36 units in upper division nursing or equivalent	125	Nursing Research	3
Informatics and Technology in Health Care	3	Nursing Theories/Scientific Foundations	3	Informatics and Technology in Health Care	3	Nursing Theories/Scientific Foundations	3
		Health Care Policy, Economics, and Political Action	3			Health Care Policy, Economics, and Political Action	3
		Advanced Pathophysiology (CM, CNL, EDU) or Organizational Theories in Health Care (ADM)	3			Advanced Pathophysiology (CM, CNL, EDU) or Organizational Theories in Health Care (ADM)	3
		Advanced Pharmacology (CM, CNL, EDU) or Change Theory and Leadership in Health Care (ADM)	3			Advanced Pharmacology (CM, CNL, EDU) or Change Theory and Leadership in Health Care (ADM)	3
		Advanced Health Assessment (CM, CNL, EDU) or Human Resources Management (ADM)	3			Advanced Health Assessment (CM, CNL, EDU) or Human Resources Management (ADM)	3
		Interprofessional Communication and Collaboration (ADM, CN, CNL) or Program Development and Evaluation (EDU)	3			Interprofessional Communication and Collaboration (ADM, CN, CNL) or Program Development and Evaluation (EDU)	3
		Functional* Specialization I with Internship	3			Functional* Specialization I with Internship	3
		Building A Budget Case and Management of Budgets (ADM, CM, CNL) or Instructional Strategies and Evaluation (EDU)	3			Building A Budget Case and Management of Budgets (ADM, CM, CNL) or Instructional Strategies and Evaluation (EDU)	3
		Functional* Specialization II with Internship	3			Functional* Specialization II with Internship	3
		Research Project	3			Research Project	3
						Optional 12-week Internship (NCLEX eligibility upon degree completion and internship)	Step-out
Total	3	Total MSN units = 36	33	Total	3	Total graduate units = 36 Total BSN and MSN = 164	33

*Functional specialization examples: Case Management (CM); Clinical Nurse leader (CNL); Supervision/Administration (ADM); Staff Development/Patient and Family Education or Nurse Educator for Undergraduate or Technical Level Nursing Programs (EDU).

TABLE 17.4 Sample Doctorate and Nonstop Graduate Entry-Level Programs

Career Stepladder Program Graduate Level: Doctorate				Nonstop Entry-level Graduate Program Doctorate (With Step-Out Options)			
Prerequisite: BSN and MSN or their equivalent with RN/Certification if Applicable				Prerequisite: Baccalaureate and graduate study with equivalent prerequisites and corequisites and nursing courses			
DNP*		DNSc or PhD**		DNP*		DNSc or PhD**	
Courses	Units	Courses	Units	Courses	Units	Courses	Units
Advanced Pathophysiology*** or Organizational Behavior	3	Nursing History and Philosophy	3	Advanced Pathophysiology*** or Organizational Behavior	3	Nursing History and Philosophy	3
Advanced Pharmacology*** or Health Care Systems Analysis	3	Nursing Science	3	Advanced Pharmacology*** or Health Care Systems Analysis	3	Nursing Science	3
Advanced Health Assessment*** **or** Human Resource Management	3	Quantitative Research	3	Advanced Health Assessment*** **or** Human Resource Management	3	Quantitative Research	3
2 cognates for specialization***	6	Qualitative Research	3	2 cognates for specialization	3	Qualitative Research	3
Translational Research	3	Seminar in Research	3	Translational Research	3	Seminar in Research	3
Evidence-Based Practice/ Administration	3	Theory Analysis, Application, Testing, Development	12	Evidence-Based Practice/ Administration	3	Theory Analysis, Application, Testing, Development	3
Health Care Economics	3	Health Care Economics	3	Health Care Economics	3	Health Care Economics	3
Advanced Informatics and Technology	3	Advanced Informatics and Technology	3	Advanced Informatics and Technology	3	Advanced Informatics and Technology	3
Analysis of Health Care Policy and Ethics	3	Analysis of Health Care Policy and Ethics	3	Analysis of Health Care Policy and Ethics	3	Analysis of Health Care Policy and Ethics	3
Residency in specialization	9	Cognates for role specialization (education, research, clinical)	9	Residency in specialization	9	Cognates for role specialization (education, research, clinical)	
DNP Project Proposal	3	Comprehensive Exam	3	DNP Project Proposal	3	Comprehensive Exam	
DNP Project Implementation	3	Dissertation Proposal	6	DNP Project Implementation	3	Dissertation Proposal	6
DNP Project Defense	3	Dissertation Defense	6	DNP Project Defense	3	Dissertation Defense	6
Total Credits	48****	Total Credits	60	Total Credits	48****	Total Credits	60

*Doctor of Nursing Practice (DNP) for Advanced Practice or Nurse Executive roles.
Examples: Nurse Practitioner, Nurse Midwife, Nurse Anesthetist, Clinical Specialist or Chief Nursing Officer, Health Care Policy Analyst, Informatics Specialist, Quality Assurance Officer, and so forth.
**Doctor of Nursing Science (DNSc/DNS) or Doctor of Philosophy in Nursing (PhD).
Examples: Research and theory development in administration, education, informatics and technology, nursing science, nursing practice, public policy.
***Credit for these courses may be transferred in from previous master's level work.
****Graduates of master's programs that include advanced practice may transfer in a total of 12 credits; thus the post-master's DNP totals 36.

TABLE 17.5 Proposed Entry-Level Doctorate Curriculum

Prenursing Freshman Year (9 Courses with 31 Semester Units or Credits)

Life, physical, and social sciences	Number of courses (units or credits)	General education, liberal arts, and humanities	Number of courses (units or credits)
Anatomy	1 (4)	Communications–Written	1 (3)
Physiology	1 (4)	Communications–Oral	1 (3)
Psychology	1 (3)	History	1 (3)
Chemistry	2 (8)		
Subtotal	**5 (19)**		**3 (9)**

Sophomore Year (10 Courses with 32 Semester Units or Credits)

Microbiology	1 (4)	Language (or elective if proficient)	2 (6)
Physics	1 (4)	Government and Politics	1 (3)
Human Growth and Development	1 (3)	Electives or General Education Requirements	1 (3)
Sociology	1 (3)		
Subtotal	4 (14)		4 (12)

Junior Year (10 Courses with 32 Semester Units or Credits)

Genetics	1 (4)	Bioethics	1 (3)
Anthropology (Sociology)	1 (3)	Economics	1 (3)
Biochemistry	1 (4)	Electives or General Education Requirements	2 (6)
Subtotal	3 (11)		4 (12)
Pharmacology I	1 (3)	Electives or General Education Requirements	1 (3)
Nutrition	1 (3)	Introduction to Business Administration	1 (3)
Gerontology	1 (3)		
Pathophysiology	1 (3)		
Subtotal	4 (12)		2 (6)
Grand Total	16 (56)		13 (39)

Graduation at the end of 4 years with baccalaureate and 125 semester units or credits.

Senior Year (10 Courses with 30 Semester Units or Credits: 1 Clinical Experience Course)

Nursing Science	Number of courses (units or credits)	Nursing Practice	Number of courses (units or credits)
Care of the Adult	1 (3)	Advanced Nursing Skills	1 (2)
Parent–Child Nursing	2 (6)	Clinical Practice	3 (9)
Subtotal	3 (9)		4 (11)

Four Year School of Nursing First Year (11 courses with 32 semester units or credits).

Mathematics and statistics	Number of courses (units or credits)	Nursing and health care	Number of courses (units or credits)
Mathematics	1 (3)		
	1 (3)		
Computer Science	1 (3)	The Health Care System and Professions	1 (3)
	1 (3)		1 (3)
Statistics	1 (3)	History of Nursing	1 (3)
		Transcultural Nursing	1 (3)
	1 (3)		2 (6)
Introduction to Research	1 (3)	The Nursing Process and Skills	1 (3)
		Health Assessment	1 (2)
		Care of the Older Adult with Clinical	1 (4)
	1 (3)		3 (9)
	4 (12)		6 (18)

Cognates	Number of courses (units or credits)	Nursing Research	Number of courses (units or credits)
Pharmacology II	1 (3)	Introduction to Nursing Research	1 (3)
Advanced Statistics and Computer Science I	1 (3)	Nursing Science and Domains	1 (3)
	2 (6)		2 (6)

(Continued)

TABLE 17.5 Proposed Entry-Level Doctorate Curriculum *Continued*

Second Year (11 Courses with 32 Semester Units or Credits)

Nursing Science	Number of courses (units or credits)	Nursing Practice	Number of courses (units or credits)
Mental Health Nursing	1 (3)	Advanced Health Assessment	1 (2)
Acute Care Nursing	1 (3)	Clinical Practice	3 (9)
Community Health Nursing	1 (3)		
Leadership and Management	1 (3)		
Subtotal	**4 (12)**		**4 (11)**

Third Year (11 Courses with 32 Semester Units or Credits)

Selected Nursing Specialty I and II	2 (6)	Role Development	1 (2)
History and Philosophy of Nursing	1 (3)	Clinical Practice	2 (6)
Health Care Issues, Ethics Policies and Actions	1 (3)		
Subtotal	4 (12)		3 (8)

Fourth Year (7 Courses with 30 to 33 Units or Credits)

Theory in selected program	1 (3)	Internship in selected specialty	1 (12)
Seminar in selected program	1 (3)		
Subtotal	2 (6)		1 (12)
Grand Total	13 (39)		12 (42)

Graduation with DNP with 126 to 129 semester units or credits.

Fifth Year (8 Courses with 30 Semester Units or Credits)

Nursing Science	Units	Nursing Practice or functional area	Units
Seminar in selected function or practice	1 (3)	Residency in selected program	1 (6)
Grand Total	1 (3)		1 (6)

Graduation with DNSc or PhD in Nursing = 156 to 159 semester units or credits.

Cognates	Number of courses (units or credits)	Nursing Research	Number of courses (units or credits)
Advanced Statistics and Computer Science II	1 (3)	Theories Analysis	1 (3)
Advanced Pathophysiology	1 (3)		
	2 (6)		**1 (3)**
Research Methodologies	1 (3)	Nursing Research I	1 (3)
		Theory Application	1 (3)
		Research or Project Proposal	1 (3)
	1 (3)		3 (9)
Two cognates to support specialty	2 (6)	Theory Testing	1 (3)
		Research project or dissertation	1 (3 to 6)
	2 (6)		2 (6 to 9)
	7 (21)		8 (24 to 27)

Cognates	Units	Nursing research	Units
Advanced Statistics III or Computer Science	1 (3)	Nursing Research II	1 (3)
Research Methodology	1 (3)	Theory Development	1 (3)
		Dissertation Seminar	1 (3)
		Dissertation Defense	1 (6)
	2 (6)		4 (15)

to predict the development of a nationwide licensing program that could help to define a unified code of requirements for licensure eligibility, these new programs would continue to meet licensing requirements. The entry-level doctorate programs could be of two types, that is, the research-focused PhD and DNSc and the practice-focused DNP.

The advantages to the entry-level doctorate program are numerous. It would facilitate high school graduates' entry into a nursing program with graduation 8 years away thus, producing expert clinicians, researchers, and educators who are relatively young in age. If these candidates choose not to pursue nursing in the first 4 years, their options are many for changing majors. The prenursing curriculum provides a strong scientific and liberal arts background for the increasingly complex professional world of nursing. Graduates of the programs will be on equal footing with other health care professionals. The 4-year nursing school would be open to applicants with baccalaureates who seek major or career changes. The 8-year total curriculum plan provides the time for in-depth education and the production of quality graduates prepared for practice, teaching, and research roles.

If the profession embraces this transformation of nursing education, then it must come to grips with the reality that there are roles for personnel such as the licensed practical/vocational nurses. The proposed model calls for an expansion of that technical model comparable to the expansion of technical and support services within the health care system. It is logical that these programs fall into the community college genre; thus, raising the specter of the "Civil War" in nursing yet again. This author leaves that debate to the nurse educators reading this text and the nursing profession over the next few decades.

SUMMARY

Chapter 17 summarized each of the previous chapters in the text and raised issues from each topic. While the world order, the national society, and the health care system change so rapidly, it is difficult to predict the future; there are prevailing trends that should have an impact on the development and evaluation of nursing curricula over the next decade. If nursing chooses not to respond to these changes, the danger is that education will not transform and instead, maintain a status quo existence much as it has in the past 60 years. This could mean that the profession will continue to be splintered with less opportunity for it to help in shaping public policy toward optimal health care for the populace. Nurse educators have a responsibility to work with their colleagues in practice and research to develop curricula that prepare nurses for the future, who are competent and caring, and who are scholars and researchers. A nursing education system for the future will have the following characteristics:

1. Clearly defined levels of education and differentiated practice based on education and experience
2. Entry into practice for staff nurse positions following a 3-month internship in a selected arena of practice
3. Quality institutions of higher education that specialize in the preparation of staff nurses for entry into practice in a timely fashion

4. Quality institutions that focus on the faculty role of excellence in teaching, community service, research, and the application of knowledge from nursing science and related disciplines

5. Quality institutions of higher education that specialize in the preparation of nurses to provide evidence-based advanced practice nursing services for families, communities, and aggregates

6. Students and faculty who are active participants in nursing and related disciplines' research activities

7. Quality institutions of higher education that specialize in the preparation of nurses for advanced practice nursing services for families and aggregates

8. Quality institutions of higher education that specialize in the preparation of nurse leaders who will influence health care policy and change the health care system for the benefit of the populations they serve

9. Academic and health science centers that specialize in nursing research and development for the advancement of nursing science through evidence-based practice; testing of theories; the development of new theories, concepts, and models; and educational innovations on the national and international levels

DISCUSSION QUESTIONS

1. Given the rapid changes in the health care and education systems and the ongoing shortage of nurses, what changes in nursing education do you envision within the next 5 to 10 years?

2. What strategies for changing nursing education worked in the past and how can these success stories apply to needed changes in nursing education today? What are the lessons from the past that prohibited nursing from moving its educational agenda forward? How can today's nurse educators use these lessons to bring about change?

LEARNING ACTIVITIES

Student Learning Activities

Synthesize the information in this text into a "Dream School of Nursing." Develop a curriculum that prepares nurses to practice 10 years hence, keeping in mind that practice and the setting in which it is delivered will be different. Let your imagination run wild!

Faculty Development Activities

Hold a faculty meeting focused on brainstorming and let creative thoughts flow freely. List the characteristics of the ideal nurse prepared to practice 5 to 10 years hence. Examine these characteristics and decide how a curriculum can be developed that provides the kind of education necessary to prepare this kind of nurse. Focus on creativity and newer theories of learning. Compare these ideas to your existing curriculum. How can it be transformed into the one you envision?

REFERENCES

American Association of Colleges of Nursing. (1998). *The essentials of baccalaureate education: For professional nursing practice.* Washington, DC: Author.

American Association of Colleges of Nursing. (2004). *AACN position statement on the practice doctorate in nursing.* Retrieved from http://www.aacn.nche.edu/DNP/DNPPosition Statement.htm

American Association of Colleges of Nursing. (2010). *The essentials of baccalaureate education for professional nursing practice.* Retrieved from http://www.aacn.nche.edu/Education/bacessn.htm

Bloom, B. S., Engelhart, M. D., Furst, E. J., Hill, W. H., & Krathwahl, D. R. (1956). *The taxonomy of educational objectives, handbook 1: Cognitive domain.* Chicago: University of Chicago.

Board of Registered Nursing. (2010). *RN programs. entry-level master's degree programs.* Retrieved from http://www.rn.ca.gov/schools/rnprograms.shtml#msn

Donley, R., & Flaherty, M. J. (2008). Promoting professional development: Three phases of articulation in nursing education and practice. *Online Journal of Issues in Nursing. 13*(3).

Edwards, K., Radcliffe, S., Patchell, B., Broussard, K., Wood, E., & Ogans, J. (2009). Outcomes: The recruitment enhancement cultural affirmation project. *Journal of Cultural Diversity, 16*(2), 64–67.

Ervin, N. (2008). Public health nursing education: Looking back while moving forward. *Public Health Nursing, 25*(6), 502–504.

Haigh, C. (2009). Legality, the web and nurse educators. *Nurse Education Today. 30*(6), 553–556.

Jeffries, P. R. (2009). Dreams for the future for clinical simulation. *Nursing Education Perspectives, 30*(2), 71.

National League for Nursing. (2008). *Research priorities in nursing education.* Retrieved from http://www.nln.org/research/priorities.htm

Oliver, B. (2008). Reforming the children and young people's workforce: A higher education response. *Learning in Health & Social Care, 7*(4), 209–218.

Porter-Wenzlaff, L. J., & Froman, R. D. (2008). Responding to increasing RN demand: Diversity and retention trends through an accelerated LVN-to-BSN curriculum. *Journal of Nursing Education. 47*(5), 231–235.

Raines C. F., & Taglaireni M. E. (2008). Career pathways in nursing: Entry points and academic progression. *Online Journal of Issues in Nursing, 13*(3).

Shaw, H. K., & Degazon, C. (2008). Integrating the core professional values of nursing: A profession, not just a career. *Journal of Cultural Diversity, 15*(1), 44–50.

Simulation Innovation Resource Center. (2010). Retrieved from http://sirc.nln.org/

Skiba, D. (2008). The year in review and trends to watch in 2008. *Nursing Education Perspectives, 29* (1), 46–47.

Speziale, H. J., & Jacobson, L. (2005). Trends in registered nurse education programs 1998–2008. *Nursing Education Perspectives, 26*(4), 230–235.

Tyler, R. W. (1949). *Basic principles of curriculum and instruction.* Chicago: University of Chicago Press.

APPENDIX: Glossary

accreditation. A process that education programs and curricula undergo to receive recognition for meeting basic standards or criteria set by national, regional, or state organizations. Although it is voluntary, most programs undergo accreditation to demonstrate their quality to the consumers of their products (students, parents, alumni, and employers).

adult learning theory, andragogy. A model of learning using assumptions of adults' autonomy, life experiences, personal goals, and need for relevancy and respect.

advance organizers. A means of preparing the learner's cognitive structure for the learning experience with activities at the onset of the lesson to help the new information be more readily connected with prior learning or help direct the learners' attention to important concepts (Schunk, 2004).

assessment. A process that gathers information that results in a conclusion such as a nursing diagnosis or problem identification.

asynchronous. Learning activities that occur at various times.

behaviorism, behaviorist learning theory. A group of learning theories, often referred to as stimulus–response, that view learning as the result of the stimulus conditions and the responses (behaviors) that follow, generally ignoring what goes on inside the learner.

body politic. The people power(s) behind the official government within a community. It is composed of the major political forces and the people who exert influence within the community.

business case. A document prepared or written and presented to generate support from the agency leadership and other key stakeholders. It identifies the need, purpose, and the relationship of the program to the overall mission of the organization. It provides the context and content around the need and lists the desired objectives, outcomes, and its advantages to the health care organization.

classical conditioning. Respondent or Pavlovian conditioning that emphasizes the stimulus and associations made with it in the learning process; these associations are often unconscious.

cognitivism, cognitive learning theory. A group of learning theories focused on cognitive processes such as decision making, problem solving, synthesizing, and evaluating.

competencies. These are very similar to objectives but are usually used to describe the skills and/or application of knowledge to practice or professional behaviors.

Skills example: At the end of the vital signs lab, the student will accurately measure, and record the vital signs of a classmate.

Knowledge example: At the end of the class on the history of nursing, the student will write a short well-organized, correct, and referenced essay describing one milestone in nursing history over the past century that had an influence on today's profession.

Application to practice example: When caring for a diabetic patient, the student will provide the patient with accurate knowledge about diabetes and self-care that is at an appropriate level for the patient's age, development, education, culture, and understanding.

community. A place-oriented process of interrelated actions through which members of a local population express a shared sense of identity while engaging in the common concerns of life (Theodori, 2005, pp. 662–663).

constructivism, constructivist learning theory. A learning perspective arguing that individuals construct much of what they learn and understand, producing knowledge based on their beliefs and experiences.

continuous quality improvement (CQI). The implementation of a system designed to provide for ongoing evaluation, analysis of findings, and implementation of plans for improvement within an organization.

critical thinking. "Critical thinking is the intellectually disciplined process of actively and skillfully conceptualizing, applying, analyzing, synthesizing, and/or evaluating information gathered from, or generated by, observation, experience, reflection, reasoning, or communication, as a guide to belief and action" (Scriven & Paul, 1987).

cross-disciplinary. Activities involving two or more disciplines in learning together and/or providing services to clients that reflect the characteristics of each of the disciplines involved.

cultural and linguistic competence. A set of congruent behaviors, attitudes, and policies that come together in a system, agency, or among professionals that enables effective work in cross-cultural situations (U.S. Department of Health and Human Services, 2001).

curriculum. The formal plan of study that provides the philosophical underpinnings, goals, and guidelines for delivery of a specific educational program.

demographics. Data that describe the characteristics of a population (e.g., age, gender, socioeconomic status, ethnicity, education levels, etc.).

discovery learning. Obtaining knowledge for oneself by formulating general rules, concepts or principles through learning activities and assignments rather than studying specific examples by reading or listening to the teacher.

disinhibition. A situation in which performing a particular behavior does not result in negative consequences.

distance education. Any learning experience that takes place a distance away from the parent educational institution's home campus.

entry-level programs. Programs that prepare students for eligibility to take the licensure examination (NCLEX) for registered nurses (RNs). The programs include diploma, associate degree, baccalaureate, master's and doctoral levels. Students entering master's entry-level programs have a baccalaureate in another field as a minimum, whereas students in entry-level doctoral programs have a master's degree in another discipline as a minimum. Students in entry-level programs *do not* have previous education in nursing.

evaluation. The determination of the worth of a thing. It includes obtaining information for use in judging the worth of a program, product, procedure, or objective or the potential for utility of alternative approaches to attain specific objectives (Worthen & Sanders, 1974, p. 19).

external frame factors. Those factors that influence curriculum development in the environment and outside the parent institution.

formal curriculum. The planned program of studies for an academic degree or discipline.

formative evaluation. The assessment that takes place during the implementation of the program or curriculum. It can also be viewed as process evaluation. In education, this type of evaluation is often linked to course or level objectives.

frame factors. The external and internal factors that influence, impinge upon, and/or enhance educational programs and curricula. As a conceptual model, they serve to collect, organize, and analyze information that is useful for the development and evaluation of curricula. There are two major categories of frame factors, external and internal factors.

generalization. A conditioned response that spreads to similar situations.

genetics. The study of inheritance patterns of specific traits (Human Genome Project Information, 2010).

genome. All the genetic material in the chromosomes of a particular organism; its size is generally given as its total number of base pairs (Human Genome Project Information, 2010).

genome project. The research and technology-development effort aimed at mapping and sequencing the genome of human beings and certain model organisms (Human Genome Project Information, 2010).

goal. Overall statement(s) of what the program prepares the graduates for. They are usually long-term and in global terms.

goal-based evaluation. Based on the stated goals of the entity undergoing evaluation. It is frequently used in education and tied to the stated goals, purpose, and end-of-program objectives of the program or curriculum.

goal-free evaluation. A method for evaluators to assess and judge some thing or entity. That person has no prior knowledge of the entity (program or curriculum) that he/she is evaluating. The person must be an expert in the field of evaluation and the type of entity that is evaluated. The value of this type of evaluation is that it is relatively bias-free.

humanism, humanistic learning theory. An approach to teaching that assumes people are inherently good, possess unlimited potential for growth, and therefore, it emphasizes personal freedom, choice, self-determination, and self-actualization.

informal curriculum. Sometimes termed as the hidden curriculum, cocurriculum, or as extracurricular activities; planned and unplanned influences on students' learning.

inhibition. Reducing the frequency of an action by receiving negative feedback for that action.

institutional accreditation. Accreditation that provides a comprehensive review of the functioning and effectiveness of the entire college, university, or technical institute. The state mandate or particular institutional mission provides the lens used to guide the review.

instructional scaffolding. A process of controlling task elements by gradually increasing expectations of complex, realistic, and relevant learning projects; initially beyond the learners' capacity (Schunk, 2004; Woolfolk, 2010).

interdisciplinary. Activities in learning together and/or providing services to clients that focus on the client served and integrate knowledge and skills from the disciplines involved. Disciplines are not specific to the professions and can include such disciplines as mathematics, the humanities, sociology, and so forth.

internal frame factors. Those factors that influence curriculum development and are within the environment of the parent institution and the program itself.

interprofessional. Activities that involve learning together and/or providing services to clients that are reflective of the individual professions but integrate the knowledge and skills of all professions involved, with the client as the focus of service.

learning. A "relatively permanent change in mental processing, emotional functioning, and/or behavior as a result of experience" (Bastable, 2008, p. 52).

learning theory. A coherent framework of integrated constructs and principles that describe, explain, or predict how people learn (Bastable, 2008, p. 52).

managed care system. A health care system with administrative control over primary health care services in a medical group practice. The intention is to eliminate redundant facilities and services and to reduce costs. Health education and preventive medicine are emphasized. Patients may pay a flat fee for basic family care but may be charged additional fees for secondary care services (Mosby, 2009).

metacognition. Cognition about cognition, or thinking about thinking; monitoring the learning progress by checking the level of understanding, evaluating the effectiveness of efforts, planning activities, and revising as necessary.

metaparadigm for nursing. Most commonly accepted terms included in the metaparadigm are nursing (practice), environment, health, and the client (Fawcett, 1996).

mission statement. The institution's beliefs about its responsibility for the delivery of programs through teaching, service, and scholarship.

multidisciplinary. Activities that involve learning together and/or providing services for clients that reflect the knowledge and skills of each discipline but provided as parallel services, not integrated.

national accreditation. Any accreditation agency that accredits colleges, universities, or technical institutes within an entire country.

needs assessment. The process of collecting and analyzing information that can influence the decision to initiate a new program or revise an existing one.

negative reinforcement. Strengthening a behavior by the removal of an unpleasant stimulus.

nonsectarian. Not associated with a religious organization.

objectives. The steps necessary for reaching the overall goal of the program that include the learner, a behavior that is measurable, a time frame, level of competency, and the topic or behavior expected.

> **end-of-program objectives.** Highest level of learner behaviors that demonstrate the characteristics, knowledge, and skills expected of the graduate and relate to the overall goal. They focus on the learner and must include a behavior that is measurable, a time frame, level of competency, and the topic or behavior expected. These can also be defined as student learning outcomes.
>
> *Example: X School of Nursing* prepares competent, compassionate nurse clinicians and leaders who serve the health care needs of the people of *State* and the health care system.
>
> **midlevel (intermediate) objectives.** Have the same properties as end-of-program objectives but occur midway through an educational program and are usually higher than the first level objectives.
>
> **course objectives.** Have the same properties as end-of-program and midlevel objectives but apply to specific courses and relate to and lead toward midlevel and end-of-program objectives.
>
> **student (individual) learning outcomes.** All of the above objectives are student or individual learning outcomes as each objective should be learner-centered and describe what behavior (outcome) is expected.
>
> *Example:* At the end of the health assessment course, the student will present a complete health assessment of a client that includes an accurate health history, a write-up of all components of the physical examination, a list of problems and actual or potential nursing diagnoses, and a plan for follow-up of the problems and diagnoses.

operant conditioning. Rewarding a behavior to strengthen its likelihood of repetition. These behaviors are emitted responses or operants, voluntary operations performed by the individual, in contrast to classical conditioning in which behavior follows a stimulus (Standridge, 2002).

outcome evaluation. Similar to goal-based evaluation, but it may include other items to measure outcomes, for example, graduation rates, NCLEX results, career success for its graduates, and so forth.

PhD program (or in the case of nursing, PhD, DNS, or DNSc). Degrees that emphasize nursing theory and research and educate nurses prepared to conduct research and foster the development of new knowledge in health care and nursing.

phenomenological field. An individual's reality, as the center of their own personal experience, that can never be completely known by another (Boeree, 2006).

philosophy. "the critical analysis of fundamental assumptions or beliefs" ("Philosophy," 2005).

positive reinforcement. Strengthening a behavior by a pleasant stimulus presented following a particular behavior.

presentation punishment. The appearance of the stimulus following the behavior suppresses or decreases that behavior.

principle of contiguity. Two or more sensations occurring together often enough will result in association (Woolfolk, 2010).

private educational institution. An institution supported through private funding.

professional degree. The Doctor of Nursing Practice (DNP) that prepares graduates for application of research to practice or another way to say it is to translate research into practice.

program approval. A process whereby regulating bodies review programs to ensure consumer safety. Nursing education programs are subject to the state regulations that are usually administered by the State Board of Registered Nursing.

programmatic or specialized accreditation. Accreditation that focuses on the functioning and effectiveness of a particular program or unit within the larger institution (e.g., nursing).

public institution. Institution whose main financial support comes through governmental funds.

punishment. Anything that decreases or suppresses behavior.

quality. A "degree of excellence" ("Quality," n.d.).

quality assurance. "…the systematic monitoring and evaluation of the various aspects of a project, service, or facility to ensure that standards of quality are being met" ("Quality assurance," n.d.).

quality control. "An aggregate of activities (as design analysis and inspection for defects) designed to insure adequate quality especially in manufactured products" ("Quality control," n.d.).

regional accreditation agency. One of six private, voluntary accreditation agencies within the United States, formed for peer evaluation and setting of standards for higher education.

regulatory. A form of approval, recognition, or accreditation required by a federal, state, or provincial government agency.

reinforcement. Any consequence that strengthens the behavior it follows.

removal punishment. Removal of a stimulus following the behavior in question to decrease the likelihood of the behavior.

research extensive institution. Institutions that award at least 50 or more doctoral degrees in at least 15 or more disciplines.

research intensive institution. Institutions that award at least 10 doctoral degree in at least 3 or more disciplines or at least 20 degrees per year overall.

response facilitation. Providing social prompts for observers to behave in a certain way.

role modeling or observational learning. Behavioral, cognitive, and affective changes resulting from observation of others.

satellite campuses. Those programs that offer the curriculum in whole or in part on off-campus sites from the institution. Although they can incorporate technology methods such as videoconferencing and Web-based instruction, the majority of teaching and learning takes place in classrooms and involves in-person interactions between the faculty and students.

sectarian. Associated with or supported by a religious organization.

self-efficacy. "People's judgments of their capabilities to organize and execute courses of action required to attain designated types of performances" (Bandura, 1986, p. 391).

single-purpose institution. An institution of higher education that focuses on one discipline.

situated cognition. Learning that cannot be separated from its context; the way individual learners interact with their worlds transforms their particular thinking.

social cognitive theory. An explanation for learning that emphasizes the importance of observing and modeling behaviors, attitudes, and emotional responses of others. Largely attributed to Bandura (1986) and earlier known as social learning theory.

specialized accreditation agencies. Accreditation agencies that focus on the functioning or effectiveness of a particular kind of program (e.g., nursing) or those that review a specialized, single-purpose college or postsecondary school.

state-regulatory agencies. Those agencies that are required to recognize or approve colleges, universities, or programs for operation with the state as governed by state statutes.

summative evaluation. Takes place at the end of the program and measures the final outcome. In systems theory, one could say that for all living systems, evaluation is formative. Summative evaluation takes place after a system terminates or "dies." In education, summative evaluation is often linked to the goal(s) or purpose of the program.

synchronous. Learning activities that take place simultaneously.

total quality management. An educational program's commitment to and strategies for collecting comprehensive information on the program's effectiveness in meeting its goals and the management of its findings to ensure the continued quality of the program.

transformative learning. Reformulating understanding of an experience with the specific purpose of transforming one's perspective; the learner "uses a prior interpretation to construe a new or revised interpretation of the meaning of one's experience to guide future action" (Taylor, 2007, p. 173).

vision statement. Outlook-oriented and reflects the institution's plans and dreams about its direction for the future.

voluntary. A form of accreditation not required by law or regulation. Voluntary accreditation processes are managed by private, voluntary organizations composed of peer member institutions or programs.

REFERENCES

Bandura, A. (1986). *Social foundations of thought and action: A social cognitive theory.* Englewood Cliff, NJ: Prentice-Hall.

Bastable. S. (2008). *Nurse as educator. Principles of teaching and learning for nursing practice* (3rd ed.). Sudbury, MA: Jones and Bartlett.

Boeree, C. G. (2006). Carl Rogers. Retrieved February 21, 2010, from http://webspace.ship.edu/cgboer/rogers.html

Human Genome Project Information. (2010). *About the human genome project.* Retrieved from http://www.ornl.gov/sci/techresources/Human_Genome/project/about.shtml

Mosby. (2009). *Mosby's Medical Dictionary* (8th ed.). St. Louis, MO: Elsevier.

Philosophy. (2005). *The American Heritage® Dictionary of the English Language* (4th ed.). Boston, MA: Houghton Mifflin Company.

Quality. (n.d.). In *Merriam-Webster's online dictionary.* Retrieved from http://www.merriam-webster.com/dictionary/quality

Quality assurance. (n.d.). In *Merriam-Webster's online dictionary.* Retrieved from http://www.merriam-webster.com/dictionary/quality%20assurance

Quality control. (n.d.). In *Merriam-Webster's online dictionary.* Retrieved from http://www.merriam-webster.com/dictionary/quality%20control

Schunk, D. H. (2004). *Learning theories: An educational perspective* (4th ed.). Upper Saddle River, NJ: Pearson, Prentice Hall.

Scriven, M. & Paul, R. (1987). Critical Thinking as Defined by the National Council for Excellence in Critical Thinking. *A statement by Michael Scriven and Richard Paul.* Retrieved from http://www.criticalthinking.org/aboutCT/define_critical_thinking.cfm

Standridge, M. (2002). Behaviorism. In M. Orey (Ed.), *Emerging perspectives on learning, teaching, and technology.* Retrieved February 15, 2010, from http://projects.coe.uga.edu/epltt/index.php?title=Behaviorism

Taylor, E. W. (2007). An update of transformative learning theory: A critical review of the empirical research (1999–2005) [Electronic version]. *International Journal of Lifelong Education, 26*(2), 175–183.

Theodori, G. L. (2005). Community and community development in resource-based areas: Operational definitions rooted in an interactional perspective. *Society and Natural Resources, 18*(7), 661–669.

Woolfolk, A. (2010). *Educational psychology* (11th ed.). Upper Saddle River, NJ: Merrill.

Worthen, B. R., & Sanders, J. R. (1974). *Educational evaluation: Theory and practice.* Belmont, CA: Wadsworth Publishing.

Index

Note: Page numbers followed by *c* indicate cases, *f* indicate figures, and *t* indicate tables.